Praise for *I Don't Want to Talk About It*

"This is a sobering, powerful book about male depression both 'covert' and 'overt.' The book moves on to new ground both in language and story. *I Don't Want to Talk About It* is exhilarating in its honesty and grief; it moves forward like a hurricane."

—Robert Bly

"The most provocative in a flood of new books on depression. . . . The only volume that speaks exclusively to and about depressed men."

—Pamela Warrick, *Los Angeles Times*

"Even in this era of managed care and Prozac, therapy is still an art. Mr. Real emerges in this book as an artist who plays his theories with the passion and skill of Isaac Stern in concert."

—*Dallas Morning News*

"A tour-de-force, this landmark book uncovers a hidden epidemic with devastating effects. In an elegant novelist style, Terrence Real traces the shadow of male depression from father to son. And in a bold, courageous way, he tells his own story of trauma and recovery, which shines like a golden thread throughout the book."

—Connie Zweig, Ph.D., author of *Romancing the Shadow*

"Riveting reading. You pick it up and can't put it down. . . . *I Don't Want to Talk About It* could get you started on a conversation with yourself that would allow you to shed a burden you've been carrying a long time."

—Jane Tompkins, *The Raleigh News & Observer*

"Terry Real writes with understanding and compassion for his own father, for himself as a father of young sons, and for the many men in his practice whose stories he tells. Like a good novel, *I Don't Want to Talk About It* pulls you in and keeps you reading. Beautifully written; it's an important book for all of us."
—Olga Silverstein, author of *The Courage to Raise Good Men*

"Boys in our culture are taught that real men are stoic. The ability to not complain, endure pain, and strive in the face of adversity is admired and celebrated in story and song. The price paid for this isolation is depression. Terry Real has produced a seminal work that is likely to be the text of choice for therapists and patients for many years."
—Pia Mellody, author of *Facing Love Addiction* and *Facing Co-Dependence*

"Clear, compelling . . . strongly reasoned. . . . The book is wise beyond its stated scope: in setting up a model, nature, and etiology and treatment of male depression, Real ends up offering—with some gender variants—an almost universal paradigm."
—*Publishers Weekly*

"This is a very beautiful book, one that can help a multitude of men, women, and children. Written with grace and graced with humor, *I Don't Want to Talk About It* goes down as smoothly as a sigh, but it carries the power to change your life."
—Edward Hallowell, M.D., author of *When You Worry About the Child You Love* and *Driven to Distraction*

"An absorbing and informative look at the hidden long-term depression that constricts or undermines the relationships of many American men. . . . An important and rewarding work."
—*Kirkus*

I DON'T WANT TO TALK ABOUT IT

*Overcoming the Secret Legacy
of Male Depression*

Terrence Real

SCRIBNER

New York   London   Toronto   Sydney   New Delhi

SCRIBNER

An Imprint of Simon & Schuster, Inc.

1230 Avenue of the Americas

New York, NY 10020

SCRIBNER and design are trademarks of Macmillan Library Reference USA, Inc.,
used under license by Simon & Schuster, the publisher of this work.

DESIGNED BY ERICH HOBBING

Manufactured in the United States of America

33 35 37 39 40 38 36 34 32

The Library of Congress has cataloged the Scribner edition as follows:
Real, Terrence.
I don't want to talk about it: overcoming the secret
legacy of male depression / Terrence Real.—1st Fireside ed.
p.   cm.
Includes index.
1. Depression, Mental. 2. Men—Mental health.
3. Masculinity. I. Title.
[RC537.R39   1998]
616.85'27'0081—dc21   97-39236   CIP

ISBN 0-684-83539-8 (Pbk)

With gratitude
this book is dedicated to my wife,
BELINDA BERMAN,
and our sons,
JUSTIN and ALEXANDER,
who remind me that hope
is the remembrance of the future.

The pebble my son
spraypainted gold

rests in my palm, a gift,
and he asks in a clear, high

temporary voice
who taught me my life

is base and needs great pain
to turn itself into gold?

And who taught them?
And for what, and whose, reasons?

—RICHARD HOFFMAN,
History

Let the dead pray for their own dead.

—JAMES WRIGHT,
Inscriptions for the Tank

Author's Note

All of the cases described in this book are composites. They have been deliberately scrambled in order to protect my clients' rights of confidentiality and privacy. No client found in this book corresponds to any actual person, living or dead.

Acknowledgments

I t is fitting that this book, with its emphasis on men's relationships, should owe so much to so many. The thoughts presented here would not have been possible were it not for the genius of two very different women, Olga Silverstein and Pia Mellody, each a legendary figure in her field. I borrowed Olga's daring in abandoning current theories of male development. It was she who first conceived of this book at all, and I see it as a companion to her superb treatment of mothers and sons, *The Courage to Raise Good Men*. As with Olga, my debt to Pia is obvious throughout the book. Not only has her work thoroughly informed my practice with clients, it has changed my own life. Jack Sternbach has taught me most of what I know about running men's groups. It was Jack who first made clear to me the revolutionary perspective of Joe Pleck, and it was Jack who introduced me to the idea of lovingly holding men accountable, of men as "wounded wounders." I want also to thank my colleagues and friends at the Family Institute of Cambridge, a teaching facility that has been responsible for training three generations of family therapists throughout New England. In particular, I wish to pay homage to my own mentors, Charles Verge, Caroline Marvin, Richard Chasin, Rick Lee, David Treadway, Sally Ann Roth, and Kathy Weingarten. Any light that passes through my work with men and their families is principally yours. I am enormously grateful.

My agent, Beth Vesel, one of the initial architects of this endeavor, has been a powerful guide, protector, and muse throughout the process, as well as a reader of extraordinary perspicacity. My early collaboration with Elizabeth Stone deserves grateful acknowledgment, as do the tenacious research efforts of Rina Amiri. I want to thank Per Gjerde of Stanford University for his warm support and guidance, Bessel van der Kolk for his wisdom, openness and clarity, David Lisak and Ron Levant for their many good thoughts.

Many editors deserve my deepest gratitude. Virginia LaPlante was coach, critic, and midwife. Gail Winston shaped the project early on with the stamp of her intelligence. Nan Graham and Gillian Blake of Scribner brought the work to fruition, giving it final form. Nan Graham's vision informs my own, and Gillian Blake brought incisive skill to the text. The insight and keen energy of these four women flow through each page.

Many kind, loving friends surrounded me and my family during this taxing period: Jeffrey and Cheryl Katz; Scott Campbell and Richard MacMillan; Rick Thomson and Judy Wineland; Denise and Kenneth Malament; Margie Schaffel and Peter Belson; Carter, Susan, and Jessica Umbarger; Jeffrey Kerr; Mora Rothenberg; Winthrop Burr; Meredith Kantor; Mel Bucholtz; Gerry Schamess; Kristin Wainwright; Joan Wickersham; Alan and Deborah Slobodnik—patient, patient friends all.

I want to thank the men, women, boys, and girls I have had the honor of working with over the years. This book is, more than anything else, a document of their heroism.

Finally, I pay tribute to my greatest source of inspiration, my soulmate, Belinda Berman. Along with the hours of hard work and support, I thank you also for your passion, depth, and unfailing intelligence. Loving you has been the most exquisite thing I have ever done. To my children, Justin and Alexander, I am grateful for your tolerance and enthusiasm. Whenever my mind went numb or my spirits flagged, your shining presence revived me.

In every step of my travels through a dark wood I have benefited from help and good company. A blessing to all my fellow travelers.

Contents

Prologue

The son wishes to remember what the father wishes
to forget.

—YIDDISH PROVERB

In high school, my father saw two boys he knew drown. One kid
got pulled out in an undertow off the New Jersey coast and his
friend evidently dove out to save him. This tragedy became one
of the central metaphors of his life. "A drowning person will grip
you," my father told me, "if you get in too close. They'll pull you
down with them. You should throw them something, a rope, a life
preserver. But don't touch them, don't go in after them." He used
to say this to my brother and me, from time to time, as if dispens-
ing advice on driving or study habits, as if drowning were an ordinary occurrence. While I heard the advice, I did not learn the story
of the two boys until much later, because my father never spoke
about himself during my childhood, only about others.

It took me twenty years to get my father to talk about his own
life. I remember the first day he did. I recall the prickly feel of our
old yellow couch as we sat together. I was painfully aware of my
father's great bulk beside me. He was a big man for his generation,
six two and well over two hundred pounds, with broad arms, a barrel chest, and a great potbelly that thrust out before him like the
bass drum of his booming voice, his laugh.

Most of my father's gestures, his expressions, were broad,
coarse, larger than life, like his body, like the clay figures he
sculpted in our garage—abstract, looming shapes with massive

limbs—or like his rage, which came as suddenly as a storm, with no particular intent or thought, like some dark animal, some bear.

My twin brother, Les, had the good sense to keep a low profile and stay close to the ground, but I was Dad's gifted child. I was the sensitive one. I was trouble. "You little brat. I'm going to beat you to within an inch of your life," my father used to say. And there were times he seemed bent on making good on his promise. His violence should have pushed me away from him, and consciously it did. But in some more primitive way it only drew me closer. As he raged, out of control, even as he beat me, I never lost touch with him. It was the vortex of *his* pathos, *his* insanity, *his* hurt that overwhelmed me, filling me, more than the physical pain, with black despair, with torpor. I couldn't wait for the ritual to end so that I could take to my bed, pull the covers up over me, and sleep.

Later, in adolescence, I began to find that same sweet release in drugs and in the thrill of risk taking. Things got worse. My life grew more dangerous. By late adolescence I started to wonder which one of us, my dad or me, was going to survive.

A skinny twenty-seven-year-old, I pull a thick afghan onto my lap and ask my father to tell me about his childhood. He begins with the usual maneuvers: he adopts surliness, then he jokes, evades. But this time I am armed with the fledgling skills of a young therapist. I have learned a few lessons in the craft of opening up a closed heart.

"You know, your mother and I deliberately made the decision to keep all this from you," he begins.

"I understand," I say.

"We didn't want to burden you kids."

"I appreciate that."

"But, I suppose you're certainly old enough now . . ." he falters. I am quiet.

He pauses. "You'll never know what it was like back then," he tells me, "the Depression . . ." He lapses into silence for a while and then he begins. He wasn't more than six or seven when his mother died of some lingering disease whose name he affects not to remember. He had only vague pictures of her in his head, hardly memories; he recalled her warmth, an infectious laugh.

After she died, things went downhill for my father's father, Abe, "a weak, passive man." Abe lost his job, bought a little mom-and-pop store; then he lost the store. Unable to support itself, the family broke up. My dad and his younger brother went to live with a cousin. "Aunt" Sylvie was mean. She was bitter before the Depression and taking in my father, Edgar, and his brother, young Phil, did nothing to slake the venom in her disposition. She was cruel in a daily, ordinary way.

"Like how, Dad?" I ask him .

"Oh, I don't know," he shrugs me off.

"Like how, Dad?" I repeat the question.

I eventually get my father to tell me about the humiliation of ragged hand-me-downs, about how Sylvie would dish out food to him with a line such as, "Here is a big piece of chicken for Steven, because he is my son. And here is a small piece of chicken for you, Edgar. Because you are not."

When he was eleven or twelve, the rage in my father, the missing of his mother, his father, filled him to the bursting point. His little brother was still young and sunny enough to adjust, but my dad began acting out. An "instigator" at school, a petty thief at home, he lasted through one or two "incidents" and then Aunt Sylvie summarily got rid of him. He found himself banished to the home of elderly grandparents in another part of town.

"What did you do?" I ask.

"What do you mean, what did I do? I went to school. I worked."

"Did you have friends?"

"I made friends."

"Did you see Phil and your father?"

Yes, he saw them. All that winter after school he would walk six miles through the snow to have dinner with them at Sylvie's house. He would linger over a cup of cocoa until Sylvie asked him to leave. Then he'd walk back again alone.

I look out of the window of our little seaside apartment, onto bare November trees. I picture that twelve-year-old boy walking back in the snow.

"How was that for you?" I ask. "What did you feel?"

My father shrugs.

"What did you feel?" I insist.

"A little cold, I guess."

"Come on, goddamn it."

"I don't hold a grudge, Terry." My father's tone levels me. "They did what they had to. All right? These were rough times. Besides," his voice becomes still, "I understand in a way. I wasn't so easy to handle."

"You were a child," I tell him.

My father shakes his head. "Yeah, well, I was pretty hard-boiled. I could be quite a little son of a bitch."

"How much of a son of a bitch could you have been, Dad?" I say. "You were twelve years old!"

He turns away. "I don't know." He slumps.

"Look at me." I take his shoulders. "I don't give a shit what you did, do you understand? You were a kid. Your mother was dead; your father was gone. You didn't deserve it, okay? Don't you get it? *You didn't deserve it.*"

My father looks up at me, his blue eyes magnified by thick glasses. "Okay," he sighs. Then, as sudden as any rage, he reaches out his thick arms and pulls me toward him. Without a word he lays his head on my shoulder, as tender and guileless as a child. Holding him, I breathe in his familiar smell, coffee and cigarettes and a touch of Brylcreem. Feeling the weight of his great head, I am physically awkward, almost repelled, but when he pulls away, I instinctively tighten my hold on him. Gingerly, reluctantly, I stroke his back, his stiff hair.

"It's okay, Dad," I murmur.

I look out past him at the trees, and wonder what will become of us, my father and me. I still neither trusted nor forgave him, but something deep inside me began to uncoil.

That night was a first green tendril piercing through a stone wall. Others followed. In the years ahead, as our closeness developed, my life became more successful, and my father's life grew ever more desperate. I watched, helpless, as financial worry, social isolation, and finally, a horrible disease whittled him, sucked the marrow out of him, pulled him under. I stayed as close, I gave as much as I could.

I buried my father in September 1991. The night before, when I left his bedside, he gave me his blessing and I gave him mine. The next morning, I walked into the hospital room to find him dead. His head was thrown back, his eyes shut, his mouth open. It didn't look like my dad. It looked like my dad's body, a thing made of clay, like his statues. I touched his eyes and kissed him. His skin on my lips tasted bitter, earthen.

I have often thought about the high school boys my father saw drown and the advice he gave me: "Don't touch them. They'll drag you under." As in so many other instances, his advice on this matter was wrong. I did not go down into that dark vortex with my father. But neither did I let go of his embrace.

CHAPTER ONE

Men's Hidden Depression

> In the middle of the journey of our lives,
> I found myself upon a dark path.
>
> —DANTE

When I stand beside troubled fathers and sons I am often flooded with a sense of recognition. All men are sons and, whether they know it or not, most sons are loyal. To me, my father presented a confusing jumble of brutality and pathos. As a boy, I drank into my character a dark, jagged emptiness that haunted me for close to thirty years. As other fathers have done to their sons, my father—through the look in his eyes, the tone of his voice, the quality of his touch—passed the depression he did not know he had on to me just as surely as his father had passed it on to him—a chain of pain, linking parent to child across generations, a toxic legacy.

In hindsight, it is clear to me that, among other reasons, I became a therapist so I could cultivate the skills I needed to heal my own father—to heal him at least sufficiently to get him to talk to me. I needed to know about his life to help understand his brutality and lay my hatred of him to rest. At first I did this unconsciously, not out of any great love for him, but out of an instinct to save myself. I wanted the legacy to stop.

One might think that I would have brought to my work a particular sensitivity to issues of depression in men, but at first I did not. Despite my hard-won personal knowledge, years passed before I found the courage to invite my patients to embark upon the same journey I had taken. I was not prepared, by training or experience, to reach so deep into a man's inner pain—to hold and confront him there. Faced with men's hidden fragility, I had been tacitly schooled, like most therapists—indeed, like most people in our culture—to protect them. I had also been taught that depression was predominantly a woman's disease, that the rate of depression was somewhere between two to four times higher for women than it was for men. When I first began my clinical practice, I had faith in the simplicity of such figures, but twenty years of work with men and their families has lead me to believe that the real story concerning this disorder is far more complex.

There is a terrible collusion in our society, a cultural cover-up about depression in men.

One of the ironies about men's depression is that the very forces that help create it keep us from seeing it. Men are not supposed to be vulnerable. Pain is something we are to rise above. He who has been brought down by it will most likely see himself as shameful, and so, too, may his family and friends, even the mental health profession. Yet I believe it is this secret pain that lies at the heart of many of the difficulties in men's lives. Hidden depression drives several of the problems we think of as typically male: physical illness, alcohol and drug abuse, domestic violence, failures in intimacy, self-sabotage in careers.

We tend not to recognize depression in men because the disorder itself is seen as unmanly. Depression carries, to many, a double stain—the stigma of mental illness and also the stigma of "feminine" emotionality. Those in a relationship with a depressed man are themselves often faced with a painful dilemma. They can either confront his condition—which may further shame him—or else collude with him in minimizing it, a course that offers no hope for relief. Depression in men—a condition experienced as both shame-filled and shameful—goes largely unacknowledged and unrecognized both by the men who suffer and by those who surround them. And yet, the impact of this hidden condition is enormous.

Eleven million people are estimated as struggling with depression each year. The combined effect of lost productivity and medical expense due to depression costs the United States over 47 billion dollars per year—a toll on a par with heart disease. And yet the condition goes mostly undiagnosed. Somewhere between 60 and 80 percent of people with depression never get help. The silence about depression is all the more heartbreaking since its treatment has a high success rate. Current estimates are that, with a combination of psychotherapy and medication, between 80 and 90 percent of depressed patients can get relief—if they ask for it. My work with men and their families has taught me that, along with a reluctance to acknowledge depression, we also often fail to identify this disorder because *men tend to manifest depression differently than women.*

Few things about men and women seem more dissimilar than the way we tend to handle our feelings. Why should depression, a disorder of feeling—in psychiatric language, an *affective disorder*—be handled in the same way by both sexes when most other emotional issues are not? While many men are depressed in ways that are similar to women, there are even more men who express depression in less well-recognized ways, ways that are most often overlooked and misunderstood but nevertheless do great harm. What are these particularly male forms of depression? What are their causes? Is the etiology of the disorder the same for both sexes? I think not. Just as men and women often express depression differently, their pathways toward depression seem distinct as well.

Traditional gender socialization in our culture asks both boys and girls to "halve themselves." Girls are allowed to maintain emotional expressiveness and cultivate connection. But they are systematically discouraged from fully developing and exercising their public, assertive selves—their "voice," as it is often called. Boys, by contrast, are greatly encouraged to develop their public, assertive selves, but they are systematically pushed away from the full exercise of emotional expressiveness and the skills for making and appreciating deep connection. For decades, feminist researchers and scholars have detailed the degree of coercion brought to bear against girls' full development, and the sometimes devastating effects of the loss of their most complete, authentic selves. It is time to understand the reciprocal process as it occurs in the lives of boys and men.

Current research makes it clear that a vulnerability to depression is most probably an inherited biological condition. Any boy or girl, given the right mix of chromosomes, will have a susceptibility to this disease. But in the majority of cases, biological vulnerability alone is not enough to bring about the disorder. It is the collision of inherited vulnerability with psychological injury that produces depression. And it is here that issues of gender come into play. The traditional socialization of boys and girls hurts them both, each in particular, complementary ways. Girls, and later women, tend to internalize pain. They blame themselves and draw distress into themselves. Boys, and later men, tend to externalize pain; they are more likely to feel victimized by others and to discharge distress through action. Hospitalized male psychiatric patients far outnumber female patients in their rate of violent incidents; women outnumber men in self-mutilation. In mild and severe forms, externalizing in men and internalizing in women represent troubling tendencies in both sexes, inhibiting the capacity of each for true relatedness. A depressed woman's internalization of pain weakens her and hampers her capacity for direct communication. A depressed man's tendency to extrude pain often does more than simply impede his capacity for intimacy. It may render him psychologically dangerous. Too often, the wounded boy grows up to become a wounding man, inflicting upon those closest to him the very distress he refuses to acknowledge within himself. Depression in men, unless it is dealt with, tends to be passed along. That was the case with my father and me. And that was the situation facing David Ingles and his family when we first met.

"So, what do you get when you cross a lawyer, a dyslexic, and a virus?" David, himself a lawyer, eases into his accustomed chair in my office.

His wife, Elaine, also a lawyer in her mid-forties, and their seventeen-year-old son, Chad, show no signs of curiosity. Elaine levels a gaze a few inches above her husband's left ear. Without looking at him, she says simply, "*No*, David." And we all sit for awhile in ponderous, uncomfortable silence. David stares at me amiably, a tall man grown pudgy in middle age, with an open, dark face and thinning black hair. Sitting across from her husband, Elaine angles her small, muscular body as far from him as possible. Chad, a beanpole in baggy pants and a T-shirt, puts on a pair of wire-rimmed John Lennon sunglasses and rotates his chair toward the wall.

"Take off the glasses," David mutters to Chad, who ignores him.

While David glares at Chad, Elaine informs me, once again, that David is really quite a good father, involved, caring.

"Take them *off*!" David repeats.

Chad grunts and slumps further away.

I had been treating David and Elaine for close to six months. Elaine first wanted me to see the two of them, not for Chad's sake but for the sake of their marriage. After twenty years she had to admit that she felt—and had felt for some time now—miserably alone. David was good-natured, helpful, cooperative. The problem was that she felt like he just wasn't there. For a while, she had wondered if he was having an affair, but David seemed too *vague* to pull off an affair. More and more, he moved through his life savoring nothing, not her, not his son, not even his own success. For years he had been working too hard. Now he had also begun drinking too much and, on too many occasions, blowing up. Elaine worried about David's anger; she worried about his health. Although she had not yet said it out loud, Elaine already knew by the time she called me that she was on the verge of leaving her husband.

David had weathered his wife's complaints before. His strategy had always been to batten down the hatches and wait until it all blew over. "Sort of an extended PMS" was how he had described her dissatisfactions. As their therapist, I informed him that this time he might have to do some changing himself. But when David showed signs of responding, Chad began acting up, so I asked them to bring in their son, "as my consultant." I was interested to hear what this boy—who was in the middle of their marriage from the day he had been born—would have to say about his parents. But Elaine had another agenda.

"David," Elaine says evenly. "You need to tell Terry about hitting Chad."

"I didn't hit him," David says sullenly.

"Whatever." Elaine shrugs this off. "It needs to be addressed."

David hovers for a moment between fighting and giving in. Then he sighs, leans back in his chair, and tells me the story.

"Chad was walking out the back door last night," he begins, "with the keys to the car in hand. Elaine and I were in the kitchen, and I asked him a few questions—Where was he going?—that sort of thing."

"Yeah *right*," snorts Chad.

His father's pointed finger shoots up at him. "Was I unreasonable?" David asks. "*Was I?*"

"All right," I calm David. "Tell me what happened."

"So, he doesn't answer. And Elaine and I follow him into the garage"—he glances reproachfully at his son,—"where he starts to give me a lot of back talk. Right?" he turns to Chad.

"Go on," I say softly.

"Well, I tell him, '*Fine. If you want to keep up the back talk, then I keep the car.*' You know, '*Hey, it's your choice, okay?*' And he throws the keys against the car . . ."

"On the *ground*," says Chad.

"Against the *car*," repeats his father, "and then I hear, 'Fuck you' under his breath." David falls silent.

I try catching his eye. "At which point you . . ." I prompt.

"I pushed him," he allows.

"You pushed him," I repeat.

"Yes. You know. I shoved him. Whatever. I pushed him." David stares intently at the spot of rug between his feet.

"Hard?" I ask.

David shrugs.

"Hard enough," says Elaine.

I look for a moment at Chad. Behind his glasses, I cannot tell his expression, or even if he is crying. I am suddenly aware of how thin he is, how young.

I stand up, motioning David to stand beside me. "Show me how it went," I say.

In conventional individual therapy, people tell their therapist about the things that have happened to them out in the world. In family therapy, the major players in such events are often sitting together in the therapist's office. It is a tradition in family therapy to shift from reporting about tough events to having the family reenact them. Bringing the scene palpably into the room adds an emotional charge that the therapist can use to advantage.

Reluctantly, with many safeguards and assurances, David and his family let me set up the scene. Chad still wears his sunglasses. When they get to the part where Chad throws down the keys and mutters "Fuck you" under his breath, David, with alarming speed, throws his son against the wall of my office so hard that he knocks a picture off one of its hooks, leaving Chad winded. David has pinned his forearm against his son's throat. His muscles are taut and his breathing is hard. "Say it again!" he threatens. "Go ahead. Say it again!"

Chad is gasping for breath. He is scared. Elaine is scared. My heart is pounding as well.

"David." I touch his shoulder gently while looking at Chad. "It's okay." I can feel his muscles relax under my touch. "I get it," I say. "Really clearly. Good job."

Everyone takes a deep breath and after a while our hearts stop hammering. I ask Elaine if she would role-play David, and she agrees. Now I mold her into position as David, with her forearm against Chad's throat. Then I walk with David to the far end of the room, and I ask him to take a good look at this tableau. We stand for a long time together, our shoulders almost touching. Whether it is my imagination or not, I can feel sadness radiating from him, like heat, as we stand side by side.

"What do you see, when you look at this?" I ask him. "What do you feel?"

David drops his head. After a long while he speaks. "I guess it's not right," he offers, ever so meekly.

"Pretty grim," I agree. After a pause, he nods. "Tell *him*," I say, nodding toward Elaine, who is role-playing David, still with an arm pressed against Chad's throat. "Tell him what he needs to hear."

David shuffles about uncomfortably. "You're a jerk," he cracks, halfheartedly.

"No, I mean it." I say, standing close. "*Tell* him."

David pauses for a long time, then he lifts his head and addresses his role-played self. All traces of self-mockery or humor have left him. "Don't do it," he says quietly.

"Don't do what?" I push him.

"Don't treat him that way." His voice is small, flat.

"Is that enough force to stop this guy?" I ask.

"No," he agrees.

"It's going to take some conviction," I tell him. "Some *oomph*, you know what I mean?"

David nods.

"You want to try it again?" I ask.

Without answering in words, David obediently squares off. This time he reaches deeper in and his voice carries some weight. "Don't treat him this way," he says.

"More," I say. "*Louder.*"

"*Don't* treat him this way," David repeats.

"Good!" I say. "Do it again. Tell him why."

"Don't fuck with him," David begins. "Just don't . . ." and then the dam breaks. "He's your *son*, for Christ's sake!" David yells, thoroughly enrolled. "For Christ's sake! He's your *son.*"

David suddenly deflates, crestfallen and profoundly sad. I have not seen him look this way in the months we have worked together. This is an opening.

As his sadness grows in the space between us, I ask, "Tell me, who else are you talking too, right now? Is there anyone else standing beside this guy as you say this? Friend? Teacher? Mother? Father?"

David looks absolutely defeated. "I guess," he allows.

"So, who is it?" I ask softly.

Embarrassed and angry, he says, "My father."

"Tell me about him," I ask.

David sketches the portrait of a responsible, taciturn, working-class man who put in long hours to provide for his family, who loved them all—though he rarely spoke it—whose sudden temper sometimes got the better of him.

"I guess the apple hasn't fallen too far from the tree," David says with a sheepish smile.

"We're working on it," I assure him. We look together at the frozen tableau facing us across the room, both of us thinking.

"Don't treat him this way," I repeat, musing. "David, can you give me a particular memory, a scene, a vignette that would capture that feeling with your dad?"

At first David does not remember any, but then he begins to tell me.

David recalls himself as a boy of seven or eight handing his father a report card with a bad grade. He is nervous because of the D he got in some subject or other.

"We don't get D's in this family," his father intones, in David's memory. And then, in a sudden, raw temper, his father reaches out, grabs the report card, and rips it to pieces.

"Take that back to your teacher," his father says.

Frightened and angry, young David grabs at his father's hands. "What did you do that for!!!" he screams. Without a word his father draws back his huge fist and lands it squarely on the boy's chest, knocking him to the ground.

"I haven't thought about that for years," says David.

Again, I get up. "Show me," I ask him.

David and I act out the scene first. And then Chad and Elaine agree to reenact it. David and I step to one side, as we watch Chad playing the young David, with Elaine playing David's dad.

"We don't get D's in our family!"—once, twice, three times the fist goes out until the scene feels real enough that violence is palpable in the air.

"Okay, David," I say. "Fix this scene. Make it right."

David looks down at me for a moment, quizzically, and then,

without a word, signals the players to begin. Again, the frightened boy offers the offending report card. The father destroys it. The boy protests. The father leans into his swing—but at just that moment David steps forward, catching the fist in his own large hand and enveloping it.

David looks his "father" in the eye and says very quietly but with full conviction, "Don't do it, Dad. Don't touch the boy." I notice he is shaking as I step in behind him.

"Don't hurt him, Dad," I prompt.

"Don't hurt him," David repeats. He has begun to tear up.

"He's just a little boy," I prompt.

"He's just a little boy." David bends over and cries. It is a strangled cry without sound that lifts his shoulders.

"Don't hold it back, David," I say. "You'll just give yourself a headache."

David sits down, still crying, his face hidden in his hands. Elaine pulls her chair next to him, rests her palm on his thigh. I ask Chad to pass his father the tissues. As he does, for just a moment, briefly, almost furtively, David grasps his son's hand. Chad takes off his sunglasses and folds them into the pocket of his shirt.

David did not know it, but he was depressed. Along with whatever biological vulnerabilities he may have carried, David's depression was born from the pain of that little boy—not just from this one incident with his father, but from hundreds, perhaps even thousands of similar moments, small instances of betrayal or abandonment, perhaps more subtle than this one but just as damaging. For those with a biological vulnerability to the disorder, such moments can become the building blocks of depression, a condition which, conceived in the boy, erupts later on in the man. David's unrecognized pain ticked inside like a bomb, waiting for its appointed time. The force of that ticking pushed him from his family. It sped him toward mood buffers and self-esteem enhancers like work, alcohol, and occasional violence. By the time I first met him, his son was on the edge of school failure and his wife was on the verge of filing for divorce. The bomb inside was due to release itself and his life was about to explode. And neither he nor anyone close to him would have understood why. But I knew why.

I knew what it felt like to have the breath knocked out of you by your own father, what it meant to be thrown against a wall and dared to fight back. Intimacy with the sticky threads of loving violence that bind parents to sons across generations helped me recognize David's secret. Deep inside his bullying and drinking, his preoccupations and flight, lay that little boy. The depressed part of David, his unacknowledged child, waited in darkness, resentfully, for its moment in the light, wreaking havoc upon anyone near. Showing great courage, David allowed, on that afternoon in my office, the pain he had carried within for decades to break through to the surface. His vulnerability drew the people he loved back toward him. The appearance of his hidden depression permitted him to touch and to be touched after a long, bristling time behind armor. In his struggle, David Ingles is not alone.

In order to treat a man like David, I must first "get at" him, "crack him open." The patient needs help bringing his depression up to the surface. Depressed women have obvious pain; depressed men often have "troubles." It is frequently not they who are in conscious distress so much as the people who live with them.

If you had asked David what was bothering him, before that session, it is uncertain what he would have answered, or even if he would have given an answer at all. Like a lot of the successful men I treat, David was unpracticed in, even wary of, introspection.

What David might have told you was that he was unhappy at work, where he had a new senior partner to deal with, whom he neither liked as well as his old mentor nor felt particularly favored by. He might have told you that over the last several years he had grown increasingly restless—to the point where it had become difficult for him to sleep at night without pills and hard to get through a dinner at a friend's house without a few cocktails. David knew—though he would not have bored anyone other than Elaine with the details—that he was bothered more and more by stomachaches and by backaches, which his internist chalked up to "stress," a medical opinion that David dismissed as "the great twentieth-century catchall."

David's physician was right, however, although his diagnosis did not go nearly far enough. David was "stressed." At forty-seven, he had begun to feel old. He did not like the spare tire that no amount of racquetball seemed to touch. He did not like the receding hairline. And he did not like looking at the kind of women he had always admired only to have them now look away with disinterest or sometimes with outright disdain. If asked, David would gladly have unloaded his feelings of disappointment about his difficult son, Chad. He might even have voiced his sense of betrayal by Chad's "overprotective mother," who, from the day of Chad's birth, had undercut his attempts to be firm with the boy. Toward the end of an evening, after a sufficient number of drinks, David might have confessed his unhappiness in his marriage—how unsupported he felt, how much like a stranger in his own home. Not once would it have occurred to him that he might be suffering from a clinical condition. But the depression David neither felt nor recognized was close to fracturing his family. It was eating away at his relationship with his son and eroding his marriage. In his efforts to escape his own depression, David had let himself sink into behaviors—like irritability, dominance, drinking, and emotional unavailability—that pushed away the very people whom he most loved and needed. As Elaine described it, he was no longer himself. Like Shakespeare's Lear, David, without realizing it, had lost his estate. "What do you see when you look at me?" demanded the broken king of his fool. And the fool replied, "Lear's shadow." Depression was whittling David, fading him to a shadow state as surely and inexorably as a physical disease like cancer or AIDS. As one of my clients put it, depression was "disappearing" him.

We do not generally think of driven men like David as being depressed. We tend to reserve the concept of *depression* for a state of profound impairment, utter despair, thorough debilitation. A truly depressed man would lie in bed in the morning, staring up at the ceiling, too apathetic to drag himself off to another meaningless day. By comparison, what David faced seemed barely to qualify as midlife malaise. As Thoreau once wrote: "The mass of men lead lives of quiet desperation." Others, not so quiet. When we think of depression, it is to those "others, not so quiet" that our thoughts usually turn.

For close to twenty years, I have treated those others—men with the kind of depression most of us easily discern. I call this state *overt depression*. Acute and dramatic, the pain inflicted by overt depression is writ large. In contrast, David's type of depression was mild, elusive, and chronic. The kind of depression from which David suffers is not even referenced in most of the literature about the disorder. The guidebook for diagnosis used by most clinicians throughout the country is the American Psychiatric Association's *Diagnostic and Statistical Manual of Mental Disorders* (DSM IV) which labels a person as having a clinical depression only if he or she shows, for a duration of at least two weeks, signs either of feeling sad, "down," and "blue," or having a decreased interest in pleasurable activities, including sex. In addition, the person must exhibit at least four of any of the following symptoms: weight loss or gain, too little or too much sleep, fatigue, feelings of worthlessness or guilt, difficulty making decisions or forgetfulness, and preoccupation with death or suicide.

The condition described in the DSM IV is the classic form of depression most of us think of. Although many men may be reluctant to admit that they are suffering from overt depression, the disorder itself has been recognized since ancient times. As early as the fourth century. B.C., Hippocrates, "the father of medicine," reported a condition whose symptoms included "sleeplessness, irritability, despondency, restlessness, and aversion to food"—a description of overt depression easily recognizable today. Hippocrates saw the malady as caused by an imbalance of black bile, one of the four humors, and he therefore named the disease simply "black bile," which in Greek reads *melanae chole,* or *melancholia.*

Overt depression preys upon men, women, and sometimes children from all walks of life, all classes, all cultures. Epidemiologists have found descriptions resembling overt depression throughout the world—both in developed and in developing societies. And the number of overtly depressed people seems to be on the rise. Researcher Myrna Weissman and her colleagues checked medical records going back to the beginning of the century. They calculated that, even allowing for increased reporting, each successive generation has doubled its susceptibility to depression. Such trends were corroborated worldwide in a random sampling of 39,000 subjects from such diverse countries as New Zealand, Lebanon, Italy, Germany, Canada, and France. Researchers have found depression in greater numbers and at earlier ages than ever before throughout the world.

The National Institute for Mental Health reports that in the United States somewhere between 6 and 10 percent of our population—close to one out of every ten people—are battling some form of this disease. And yet, as sobering as these figures may be, I believe they greatly underestimate the full impact of depression in men's lives. A man like David Ingles, whose condition manifests itself in ways more subtle than those described by the DSM IV, would not have been included in these figures, even while the effects of his less obvious disorder are powerful enough to threaten his health and break up his family. Why is it that not only the general public but even the medical and psychiatric community give credence to depression in only its most obvious and most severe form? In a recent national survey, over half of the people questioned did not see depression as a major health issue. In another survey, in which 25 percent of the respondents had themselves experienced depression, and another 26 percent had observed it in family members, close to half of the respondents still viewed the disorder not as a disease or a psychological problem deserving of help, but rather as a sign of personal weakness.

Our current patterns of judgment and denial about depression are reminiscent of the older moralistic attitudes toward the disease of alcoholism, and the source of our minimization is much the same now as it was then. The issue is shame. While depression may carry some sense of stigma for all people, the disapprobation attached to this disease is particularly acute for men. The very definition of manhood lies in "standing up" to discomfort and pain. It is sadly predictable that David would be more likely to react to depression by redoubling his efforts at work than by sitting still long enough to feel his own feelings. Until therapy, "giving in" to his pain would have been experienced by David not as a path toward relief, but as a humiliating defeat. In the calculus of male pride, stoicism prevails. All too often, denial is equated with tenacity—"Under the bludgeonings of chance / My head is bloody, but unbowed."

When David Ingles runs from his own internal distress, he plays out our culture's values about masculinity. As a society, we have more respect for the walking wounded—those who deny their difficulties—than we have for those who "let" their conditions "get to them." Traditionally, we have not liked men to be very emotional or very vulnerable. An overtly depressed man is both—someone who not only has feelings but who has allowed those feelings to swamp his competence. A man brought down in life is bad enough. But a man brought down by his own unmanageable feelings—for many, that is unseemly.

This attitude often compounds a depressed man's condition, so that he gets depressed about being depressed, ashamed about feeling ashamed. Because of the stigma attached to depression, men often allow their pain to burrow deeper and further from view. Physician John Rush spoke in an interview about the stain of "unmanliness" attached to the condition and its possible consequences:

> [Depression] doesn't mean I'm weak, it doesn't mean I'm incurable, it doesn't mean I'm insane. It means I've got a disease and somebody better treat it. One of my friends says, "Depression? Hell, boy, that's wimp disease." Wimp disease? Oh, yeah, it's wimp disease. And I guess the ultimate wimp kills himself.

What John Rush implies is correct. For many men—ashamed of their feelings and refusing help—"wimp disease" can kill. Men are four times more likely than women to take their own lives.

Over the last twenty years, researchers have investigated the relationship between traditional masculinity and physical illness, alcohol abuse, and risk-taking behaviors—and have demonstrated what most of us already know from common experience: many men would rather place themselves at risk than acknowledge distress, either physical or emotional. In *The Things They Carried*, Tim O'Brien gives a clear example of the force of men's shame, when he remembers his fellow "grunts" in Vietnam:

> They carried their reputations. They carried the soldier's greatest fear, which was the fear of blushing. Men killed, and died, because they were embarrassed not to. It was what brought them to the war in the first place, nothing positive, no dreams of glory or honor, just to avoid the blush of dishonor. They crawled into tunnels and walked point and advanced under fire. They were too frightened to be cowards.

Preferring death to the threat of embarrassment, the men O'Brien describes remind me of Harry, the old-fashioned Irish father of one of my clients, who was too ashamed to see a doctor until cancer had eaten away half of a testicle.

The theme of the "manly" denial of vulnerability was epitomized by my patient Stan, a twenty-one-year-old undergraduate whom I saw for a short time. One hot night in Fort Lauderdale during spring break, Stan let himself be drawn into a Hollywood-style barroom brawl with some locals. After "too many brews" and "with a bunch of sweaty pals" to show off to, Stan started swinging just like they do in the movies. Stan bragged to me that he "did a lot of damage that night." Evidently someone did some damage to him as well. One punch was enough to sever a nerve in his cheek and cause paralysis in almost half of Stan's face. The skin hangs like leather. Stan, having seen so many celluloid heroes take a drubbing only to stand up and dust themselves off again, never considered that another man's punch could do such a thing to his face.

Men's willingness to downplay weakness and pain is so great that it has been named as a factor in their shorter life span. The ten years of difference in longevity between men and women turns out to have little to do with genes. Men die early because they do not take care of themselves. Men wait longer to acknowledge that they are sick, take longer to get help, and once they get treatment do not comply with it as well as women do.

For generations, we have chosen male heroes who literally are not made of vulnerable flesh—Superman, "the man of steel," Robocop, Terminators I and II. And our love of invulnerability shows little sign of abating. Both celebrities and ordinary men across the country have developed a new fascination with muscle. Every one of 256 nonmuscular adolescent boys studied by psychologist Barry Glassner demonstrated either mood or behavioral disruptions related to feelings of inadequacy. And a national survey of 62,000 readers conducted by *Psychology Today* showed a direct correlation between self-ratings of high self-esteem in men and self-ratings of muscular physiques. Men's preoccupation with "hard bodies" is fast encroaching upon traditionally female domains such as anorexia and bulimia. For the first time, a significant number of men have begun to join women in developing obsessive concerns about the size and shape of their physiques. In America, it seems, a woman cannot be too thin and a man cannot be too hard.

Trends like these underscore that, despite current talk about the "new man," and the "sensitive man," any slippage in the strict code of masculine invulnerability may be little more than window dressing. While some aspects of traditional masculinity may be changing, the code of invulnerability remains much as it was twenty years ago when Pat Conroy wrote his autobiographical novel *The Great Santini*. Colonel Frank Santini, after emotionally brutalizing his son, goes on to give the boy a critical piece of advice.

"Above all else," Santini tells him, "you must guard your six. Remember, *always protect your six.*"

Your "six," in the pilot's jargon Dad spoke, was a fighter plane's vulnerable back engine—its rectum, its Achilles heel. As a family therapist, I read such a scene between father and son with mixed emotion. Santini's code of invulnerability perpetuates pain. And yet, until that code changes, we cannot dismiss his advice as altogether stupid. The world of men and boys can be a tough one. It turns out, for example, that depressed men are not being altogether paranoid when they fear the reaction of others to their admission of turmoil.

Researchers Hammen and Peters tested hundreds of college roommates on exactly this issue. They found that when female college students reached out to their roommates for support about being depressed, they met with nurturing and caring reactions. In contrast, when male students disclosed depression to their roommates, they met with social isolation and often with outright hostility. The "roommate study" was later repeated on campuses all over the country with much the same results. It is true that men do not easily disclose their depression. But it also seems true that many may have good reason to hide.

"My first therapist told me to reach out to people," said Steven, a patient of mine in his thirties. "I was in medical school at the time—which, by the way, my shrink had been through himself, so you'd think he might have known better. 'Reach out,' he says. So good old Stevie–who always does as he's told—began reaching out. Boy, was I naive! Reach out and get crushed by someone. I think my friends would have stayed closer to me if I'd said I had AIDS. My brother decided he was too busy to talk to me for the next seven months. You know those depressed guys you read about who have this delusion that they put out a stink—you know, that they smell? Well, I think I get how they feel."

The stigma surrounding depression often affects both the distressed man and his family. For family members, there may be an impulse to "protect the male ego" by colluding in the man's obfuscation. In one session, Elaine spoke to me of not wanting to "show David up" by addressing the pain she felt radiating from him. Partners of depressed men often express fear that naming the man's condition will only make matters worse. It is better just to "get on with it" and "not dwell on the negatives." But when we minimize a man's depression, for fear of shaming him, we collude with the cultural expectations of masculinity in a terrible way. We send a message that the man who is struggling should not expect help. He must be "self-reliant." He must resolve his distress on his own.

In the same way that family members and friends may feel awkward or even cruel in confronting a depressed man's condition, so too may medical care providers, who are not immune to our culture's prejudices. John Rush put it this way:

> Doctors are still reluctant to make the diagnosis [of depression] because they, too, feel like, "Oh, you must have done something wrong. How did you get yourself into this pickle?" which sort of means the patient is to blame. It's okay if you have a neurological disease—Parkinson's, Huntington's, urinary incontinence, a busted spine because you got into an auto accident—but once you move up to the higher cortical areas, now you don't have a disease anymore; now you have "trouble coping"; now you have a "bad attitude."

In one session Elaine reported that, worried about her husband, she had insisted that David "check in" with their family doctor, a man who over the years had become a friend. David described the visit to me as a case of "the reluctant leading the awkward."

"I'm very fond of Bob," David said, "but let's face it. He's a lot more comfortable talking over test results than asking about the state of my mind."

"Or your drinking," Elaine piped in.

"Or my drinking," David allowed.

Mental health professionals, who presumably are trained to see beyond a man's report of unease or bodily complaints, are not much more successful than general practitioners with this issue. Many psychotherapists, particularly in the current, managed care environment, would treat the manifestations of David's depression—his drinking, marital tensions, or troubles at work—in short-term, focused therapy without identifying these symptoms' underlying cause.

One factor mitigating against the recognition of David's condition is that mental health professionals, no less than anyone else, tend to look for what they expect to find. The conventional wisdom that women are depressed while men are not leads some therapists away from an accurate diagnostic assessment.

A number of studies looking at who gets labeled as being depressed have been carried out nationwide. Some, like the Potts study involving no less than 23,000 volunteer subjects, have been conducted on a massive scale. The results of most of them show a tendency for mental health professionals to overdiagnose women's depression and underdiagnose the disorder in men.

In a study of a different nature, psychologists were given hypothetical psychiatric "case histories" of patients with a variety of complaints. Only one variable was changed, the sex of the client. Consistently, psychologists diagnosed the depressed "male" clients as more severely disturbed than depressed "female" clients. On the other hand, women alcoholics were viewed as being more severely disturbed than their male counterparts. These conflicting results show that an overlay of gender expectations complicates the judgment of clinicians. It seems that they are punishing clients of both sexes with a more severe diagnosis for crossing gender lines. If it is unmanly to be depressed and unwomanly to drink, then a depressed man must be *really* disturbed, just like an alcoholic woman.

While a great many men conceal their condition from the outside world, and while those close to them—loved ones, doctors, even psychotherapists—may miss a diagnosis of overt depression, a man like David Ingles goes even further with the deception. David not only managed to camouflage his condition from those around him; he managed to hide it even from himself. A great many men never make it into the official roll call of the depressed because their overt depression remains undiagnosed. But other men, like David, fail to get help because their expression of the disease does not fit the classic model as described in the DSM IV. David suffers from what I call *covert depression*. It is hidden from those around him, and it is largely hidden from his own conscious awareness. Yet it nevertheless drives many of his actions. David Ingles buries himself in work; he wraps his disquiet in anger and numbs his discontent with alcohol. Everywhere in his life, the prohibition against bringing his vulnerable feelings into the open fosters behaviors that leave him and the people around him ever more disconnected. An unrecognized swell of abandonment washes over David when Elaine does not respond to him and causes him to wall her off in subtle retaliation—throwing the couple into an escalating cycle of alienation. David's unacknowledged desperation to be involved with Chad—to be the kind of father his father was not—leads him, paradoxically, to bully his son, to reenact the very drama he wishes to avoid. My work with families like the Ingleses has convinced me that many of the difficult behaviors one sees in men's relationships are depression driven.

Under the names of "masked depression," "underlying characterological depression," and "depression equivalents," the kind of disguised condition David suffers from has been written about sporadically for years. But it has rarely been systematically studied. Researcher Martin Opler observed as far back as 1974: "Masked depression is one of the most prevalent disorders in modern American society, yet it is perhaps the most neglected category in psychiatric literature." That neglect continues. If *overt depression* in men tends to be overlooked, *covert depression* has been rendered all but invisible.

CHAPTER TWO

Sons of Narcissus: Self-Esteem, Shame, and Depression

He is the longed-for, and the one who longs; he is the arsonist—and he is the scorched.

—Ovid

While psychiatry has put little effort into exploring the nature of covert depression, art, poetry and drama have all drawn rich material from this human condition. The myth of Narcissus stands out as an archetype of the disease, telling the story of an adolescent son of a river nymph, who spent his wild boyhood running and hunting alone in the forest—until the day he himself became snared.

"Narcissus was loved by many," the poet Ovid introduces his tale. "Both youths and young girls wanted him; but he had much cold pride within his tender body: no youth, no girl could ever touch his heart." Narcissus is a radiant, energetic young man who excites the passions of the nymphs, all of whom he rejects. One of his spurned admirers, in vengeance, prays that Narcissus might himself someday know the torment of unrequited love. The nymph's wish is fulfilled when Narcissus, hot and thirsty from hunting, stumbles upon a clear pool in the woods. He leans forward to drink and instantly becomes enchanted with the beautiful face staring back at him. Narcissus brings his lips near to take a kiss and plunges his arms in for an embrace. But the image he longs for flies from his touch, only to return again each time he withdraws. When Narcissus cries in frustration, his falling tears disrupt the figure in the water, and he beseeches the spirit not to abandon him. " 'Stay, I entreat you!' he cries. 'Let me at least gaze upon you if I may not touch you.' With this," the tale concludes, "and much more of the same kind, he cherished the flame that consumed him." Narcissus loses all thought of food or sleep. Transfixed, he pines, withers away, and dies.

To understand this strange case history we must grasp the true nature of the young man's malady. People often think of Narcissus as the symbol of excessive self-regard, but in fact, he exemplifies the opposite. As the Renaissance philosopher Marsilio Ficino observed in the 1500s, Narcissus did not suffer from an overabundance of self-love, but rather from its deficiency. The myth is a parable about paralysis. The youth, who first appears in restless motion, is suddenly rooted to one spot, unable to leave the elusive spirit. As Ficino remarked, if Narcissus had possessed real self-love, he would have been able to leave his fascination. The curse of Narcissus is immobilization, not out of love for himself, but out of dependency upon his image.

Like Narcissus's obsession, covert depression is at its core a disorder of self-esteem. Healthy self-esteem is essentially internal. It is the capacity to cherish oneself in the face of one's own imperfections, not because of what one has or what one can do. Healthy self-esteem presupposes that all men and women are created equal; that one's inherent worth can be neither greater nor lesser than another's. Such a vision of intrinsic worth does not require us to lose our capacity for nuanced discrimination. We can still recognize our gifts and limitations, as well as those of others. But our basic sense of self as valuable and important neither rises nor falls based on external attributes. Parents display the basics of healthy self-esteem when talking about their young children. A parent may note that Sally is brilliant while brother Bill has only average intelligence, or that Bill is a fine athlete while Sally is uncoordinated. But no healthy parent would value one child over another because of such qualities. Developmental theorists call this crucial component of healthy parenting "unconditional positive regard." The parent's warm regard, the "gleam in the mother's eye," is internalized by the young child and becomes the seed of his own capacity for self-regard.

What comes naturally with children is often lost sight of in relation to adults, including ourselves. Society bids many of us to forget about inherent worth and, instead, to supplement the deficiency with external props such as wealth, beauty, status. The greater the scarcity in true self-esteem, the greater the need for supplementation.

Narcissus, "full of cold pride," presents an appearance of untouchability. But the myth understands his secret vulnerability. Lacking the capacity for an authentic relationship, he becomes enthralled and eventually enslaved by his own reflection. Clinically, one would guess that this young man had never developed the capacity to metabolize love, to take it in and make it his own. A therapist would speculate that in Narcissus's early development he was not cherished, never took the warmth of unconditional regard deep inside. Rather than an internal sense of worth, he becomes obsessed with his own adoration reflected back to him from without. This can never replenish him, because no amount of external validation or prestige or nurture can substitute for his own.

Narcissus in love with his image is like a man in love with his bank account, his good looks, or his power. Narcissus is an emblem for all men enthralled with just about anything other than their own deepest selves. Since the hidden depression in such men stems from a lack of internal vitality, the defense of reflected glory rarely succeeds. Each time Narcissus reaches out to embrace the object of his desire, he only causes it to withdraw. Even his tears, his expression of pain, disrupt the beautiful image and cannot be permitted. Narcissus must lay all of his authentic feelings, all of his needs, upon the altar of his worshiped reflection. He must "cherish the flame that consumes him." As inexorably as any addict, Narcissus is caught in a cycle from which he cannot break free, even to the point of death. These are the essential dynamics of covert depression.

On the surface, fifty-six-year-old Thomas Watchell, a rotund, balding executive, seemed as far removed from radiant Narcissus as a person could be. And yet, at the time I first met him, the fascination of this most ordinary man for his own reflected glory had thoroughly ruptured his family and delivered him to the brink of despair.

Thomas contacted me only after several bruising months of *overt depression* had robbed him of sleep, peace of mind, even the capacity to concentrate. He felt worried and helpless, worthless and deficient. He did not realize that his immediate crisis, his acute *overt depression*, was little more than the final eruption of a long-term chronic *covert depression*. When he first approached me, Thomas claimed to have no idea why he was in a state of such intense anguish. He was the chief financial officer of a huge international retailer with a salary of close to "four hundred thousand plus perks." He had risen from a "mean," blue-collar background to provide his three daughters with everything he never had. Thomas worked hard for his daughters, and in their pampered, opulent life, the only thing his family had ever lacked was their father. His style at home—on the infrequent occasions he was at home—was distant and dictatorial. His meteoric rise required him to uproot his family eleven times during the course of their upbringing as he followed each new career opportunity. He had neither given much thought to the impact of so much change on his wife and children nor invited anyone in the family to discuss the matter. He simply assumed that what was good for Thomas Watchell would be good for the Watchell family.

For over three decades, Thomas had logged an average of eighty hours of work per week, including evenings and weekends. And over the years, Thomas and his wife found themselves "drifting apart." By the time he had reached his mid-fifties, the demise of

Thomas's marriage struck him as no great surprise nor as any great cause for alarm. He soon found a younger, prettier, more affectionate partner. What did bother Thomas, however, what pierced him unexpectedly, was the almost complete alienation of his three daughters, all in their twenties, all of whom "sided with" their mother. According to Thomas, none of his children, except when needing money, expressed much interest in him.

It is hard for many successful men, like Thomas, to see the harmful effects of compulsive work until the relational bill comes due. Thomas's feelings of abandonment by his daughters hit him with surprising impact and triggered a drop into acute despair. Like a modern King Lear, he felt horribly betrayed by his daughters, unknown by them, despised for the very gift of his hard work and generosity. Yet, in an initial meeting with the family, Thomas's grown children revealed that they did not, in fact, feel great hostility toward their father. They just didn't feel much of anything. Having flourished throughout childhood, in a close, loving relationship with their mother, the girls had learned to grow up without him. One daughter described Thomas as an "occasionally visiting autocrat"; another called him "a blank check and a smile."

"What did you mean by 'mean'?" I ask Thomas one session, as he and his daughters—all of whom share their father's physique and posture—slouch in their chairs.

"Pardon?" Thomas looks up through large, round glasses, ever polite.

"At the end of our last session," I remind him, "you said something about growing up working-class. Remember?" I ask.

Thomas nods perfunctorily.

"When I asked you about it, your answer intrigued me." I try unsuccessfully to catch his eye. "You said you'd grown up 'blue-collar mean.' Do you remember that phrase?" I inquire.

Thomas drums his stubby fingers over thick worsted wool slacks. He looks out my window.

"Did I?" he muses, evading me. "Did I say that?" He falls silent.

Diane, the eldest, and the mouthpiece for the family's anger, shifts impatiently in her chair.

"Dad," she begins, but I cut her off, gently, with a raised hand.

"Give him a minute," I ask her. Diane and her sisters have already made their feelings about their father's elusiveness abundantly clear in our previous sessions. Thomas listened to their complaints, seemingly unperturbed, demonstrating in the office the very emotional unavailability they were berating him for. I judged that the children had said enough for the moment. It was time for something else to happen.

"*Mean*," I repeat, gently insistent. "Remember, Thomas?"

He frowns, still looking out the window. "I just don't recall . . ."

"Then, why don't you take it from scratch," I suggest, "if you can't reconstruct the conversation from a week ago? How about telling me what you *imagine* you meant by it?"

Thomas crosses his legs. He considers. "You know," he begins, "the girls don't know much about this."

"That doesn't surprise me," I answer. "It's partly why I'm asking you now."

Again, he fidgets, shifts about in his chair. Finally, after a substantial pause, he turns full around and faces me.

"All right." He squares off, looking me in the eye. "What is it that you want to know?"

"Well," I answer slowly. "You might start with whatever it was that made you decide family life was something you'd be better off running from."

Hearing these words, Thomas looks startled. He draws in a breath, offended, puffing himself up for an argument, and then he pauses—and suddenly smiles.

"So *this* is therapy," he says, amused.

"Welcome to the rich, new world of introspection," I reply.

Thomas clasps and unclasps his hands. "Frankly, I didn't expect to get into all this," he tells me, serious again.

"I understand," I answer, sympathetic to his awkwardness, his instinct toward protectiveness. I glance over at his three daughters, all of them poised, waiting, suspending judgment for a moment.

"Thomas," I ask, "how well do you think your daughters know you?"

"As well as most, I suppose," he begins.

"*Dad!*" both Diane and Patricia, the youngest, burst out in unison.

"Well, maybe not," Thomas allows, begrudgingly. "Maybe not as well as I thought."

"That's why they're here, isn't it?" I ask him. "Your daughters have come to learn something about who you are."

"Which doesn't mean, by the way—" Diane, imperious, draws herself up, looking, in her momentary belligerence, just like her father.

"Which doesn't mean anything," I both reassure her and head her off. "It means what it means. Now, listen. How much do you kids know about your dad's childhood?" For a moment, they all stare at me blankly.

Caroline, the middle one, just shakes her head.

"Not *much*," Diane finally snorts.

We all look at Patricia, the youngest, who, without speaking, spreads out her hands and suddenly begins to tear. Diane hands her a tissue. Tricia opens her mouth, but nothing comes out.

"Why are you crying, honey?" Caroline asks.

She shakes her head violently. "I just," Patricia begins, "I always feel so . . . I get *sad* when I think of Daddy, that's all."

I lean in toward her. "Tricia," I ask, "how much do you know about your father's childhood?"

"I don't know *anything* really." She reaches out for a wad of tissues. "I just know . . . Oh, God, I don't know . . ."

"Sure you do, Tricia. Go on," I urge.

"I just . . ." she stammers. "I'm not sure, *exactly.* The thing is . . . I just know it was *bad!*" Tricia folds in on herself. For no reason she could begin to articulate, she bends forward and cries.

Thomas glances at his daughter, worriedly. He looks at her sideways, afraid to meet her full in the face.

"That's yours, you know," I tell him. He looks up at me. "That pain she's expressing right now," I explain. "It's yours."

*   *   *

Two sessions later, evidencing consummate courage, Thomas Watchell sits comfortably back in his chair, eyes closed, as I have requested, thick hands folded neatly upon his wool-covered lap. Caroline, Diane, and Patricia sit flanking the two of us. Each of them slump in various states of repose. But their breathing is shallow, and their eyes are riveted on their father's face. Thomas, in a state of deep relaxation, of light hypnotic trance, has begun to explore a charged memory, a "critical image" from his childhood. Unable to speak much about his own past using ordinary forms of conversation, I have asked Thomas to intensify the process by shutting his eyes and allowing himself to drift back, to reexperience rather than merely report. In this technique in trauma recovery, Thomas first selects, and then, emotionally, comes to inhabit a primary scene, an emblem of his childhood. I see beads of perspiration collect on his forehead and neck. He is describing the "mausoleum" of his mother's bedroom as seen through his eyes as a boy.

"The main thing," Thomas recalls, "is the airlessness."

"Airlessness?" I ask.

"Yes," he nods. "All the drapery is closed."

"Keep going," I prompt.

"Well, more than just drapery. That doesn't convey it. These huge, heavy brocade things. Masses of it. Billowing all over the place. On the walls, over the bed. Pillows and flowers and—what are those things called? Sachets." He pauses, as if smelling it all again.

"Thomas, how old are you?" I ask.

"Oh," he says, "Little on up, I suppose." Then, "Four, maybe five, six, seven."

"Go on," I urge gently. Thomas sits with his eyes closed, feet flat on the floor, hands at rest, like a child's.

"You want to know what it's like?" he asks.

"Yes." I nod, even though he can't see me. "Give me details."

"Well, it's hot. In my memory, it's amazingly hot. Everything's drawn shut, you see. Windows. The blinds. Understand, now, it's August."

"Go on," I prompt. "What does it smell like?"

He wrinkles his nose. "I really don't care to. . . ."

"Were there smells you associate with her, though?" I ask, nudging him toward memories of his mother. "Her clothes, her breath?"

Thomas smiles, still with his eyes closed, as if he knows my game. "Her clothes, her breath?" he repeats. "Her *booze*, you mean?" he chides me for leading the witness. "No," shaking his head. "You are right, of course, but there isn't an odor. Straight vodka was her drug of choice. It didn't leave a strong smell. Maybe a little antiseptic, but I liked that, to be honest. It reminded me of the nurses in our school Infirmary."

"Is she moving? Talking?" I ask.

"In my conjured vision?" he clarifies, then shakes his head. "Oh, no. No. She's completely passed out. Totally out of it. Lying across the bed, snoring like a babe." He drifts off.

"And you, Thomas?" I try bringing him back.

"Me?" he waits, then drifts once again.

"Thomas?"

"I'm just there," he shrugs, at last. "You know. Just sitting there. An outpost."

"Excuse me?"

"Like a guard," he explains. "A soldier on watch. Mommy's little tin soldier." He sits up in his chair, "Ramrod straight, I am," he tells us. "Staring."

"Staring," I repeat. "Staring at what?"

"Well, at *her*, I guess," Thomas answers. "At her breathing, you know. Just, her chest, up and down, up and down." He pauses again. "It was peaceful, really."

"There was nothing peaceful about it," I counter, emphatic. "It was your *job*."

"What?" he says.

"Sitting there like that. Checking her." I notice my voice sounds almost angry. "Checking her breathing."

"Well, I don't know." He grows defensive. "Just checking in general, I'd say. Making sure she was okay, that's all."

"Making sure she was still alive," I answer.

*   *   *

When I ask Thomas how often he sat vigil like that over his drunken mother, he answers, "Every day," as if the question were stupid. But when I ask him to imagine how that little boy in his memory feels, sitting like that beside her, Thomas finally, after many sessions together, ever so quietly, lets fall a tear.

"Empty," he allows at last, after a long, awkward pause. "Really rather empty." And then he adds on his own, "Sometimes I would curl up next to her, you know. Put my head down on her, just to feel her. . . ." Even though his eyes remain closed, Thomas turns away from us toward the wall, and we know enough to leave him alone. Quietly, so as not to disrupt their father's delicate work, his daughters cry.

"So?" Thomas, looking a little rumpled, asks as all five of us hoist ourselves to our feet at the end of the session. "Was anything accomplished here today?"

His girls squeeze in close to him.

"Oh, Dad." Caroline slips her arm into her father's. "You're so clueless."

I am enormously pleased with Thomas's single tear and with his hard work of remembering. Two months ago, he would not have allowed himself to be known like that by his children. Three months ago, he had been in his neighborhood emergency room bullying some young resident on graveyard duty into giving him something that might help him sleep. Thomas thinks we are meeting to straighten things out with his children, and we are. But our goal is also the treatment of his recent acute *overt* and chronic *covert depression*.

Thomas's overt depression was a problem just waiting to happen, like that of David Ingles, though for different reasons. A lifetime of inattention to his emotions and his relationships was perched precariously over a childhood of profound psychological neglect. While Thomas kept a clear focus on his "life goals," the future he wanted, he had utterly disregarded his history. He had turned his back on the past he no longer wished to be a part of. The problem with his strategy of disowning pain was that his feelings did not cooperate very well. David Ingles turned his back on the depressed, vulnerable boy inside himself, only to wind up replaying the scene of his injury with his own son. Thomas, in one of those many dark moments by his mother's bedside, had no doubt made a vow never to subject his future family to anything like his own experience. But the life he provided his family turned out to be almost as out of balance in its own way as the life from which he had escaped. While David's disavowal pushed him toward violent engagement, Thomas's disavowal pushed him toward neglect. Both men, with no malevolent intent, inflicted on their families a version of what they themselves had been through.

Thomas's long-standing covert depression changed into acute, severe *overt depression* when his brittle sense of self-worth splintered against the sharp edge of his daughters' rejection. The concealed depression he had carried inside for so many years finally erupted. But, as Thomas himself finally admitted, it had always been with him, a feared presence lurking in the background.

"It wasn't as though I were *enjoying* myself, particularly," Thomas confessed later on in the therapy. "It was more like I was staving off a disaster. Each new success only left me breathing a little bit easier. But there was always the fear of whatever waited around the next corner. Under the rocks. I never felt much relief, really."

With few friends, no outside interests, and moving like a stranger inside his own household, Thomas comforted himself with food, kudos at work, and an "important" portfolio.

"I guess it wasn't much of a life, now that I look at it," he admitted regretfully.

Whether he knew it or not, Thomas was running. Running toward the goal of financial security, to be sure, but also running from the pain and emptiness he had felt as a child, escaping the sense of unworthiness and emotional impoverishment that had haunted him throughout much of his life.

Until his current crisis, Thomas had managed to salve his psychological wounds partially with ample amounts of external self-esteem supplements—money, prowess, prestige. These were the drugs that sustained him, taking the place of authentic relationships. Like most covertly depressed men, Thomas had trouble bearing real intimacy with others because he could not afford to be emotionally intimate with himself. Liriope, the mother of Narcissus, once asked a sage if her son would enjoy a long life. "Yes," came the ironic reply. "So long as he never knows himself." Like Narcissus, covertly depressed men do not dare know themselves; the man's own experience, the pain of depression, is avoided. It is managed and denied. Both David Ingles and Thomas Watchell had pain, but neither allowed himself to feel it.

For David and Thomas, the pain they had but refused to feel stemmed from a toxic relationship to the self, what psychiatry labels a *self disorder*. I call depression, in both its overt and in its covert forms, an *auto-aggressive disease*. Like those rare conditions which causes a person's own immune system to assault itself, depression is a disorder wherein the self attacks the self. In *overt depression*, that attack is borne; in *covert depression*, the man attempts to ward it off. But such attempts are never fully successful. The underlying assault on the self always threatens to break through the defenses.

Sigmund Freud was the first to suggest that depression was a form of internalized violence—of "aggression turned against the self," as he put it. In his classic paper "Mourning and melancholia," Freud detailed the savagery of depression's assault in a tone of bewildered alarm:

> The patient represents his ego to us as worthless, incapable of any achievement and morally despicable; he reproaches himself, vilifies himself and expects to be cast out and punished. He abases himself before everyone and commiserates with his own relatives for being connected with anyone so unworthy. He is not of the

opinion that a change has taken place, but extends his self-criticism back over the past; he declares that he was never any better. This picture of a delusion of (mainly moral) inferiority is completed by sleeplessness and refusal to take nourishment, and—what is psychologically very remarkable—by an overcoming of the instinct which compels every living thing to cling to life.

In psychiatry today, the self-attack Freud describes would be called *shame*, an acutely uncomfortable feeling of being worth-less, less than others. For many overtly depressed men, such a state of shame is itself shameful, adding to their distress and pushing them to conceal their depression from others. But covertly depressed men like Thomas and David go further still, concealing their depressions, not only from those who care about them, but also from themselves. Until undergoing therapy with me, neither man was willing to reach inside his own pain or reach out to others for help. Both were truly cut off, not merely from the possibility of comfort, but from the reality of their own conditions. While many of the men I treat report the classic symptoms of overt depression, feelings of hopelessness, helplessness, and despair, many more experience depression as a state of numbness, which is known in psychiatry as *alexithymia*. This experience of depression is not about feeling bad so much as about losing the capacity to feel at all. They are like the souls in the lowest rung of Dante's Inferno, who were not seared in fire but frozen in ice.

In overt depression, the anguish of shame, of the toxic relationship to the self, is endured. In covert depression, the man desperately defends against such an onslaught. A common defense against the painful experience of deflated value is inflated value; and a common compensation for shame, of feeling less than, is a subtle or flagrant flight into grandiosity, of feeling better than. Quite a number of theorists have noted the "narcissistic defense" of using grandiosity to ward off shame. One research team administered psychological tests measuring grandiosity and shame to a sample of one hundred college students. Their results validated long-standing clinical observation. Those subjects who scored high on grandiosity scored low on shame, and vice versa. The researchers conclude:

> There are two patterns that shame and grandiosity take in pathological narcissism: one in which the grandiosity is in the forefront of consciousness wherein shamelike feelings are denied and an opposite pattern where shame feelings are more conscious and grandiose feelings are dissociated. The central point is that grandiose behavior is a defense against images of the self as worthless and inferior.

The authors also note that the men in their sample scored significantly higher than women in grandiosity, while women subjects scored high in shame. The flight from shame into grandiosity lies at the heart of male covert depression. The means one might use to effect such a shift from shame to grandiosity are as varied as human creativity will allow, as dissimilar in style as the difference between Thomas Watchell and Brad Gaylor.

At the Family Institute of Cambridge, where I teach and practice, Brad caused a commotion by the simple act of walking down the hall. With his blue eyes, dark auburn hair, and bulging muscles, he was, as one student put it, "an ultra-hunk." Young, charming, and obviously intelligent, nevertheless Brad had, by the time I first met him, already attempted suicide six times.

In his childhood, Brad had not been actively abused by his parents; they had been too busy to bother with him one way or another. Like many children in negligent households, it was not violence at the hands of his parents but routine beatings by an older brother that turned Brad's home into a place of dread and anger. At the age of fourteen he took up bodybuilding. Like a lot of physically abused boys, Brad wanted to become invulnerable, to "get big." Brad learned to protect himself from physical assault, but his bulk did little to assuage his internal anguish. From childhood on, Brad fought to ward off a savage depression.

By nineteen, with the help of an inhuman workout schedule and gradually increasing steroid abuse, Brad had won national and even a few international competitions. But no matter how "big" he became in physique or reputation, anxiety continued to eat away at him "like a cancer." While success as a bodybuilder might ameliorate Brad's underlying depression, it could not remove it. At twenty-seven, with boundless naïveté, he imagined that becoming a movie star could subdue the ferocity he had been trying to defend against his whole life. If he were known and loved by a few million people, he thought, he might finally earn peace. And so Brad flew to Los Angeles to become rich and famous. But, like others before him, he succeeded only in becoming a prostitute to the rich and famous. He did not feel depressed during that time; he did not feel much of anything. Later, when he began to understand that, despite the "scenes" and apparent intimacies, he was still going nowhere, the despair he had held back all those years finally overwhelmed him, swamping his illusions and schemes. Five suicide attempts in two years followed this realization, all of them serious, workmanlike. Brad was tranquilized, hospitalized, even given electroshock therapy. Then one day, he finally let go of his dreams of adulation, his version of Narcissus's sprite. He moved back to Boston, tried to kill himself one last time with "almost a sense of nostalgia," and then managed to get himself into ongoing therapy.

It was clear to both of us that Brad could either give up his dreams of love from without, replacing them with the hard discipline of learning to love from within, or he would most likely die from AIDS, drugs, or suicide. After six months of intense work in therapy, Brad now has a "straight" job. He is trying, as he puts it, to "live clean." He has given up hustling and, for the moment, he has let go of his need for fame—although he tells me it's all he can do, at times, to keep himself from jumping on a plane back to L.A. and the high life he has forsaken. Neither of us knows, really, if Brad will survive.

As Narcissus was to his reflected image, as Thomas was to his work performance and bank account, so Brad was to muscle, fame, and sex, in that order. From a frightened little brother, he built himself up to become a physically imposing man. He sought out fame and adoration and settled for the illusion of tenderness in sex. When these substitutes for self-esteem failed him, the violence Brad leveled against himself was swift and determined. These are the dynamics of covert depression.

CHAPTER THREE

The Hollow Men: Covert Depression and Addiction

> Remember us,—if at all—not as lost
> Violent souls, but only
> As the hollow men
> The stuffed men.
>
> —T.S. ELIOT

The relationship of Brad or Thomas to their self-esteem props, like the relationship of Narcissus to his reflection, is an addictive one. The turning to any substance, person, or action to regulate one's self-esteem can be called an addictive process. In this framework, the terms *addition, narcissistic disorder,* and *the defenses in covert depression* are all synonyms. When a covertly depressed man's connection to the object of his addiction is undisturbed, he feels good about himself. But when connection to that object is disrupted—when the cocaine runs out, the credit cards reach their limit, the affair ends—his sense of self-worth plummets, and his hidden depression begins to unfold. Such "withdrawal" drives him back to the drug, the achievements at work, or the next sexual conquest.

Almost anything can be used defensively in covert depression to enhance self-esteem. The covertly depressed man may try to right his floundering sense of self-worth by chemically altering his moods. He may bolster failing esteem by garnering it from others, in his profession or in his romantic attachments. He may turn to a variety of compulsive activities, like sex, gambling, spending, or even something as benign as exercise.

The difference between the normal and the addictive use of these substances or activities is the difference between enhancing an already adequate sense of self-esteem and desperately propping up an inadequate one. Most of us are thrilled if we win an award, find out about a financial windfall, or arouse interest in someone attractive. But in normal circumstances we do not rely on such things in order to feel good about ourselves. We begin from a baseline feeling about ourselves that is reasonably positive or at least neutral. The covertly depressed man, in contrast, relies on such external stimulants to rectify an inner baseline of shame.

Nondepressed men turn to mood-altering behaviors like drinking, gambling, or sex for relaxation, intimate sharing, or fun. Covertly depressed men turn to such substances or activities to gain relief from distress. G. Alan Marlatt, director of the University of Washington's Addictive Behavior Research Center, found that both addictive and recreational drinkers felt a positive enhancement of mood from the physiological effects of alcohol. The difference between the two groups was that normal drinkers began with relatively good feelings from the start, while alcoholics started off with an experience of internal pain. However, the relief in such defensive maneuvers is illusory. After the wave of intoxication passes, the covertly depressed man finds himself back in the same distressed state where he began, or worse. Like wheels within wheels, this cycle of bad feeling, relief, then worse feeling is played out over days, weeks, even years.

Novelist William Styron describes a relationship between alcohol and depression that, for him, stretched across decades:

> Alcohol was a central factor, to the best of my knowledge, in my depression. I believe that many people who are by nature depressive, or have a depressive bent, use alcohol throughout most of their lives to, paradoxically, alleviate the depression. . . . You use alcohol

as a kind of medication to keep your demons at arm's length. But all of a sudden I was unable to drink. I developed a severe intolerance to alcohol. . . . In the absence of this mood bath, as I call it, that I would have every day in the evening, now I had a new experience of not having alcohol there to give me that sensation of euphoria. And that allowed the depression to crowd in.

Addiction experts call Styron's "mood bath" self-medication. Depressed people who use alcohol to "keep their demons at arm's length" are abusing the drug in a misguided, often unconscious attempt to dose themselves with a socially accepted, over-the-counter antidepressant—a "cup of cheer." Styron alleviated his lifelong covert depression with the "euphoria" of alcohol on a daily basis for years, and then, in his sixties, he suddenly developed a physical intolerance to the drug, a common occurrence for heavy drinkers late in life. At that point, the depression he had hidden for decades erupted with near lethal force.

Theories about exactly what those who self-medicate are medicating vary, some focusing on the enhancement of self-esteem, others on the regulation of feelings, still others on self-soothing. An addict's choice of drug may rest on that drug's particular medicating properties. Alcohol, for example, relieves a sense of inner emptiness and coldness by warming and disinhibiting, often making one more sociable. The first person on record to recognize these qualities was Aristotle, who reasoned that since the cause of depression, the humor bile, was dry and cold, depressed people used drink to bring heat and liveliness into their systems. From a psychological perspective, Aristotle's observations about the effects of alcohol are not far off the mark. By contrast, opioids, like heroin, do not warm one up so much as calm one down, tranquilizing the ferocity of depression, the agitation and self-hatred. Cocaine brightens a person, giving them energy; it breaks through the numb, dead feeling of alexathymia. It may be that the particular aspect of depression a person feels most strongly—such as emptiness, agitation, or numbness—determines that person's choice of a particular drug. While research on this subject remains more suggestive than conclusive, some day we may be able to map out a topography of addictive choices.

While the addiction to substances has long been recognized as having a relationship to depression, we are just now beginning to explore the relationship of depression to other addictive choices, like the addiction to persons, called erotomania or love addiction, and addiction to activities, such as gambling, spending, or violence. In 1993, Judge Sol Wachtler, a former assistant attorney general for the state of New York and a married man with four children, was accused and finally convicted of stalking an ex-girlfriend. What could have possessed a man of such high position to throw it all away? During Wachtler's trial, psychiatrist Robert Spitzer testified that Wachtler was actually suffering from severe hidden depression. Wachtler's compulsive behavior screened symptoms of loss of pleasure, loss of appetite, inability to concentrate, harsh self-criticism, and despondency. In related work, researcher Lewis Staner reported that antidepressant medication ended one patient's stalking behavior. The stalking returned when the medication was interrupted and quieted once again when treatment was resumed. There is no one answer for complex problems like violence toward women, but if Judge Wachtler had managed to receive effective treatment for covert depression, his utter ruin, and the damage done to his family, might have been averted.

Addictive choices like hustling or stalking are easy to spot because they are socially condemned and potentially life threatening. Other addictive choices, like workaholism for men or obsessive weight reduction for women, are less obvious because they are not only tolerated by our culture but often actively rewarded. Even the language of addiction in such instances can seem overblown and easy to dismiss. But the persistence of any behavior in the face of known harmful consequences qualifies as an addiction. Just because a supplement for self-esteem is socially rewarded does not mean that it will not have disastrous consequences for the individual who relies on it. Thomas Watchell and his daughters, while infinitely closer than they might have been, will never experience the closeness of the daughters and their mother. While workaholism in men may be socially acceptable, it can still wreak havoc upon their personal lives, and erode their physical health as well.

In theory an addictive relationship can be established with just about anything, so long as the substance, person, or activity relieves the threat of overt depression. To accomplish this, the defense must transform one's state from shame to grandiosity, from feelings of worth-less-ness to feelings of extraordinary worth and well-being. In common language, this sudden shift in consciousness is called intoxication. Along with the obvious effect of drugs or alcohol, one can also get "high" from the rush of physical violence, the applause of an audience, a sexual conquest, a killing in the stock market.

In covert depression, the defense or addiction always pulls the man from "less than" to "better than"—rather than to a moderate sense of inherent value. Defensive compensations for underlying depression can never move one directly from shame to healthy self-esteem, because such a shift requires confrontation with, rather than avoidance of, one's own feelings. The covertly depressed person cannot merely vault over the avoided pain directly into wholeness, as hard as he may try. The only real cure for *covert depression* is *overt depression.* Not until the man has stopped running, as David did for a moment that day in my office, or Thomas did when he let himself cry, can he grapple with the pain that has driven his behavior. This is why the "fix" of the compulsive defense never quite works. First, the covertly depressed man must walk through the fire from which he has run. He must allow the pain to surface. Then, he may resolve his hidden depression by learning about self-care and healthy esteem.

In the defensive structure of covert depression, the ordinary limits of the self are transcended through intoxication in one of two ways. In the intoxication experience that I call *merging,* the usual boundaries around the self are relaxed or even dissolved, causing feelings of boundlessness and abundance. In psychoanalysis this experience is called "oceanic bliss." The relaxation of self-boundaries lies at the core of intoxication with drugs like alcohol, morphine, and heroin. Various forms of bingeing—eating, spending, sex—can provide this same sense of expansion. Such ecstasy can also be achieved in love addiction, where the love object is felt to be godlike and thus fusion with that person brings rapture. In such cases, one projects omnipotence, or divine abundance, onto another person and then depends on that person to validate one's own worth. Engaging in such a fantasy is to some degree a universal and celebrated part of falling in love, but the love addict falls in love with the intensity of infatuation itself. Romance is not a prelude to intimacy, but a drug administered to soothe unacknowledged pain. From *Gone with the Wind* to *Basic Instinct* or *Damage*, few subjects are more compelling and disturbing than sexual obsession. But while films and romantic novels may extol the virtues of savage passion, the actual state of love addiction is often not pretty.

In the film *Camille Claudel*, director Bruno Nuytten captures both the initial exhilaration and the ultimate degradation of a severe love addiction. Based on a true story, the film traces the affair between the sculptor Auguste Rodin and his gifted student Camille Claudel. Camille moves from attraction and infatuation to horrible obsession, sinking deeper into fantasy and ultimately, psychosis. Near the film's end, Camille crouches in the mud in the pouring rain outside Rodin's house, screaming for him to come talk to her while she holds a shawl-draped stone that she claims is their baby. The final frames show her leaning against the wall of an insane asylum, where she spent the last years of her life. In severe love addiction, when the love object becomes unavailable, the experience of withdrawal can produce symptoms as horrible as in any drug detoxification, including panic attacks, depression, obsession, psychotic breakdown, stalking, murder, and suicide.

In the other type of intoxication experience, which I call *elevation*, the man's sense of power becomes inflated, so that he feels supremely gifted, special, even godlike. The purest form of this kind of intoxication is mania. The *elevating* intoxication in covert depression differs from mania primarily in that mania requires no external object to trigger the grandiose defense against shame. While the covertly depressed man must consume something or do something to shift the state of his self-esteem, a man with manic-depressive illness flips back and forth between grandiosity in the manic phase and shame in the depressed phase at the seeming whim of the disease. Manic-depression is otherwise simply a more extreme version of elevation in covert depression, in that both rely on the rush of inflated self-esteem to ward off depression. The gambler feels such a sense of chosenness when he believes he is "hot" or "on a roll." The sex addict feels that same specialness through his seductive prowess. Perhaps the most unadorned form of *elevating* intoxication is addiction to violence, when the man plays out his position of superiority by hurting and controlling others.

These two forms of addictive intoxication differ in that *merger* gives the illusion of fusion with a force that is larger than life, while *elevation* gives the illusion of becoming such a force oneself. Both are forms of grandiosity. Ernst Becker called these two possibilities the *masochistic* and the *sadistic* positions. In the masochistic position the person seeks transcendence through submerging the self in an abundant other. A person in the sadistic position also seeks transcendence, but rather than merging with the divine, he seeks to become divine, to be over nature. The exercise of illusory control and the capacity to torture are two prominent motifs of this position. Psychiatrist Judith Herman shows in *Trauma and Recovery* that the elevation of self through the medium of control over others is a central theme uniting most forms of abuse—from child molestation to wife battering and even political torture. In a totalitarian state, such exercise of control cripples dissent and protects dictatorial power. In a totalitarian family, the man imposes his will on other family members and their subservience provides the platform for his grandiosity. In severe or mild forms, both alone and, more commonly, in combination, the addictive intoxications of *merger* and *elevation* provide the means by which the covertly depressed man desperately tries to hold back his pain.

*   *   *

Jimmy, like most of the male batterers I have encountered, suffered from both forms of addictive intoxication: the need for merger with an abundant other and the need to wrestle nature, as represented by his wife, into submission. Shirley helped me see the connection between the two forms of intoxication in a couple's therapy session when she offered a suggestion.

"If you really want to be of use to somebody," Shirley proposes, folding out the wrinkles of her fashionable miniskirt, "what you should do is write yourself up some little grant, you know, some little research project, and figure out what happens to guys when their girlfriends spend time on the phone. I never met a man yet who didn't go berserk when I was on the phone for more than ten minutes."

Jimmy sputters, "Hey, listen. The baby was crying. I'm trying to get your attention. You're yappin' away on that damn . . ." He gives up, waving his hand. "It gets me upset."

At the time, Jimmy had expressed his "upset" by ripping the telephone out of the wall and handing it to Shirley. A year ago she would have gone berserk, and the fight would have escalated until the police arrived. With a half year or so of therapy under her belt, Shirley simply put down the phone, gathered up the baby, and went to her mother's with instructions for Jim not to call her until after he had spoken to me. And with six months of therapy under Jim's belt, including a batterers' program and addictions work on his drinking, he was able to let Shirley go instead of blocking or attacking her. A few sessions later, after things calmed down, I asked Jim to describe the feelings that had flooded him before he gave in to the violence. As is common with batterers, he described a momentary sense of total abandonment.

The origins of Jimmy's hypersensitivity to feelings of desertion were not hard to ascertain. His mother had died of a cocaine overdose when he was twelve, and his father spent much of Jimmy's life in and out of prison. Jimmy was raised for the most part by loyal members of his neighborhood gang. Certain that he would live a short, violent life, he once told me, "My motto was, 'Die young. Stay pretty.' " Jimmy reacted to his own surprising survival with depression in his twenties, soon followed by serious drinking and crime. Like a sprinter, Jimmy could hold his pain at bay as long as he thought it was for the short run. Once he realized he might have a future to face, he collapsed. Then Jimmy met Shirley, a social worker with whom he had grown up and, in a rare moment of good judgment, he allowed her to love him. Sober now, with a good job and a baby, he was as dismayed as she when he succumbed to fits of rage. The telephone, for him, was a cipher for being shut out, betrayed, abandoned. To call the feelings that surged up in him mere "upset" was too mild; "volcanic" was more like it; "panicked" might be better still. Jim felt victimized and alone in the minutes before he erupted—as if he were back in the chaos of his own childhood.

"I felt," he says, "as if I could stand there and slit my own throat and she'd just go right on talking."

"You felt that uncared about," I reflect back to him.

"Like she just couldn't give a shit," he replies.

Jimmy was in a momentary but profound instance of love addiction. When his connection to Shirley was disrupted by the telephone, the abandonment that inundated him, the transitory but intense depression that engulfed him, were literally more than he could bear. Jim then reached out for another addictive defense—violence—to pump up his plummeting self-esteem. Like alcohol or drugs, violence operated for Jimmy as a magic elixir transforming his shame into grandiosity, shifting him from a sense of helplessness to a sense of omnipotent control. In place of healthy self-esteem, Jim had habitually turned to Shirley for comfort. When Shirley, even for a few minutes, "betrayed him" by focusing elsewhere, he found himself becoming enraged. When Jimmy's defense of *merger* failed him, he turned to the defense of elevation. Rage never abandoned Jimmy. Like an ideal wife, rage was always available to him, night or day, at a moment's notice. These are the common dynamics of domestic violence.

When Jimmy lashed out at Shirley, he was, as one abuse expert terms it, "offending from the victim position." This is perhaps the most common pattern of male violence toward women. Flooded with depression and feelings of victimization, Jimmy used rage to physiologically pump up his sense of deflation. Research shows that rage simultaneously releases adrenaline, which speeds up the autonomic nervous system, and endorphins, which act as the body's own opioids. This is a powerful internal cocktail, which tragically, like any other form of intoxication, can offer short-lived relief from the pain of depression.

The pattern in males of moving from the helpless, depressed, "one down" position to a transfigured, grandiose, "one up" position has become one of the most powerful and ubiquitous narratives in modern times. The hero, a meek, quiet, strong man of principle, is bullied and pressed to the wall. He is humiliated and abused, often physically. Then comes the turnaround. Clark Kent rips off his business suit to become Superman; David Banner transforms when angered into the Incredible Hulk. The "weakling" stands up. In a recurring scene that lies at the heart of the film *Taxi Driver*, Robert De Niro stares into a mirror and challenges an imagined enemy. "Are you looking at me?" he threatens. "Are *you* looking at *me?*" We invariably laugh, the first time this scene is shown, as we recognize the braggart boy of our own past posturing before the looking glass. But as the scene is replayed, De Niro appears each time better armed and more psychotic, until, in the last repetition, he emerges wholly transformed and wholly mad. His head is shaved, he is covered with tattoos, and he carries enough weapons to attack a small fortress. The question he repeats one final time— "*Are you looking at me?*"—now sends an unholy chill through the audience. De Niro stands before the mirror like a deranged Narcissus bent over a well of darkness.

This theme of male transformation harkens back to our archetypal heroes, like Odysseus, Orpheus, Siddhartha, and Jesus. As mythologist Joseph Campbell elaborated, the hero's journey usually leads from some difficult trial, often involving pain and humiliation, through an experience of transformation to a triumphal return. Throughout most cultures and in most ages, this mutation from a state of helplessness to sublimity has been effected by a spiritual awakening. In modern Western mythology, the same transformation is most often effected through the forces of rage and revenge. In the film *Falling Down*, Michael Douglas, a repressed, buttoned-down nerd, fulfills our own dark fantasies by decompensating in the middle of a traffic jam and going on a bloody rampage. All of the popular *Rambo* movies follow this pattern of ritual wounding followed by grand revenge. In *Rambo I*, Stallone is unfairly pursued and shot at by bigoted police officers. In *Rambo II*, he is tortured with electricity. In *Rambo III*, his right side is lacerated by flying shrapnel. In each, he emerges stronger than ever and ready for vengeance. In *The Unforgiven*, Clint Eastwood is savagely beaten and crawls out of town, only to return and kill his abuser. In fact, almost every recent Hollywood adventure plays out this theme of revenge in some fashion.

These scenes of ceremonial injury hark back to the crucifixion and dismemberment of Dionysius, Mithras, Jesus, and other heroes of the great mystery cults. But for the spiritually rich heroes of antiquity, it is their egos, their ordinary selves, that are rent in order to give way to the sublime. In our modern version, the hero's self is not transmuted by spirit but inflated by violence. This is a dangerous direction for heroism to take.

The same shift from shame to grandiosity through violence that is celebrated in film invades our homes in the form of rampant domestic abuse. Research shows that one distinguishing characteristic of battering men is a markedly increased sensitivity to feelings of abandonment, which can often translate into love addiction. Battering men like Jimmy use connection to their sexual partners to help medicate covert depression. Without acknowledging it, these rough macho guys depend on union with their women to supplement deficiencies in self-esteem. When their partners "fail them," they are flooded by depression and shame. Rage psychologically and physiologically "medicates" their dip into the experience of depression. Helpless feelings vanish with the illusion of inordinate power. The grandiose entitlement to lash out at another human being rights their floundering sense of self-worth—and they strike. Underneath it all lies the depression, like Jimmy's, which sets a man up to be vulnerable to abandonment in the first place. With some men these dynamics are violent and obvious; with others they are violent and subtle. Damien Corleis was one of the latter.

Damien Corleis was a good-looking, successful architect—as far from the common image of a batterer as a person can get. His wife, Diane, was beautiful and bright. Both had risen from tough, working-class backgrounds. Diane had parlayed her husband's earnings into significant wealth through clever investing, and now, in their late forties and with their four kids grown or in college, they should have been on easy street. That's where Damien thought they were until Diane suddenly moved out last summer. At first, he believed she had simply gone mad. But by the time they came into my office, almost two months into the separation, Diane had managed to share a few thoughts with him that either she had been too timid to speak about before or Damien had been too walled off to hear. The issue was sex.

Diane explained to me that if she did not have sex with Damien every two or three nights, he became anxious, irritable, and sulky. If three nights stretched out to four or five, Damien started pressing her for sex, while at the same time verbally attacking her. Soon there were stormy fights, not ostensibly about sex but about anything else. Often the scenes were public. Often he humiliated her. Damien "flipped out" when they were seated in the smoking section of a restaurant. Damien "flipped out" if he didn't like the service at their hotel, if Diane "made them" late, or if she interrupted him too often at dinner. Always, there was the threat of rage, complaints of not being loved, meanness mixed with insistence on attention.

"But," Diane concludes, "Damien is not a bad man. I know he loves me. He is a good father, a great provider. I know he means well."

"So how do you cope with all this?" I ask her.

Diane looks down at the floor, her eyes welling up. "I *said* I wasn't going to do this!" she mutters, annoyed with her own tears.

"Some women cry when they're angry," I offer.

"Oh, I'm angry, all right," she answers. "You don't need a degree to know that I'm angry."

"So, how have you coped?" I ask her again, already pretty sure of the answer.

"I give in, of course." She cries in earnest. "I let him have what he wants. For twenty-three *fucking* years. *Shit*," she mumbles reaching for Kleenex. "*Tell* me why I wore mascara."

Damien has sat still for as long as he can bear it. He looks like a panther on a leash. Underneath his nice-guy exterior, good looks, and good manners, Damien does feel a little scary to sit with.

"What *I* don't get—" he starts, but I cut him off. "The key thing now, Damien—may I call you Damien?" He nods, leaning forward, impatient for me finish so he can argue with Diane. "The key thing to me is that your wife seems like she's on the brink of divorcing you. That's what strikes me. Am I exaggerating?" I ask Diane. She shakes her head. "So, I need to hear from her right now, because . . . that's assuming you want her back. Do you?"

Damien looks at me, startled. "Desperately," he says.

I look at him for a while, at his tanned, handsome face, at the eyes that do not turn away from mine. Behind his bluster, he seems hurt and jumpy.

"I believe you," I say softly, still holding his gaze. "You *look* desperate enough." I turn to Diane. "Does he always interrupt you like that?" I ask.

"Always." Emphatic.

"No, I don't," Damien protests.

"*Always.*" Her voice is raised.

"Fuck this!" Damien rises fully out of his chair.

"Listen," I say softly. "I'm on your side. You want her back. I want you to have her. Now please, Damien, *sit down.*"

Damien looks at me for a long fifteen seconds, as if he might have enjoyed extracting my windpipe. Then he blows out a huge stream of breath and sits back in his chair.

"What do I need to do?" he asks. For the moment, he has decided to let me win.

"Turn your chair this way so that you're facing Diane," I begin. "Put your hands in your lap, breathe through your nose, and listen."

Watching her husband lurch his big frame toward her, Diane cracks up. She has a thoroughly infectious laugh.

"Am I happy to be here?" Damien grins at her.

"Do you need to be somewhere else?" Diane shoots back.

"Can we begin?" I ask both of them.

Listening to Diane, I was sure she was right. Damien was used to getting his way, and not just about lovemaking but about what kind of music they listened to, about what temperature they set the heat to, about where they went on vacation, and—if I had not been careful in those first ten minutes—about who was going to take charge of the couple's therapy.

Diane was also right about sex. Damien was a mild and relatively contained sex addict. It might be jarring to hear him called that. It certainly shocked Damien, although Diane found it both odd and relieving. As with all other addictions, we tend to think of sex addiction only in its most severe form. But not all sex addicts are completely out of control like Steve, a forty-year-old executive I treated who couldn't get through a long business meeting without running off to the Fenway to cruise. Similarly, we do not generally think of a sex addict as someone who is monogamous, but it is quite possible to be sexually addicted to one partner. A university law professor, now years in recovery, saw me with his wife to heal from a time, years earlier, when he was so severely sex addicted that he at first cajoled and then eventually raped her on the day following her double mastectomy.

Damien wasn't nearly so disturbed. He was in most ways a loving man. In bed, he was a generous and considerate lover. Out of bed, there were often flowers from the office, little gifts, surprise outings, so long as, in his words, his "needs were met." It took a while to convince Damien that sex was not about meeting his needs, that sexually Diane had to be more than a well-treated appliance, that, for example, she had the right to say no. It took a while, by the way, to get the same message—called "setting a sexual boundary"—through to Diane as well. Along with her resentment, Diane's fear that any sign of affection might arouse Damien had kept her physically distant and unaffectionate for decades. While she never refused sex, she had not had an orgasm with him since their children were born.

Not wanting to struggle over semantics, I told Damien that while we need not fuss about whether or not he was "an addict" per se, I strongly believed that his relationship to sex and to sexual energy was addictive. He used sex to soothe himself and, in essence, to medicate bad feelings. Damien said he wasn't aware of having many bad feelings. I promised him that if he stayed with me long enough, he would be.

The crisis hit about two and a half months into therapy. Damien had been doing splendidly. It was as if he had woken up from a dream. Across the board, he actively tempered his controlling behavior. As his subtle bullying decreased, his receptivity increased, and he found himself, as he put it, "adoring Diane less and loving her more." On her side Diane, feeling some control for the first time in years, began to warm up again. In this atmosphere, Damien was taken by surprise when the anxiety attacks started. They were soon followed by sleeplessness, moodiness, and intense irritability.

"What the hell is all this?" he asked me.

"Withdrawal," I answered.

Damien was scared. He began to fall apart. I saw him alone to lend support. We considered medication, which he preferred not to take. At the worst point, we even considered a brief hospitalization. Damien sank so deeply into depression that he needed Diane's help to get up and dress in the morning, even to shave himself. A preoccupation with suicide emerged and grew alarmingly strong. In one couples session Damien glared at me with reproach and anger, tears streaming down his face. He spread out his arms, helpless and disheveled, as if to say, See what you've done?

"This is what I've been afraid of," he said.

I touched his shoulder as he bent doubled over in pain. "I know," I said. "I know."

Between the ages of seven and thirteen Damien Corleis had been passed back and forth between his older brother, Peter, whom he adored, and a neighbor down the block, both of whom engaged in sex with him. Until now, Damien had not remembered. He had not recalled it even when, in his first year at college, he became so depressed that he was hospitalized and received electroshock therapy—a bit of his history he initially neglected to share with me. It became clear as he and I spoke that Damien's parents had suspected the abuse but were too ineffectual to do anything about it. They had abandoned him.

In the weeks that followed, Damien regressed until he became completely unable to function. When he was on the brink of a second hospitalization, Diane and I scrambled to arrange an emergency meeting with his family. As a family therapist, I have a distinct advantage over individually oriented therapists in such times of crisis. While individual therapists must rework early abuse issues slowly and painfully within the confines of the treatment relationship, my training allows me to invite the abusers themselves into my office—to heal as a family from traumas of their collective past. In such instances one must measure whether or not the family can be brought to the point of dealing with the truth about their own experience. After listening to Damien describe his family, which, despite its difficulties seemed to have resources of love and intelligence, I believed that there was a good chance that they could.

This was a high-risk move, but Damien was in a high-risk state. His parents flew in from Detroit, his brother from Washington State, and a younger sister from Georgia. I met with the family for three whole days. After initial, violent protests of innocence, Peter cracked open in the middle of the second day, admitting all that he had done. Later, he said he just could not bear another minute of

Damien's inconsolable tears. Under my direction, on his knees, Peter voiced his utter remorse to his brother. At the end of these family sessions Damien agreed, at his family's urging, to try a short course of antidepressant medication. Within a month the worst had passed.

Damien Corleis had good reason to be controlling. What he unconsciously felt the need to control was the depression that had disabled him once already and, beneath that, the trauma that threatened to rip him apart. Like many adults with abuse histories, Damien's behavior—insistent sex—both soothed and, in masked form, replayed his trauma. But like David and Thomas, the means Damien chose to keep his depression at bay almost cost him his family.

Damien's treatment illustrates the principle that the cure for covert depression is overt depression. First, the addictive defense must be confronted and stopped. Then, the hidden pain emerges. Underneath Damien's addiction lay depression, and underneath his depression lay trauma. During the course of his treatment Damien courageously allowed his grandiose defense to drop, his depression to surface, and the trauma behind them both to be confronted.

At this point I was, if anything, more worried about Peter. Peter had walled off both his abuse and his crime almost totally from consciousness. By all accounts, he was a well-adjusted, if somewhat driven, man. With the reemergence of all that had happened to him as well as all he had done, Peter stood in desperate need of counseling, and we worked together to ensure that he received it back in his hometown.

Peter is not the villain in this tale. He had begun sexual relations with his neighbor at about the same age Damien was when Peter later abused him. This is a familiar pattern, in which the molested turn around and molest. My clinical experience has led me to assume that an experience of sexual abuse or at least wildly transgressed boundaries lies behind a sibling committing incest with another sibling. Children simply do not "come up" with such behavior on their own.

Peter reminded me of a case I supervised in which five British boys were lured onto a deserted beach by a local man who sodomized two of them while the others watched. True to the male norms of their culture, none of the boys said a word about their experience from that day forward, to anyone else or even to one another. What they did do, however, for the next five years or so, was take turns sodomizing one another. This was not normal homosexual play among kids, nor were all these children coincidentally gay. These boys were replaying the wound, and in a sadly convoluted way, they were comforting one another. There is something dreadful and touching about this story. By carrying on the abuse with one another, the boys were trying to normalize it, to share the burden. One wonders if a similar impulse may in part lie behind the universal brutality of boy's initiation rites into manhood. Perhaps the male community's tradition of "welcoming" a boy into its midst by hurting him is not just a test to prove the boy tough enough to be worthy of joining. Perhaps it is also a demonstration, a need to communicate the men's own sense of woundedness, a ritual dramatization of how much pain they all carry inside.

Peter passed on the wound that had been passed to him. Ironically, Damien, like his brother, learned to use the soothing of sex to manage the depression, to compensate for the fragility of self, which his sexual molestation had helped to create. That depression flooded over him within weeks of stopping the addictive behavior. Damien's story illustrates a common pattern, where the defenses to which covertly depressed men turn often compound their difficulties. Damien hurt Diane and almost destroyed his marriage. But he had no real feeling for the damage he was inflicting. Between the inordinate shame of depression and the relative shamelessness of grandiosity, there lies *appropriate shame*, feeling proportionately bad about something one has done wrong. Men who offend must first be brought from shameless behavior into the experience of their forgotten, appropriate shame. They must be thawed out. If not, the addictive defenses pull them toward behaviors that are at best disconnected and at worst irresponsible, the kind of behaviors my father engaged in throughout much of his life.

*   *   *

My father, as poor as he was, worked his way through the Philadelphia College of Art with the help of the GI bill. When my twin brother and I were born, Dad took on two jobs along with his schoolwork. For three years he slept only a few hours each night. He spoke with great pride of making "the dean's list" throughout those tough school years and of the praise he had won for his art work, particularly sculpture, which was his great passion. But my father had three hungry people to care for, and so he switched his major from fine art to industrial design. Years later, he told me that a part of him had died on the day he went to the registrar's office to make the change. Although he would have been horrified to admit it, my father never really forgave any of us—my mother, brother or me—for depriving him of his dream. From early childhood it was clear to me that Dad saw himself as our victim.

My father medicated his sense of being shackled and held back with regular doses of arrogance. He was a consistent rage-aholic. His pattern during my growing up was to get a job designing signs or warehouses and within a few months to behave so abrasively to his colleagues that he would get himself fired. Then, ostensibly miserable but in reality happy to spend all of his time sculpting in our converted garage, he would procrastinate about finding a new position. Mom held the family together with sporadic work as a nurse while our finances degenerated to a point of desperation.

Mom and Dad fought bitterly throughout most of this cycle. When working, Dad was short-fused and attacking because he felt so put upon. When Dad would get fired they both fought out of exasperation and worry. And finally, Mom fought with Dad in order to shoehorn him out of the garage to mail out a few résumés. A flurry of hope for a fresh start would come with each new job, only to have the cycle repeat itself.

Dad used notions about the status of "real art," as he put it, to justify his own irresponsibility. During the hours he spent slapping plaster of paris around in the garage, he was salving his unacknowledged depression with dreams of artistic achievement. He avoided many of the realistic demands of family life while working out there in the garage, away from us, reliving his golden moments in college and fantasizing about winning awards once more. Dad never did win many accolades again, but his passion burned bright from the days of his glory. When I was about eight or nine, he took the whole family to the shrine of his past victory, the Philadelphia Museum of Art. It looked like a magnificent Greek temple. As we climbed the biggest set of steps I had ever seen, Dad held my brother's and my hands. Mom trailed behind, understood by us to be irrelevant. At the top of the stairs was a statue by Dad's favorite sculptor and sometime mentor, Jacques Lipchitz. It was a huge, rough-hewn piece showing Prometheus in torment after stealing fire from the Titans to give to man. I knew, because Dad had told us, that he himself felt like Prometheus, trying in vain to bring the light of rationality and art to the weak, stupid people surrounding him. In the sculpture, the hero emerges only partially from the stone, arms spread wide, trying in vain to hold back the eagle that mercilessly plucks at his liver. Prometheus and his nemesis merge and coalesce, blurring the line where one ends and the other begins.

In the glare of autumn sunlight, I remember looking up at Dad, who was staring at the statue, transported. Completely uncognizant of those around him, he stretched his arms out wide as he gazed. Seeing him this way frightened me.

"Let's go, Dad," I said, pulling at him. "Let's go inside." Looking up at my father's outstretched arms, his powerful shoulders and thick hands, I am not sure if I thought more of the arms of the hero or the wings of the avenging bird.

From an early age I instinctively knew, though I would not have been able to express it in words, that my father was in the grip of something big and violent, something he depended on. It was dangerous to get in its way or even come too close to it. Neither my brother nor I ever asked Dad, for example, to teach us how to draw or paint. Without being forbidden, neither of us ever explored the garage. We were too frightened to tamper with it.

With each new failure, my father became more bellicose and dismissive. And as his attitude worsened, he found it ever more difficult to succeed. The defenses one chooses to avoid shame often afford relief while breeding more shame. Addiction experts have termed this pattern a "shame cycle." The covertly depressed man's defensive maneuvers or addictions can be experienced by the man as shameful in themselves or else they can create difficulties in his life that intensify his sense of inferiority, leading in either case to an increased craving for the defenses. This cycle reminds me of a little round my friends and I found amusing when we were kids.

"Why do you drink?"

"Because I'm depressed."

"And why are you depressed?"

"Because I'm a lush."

Current research on drinking and depression gives credence to this cyclic pattern. Research indicates that depressed people may experience the effects of alcohol and other drugs more strongly than nondepressed people do and have a higher expectation that such substances will help them to feel better. Other research, however, reports that the high incidence of depression in alcoholics stems not from an underlying mood disorder but from the fact that alcohol in general, and prolonged drinking in particular, actually causes depression. The debate has been framed as: Does depression lead to alcohol abuse or does alcohol abuse lead to depression? One way to synthesize these perspectives, as well as the apparent contradiction in the findings, is to understand that alcohol *both* provides relief from depression and simultaneously creates more of it. What is true for alcoholism is true for all of the defenses used in covert depression. Addictions do to shame what saltwater does to thirst. The defenses used in covert depression tend to grow, providing ever decreasing amounts of relief while requiring ever increasing amounts of indulgence.

News anchorman Jim Jensen, who has spoken out about his struggles with cocaine and depression, describes his experience of that escalation:

You never recreate the same feeling that you had the first time, and you've got to use more and more and more and you never get back. It takes on a life of its own. Then it controls you. And when you fall off cocaine, there's the depression. And depression was the main cause of it all.

Because of the insidious capacity of self-esteem supplements to "take on a life of their own," therapy must first treat the addictive behavior as an addiction per se. Before AA and other addictions recovery programs won grudging acceptance by the medical establishment, many lives were damaged when mental health professionals tried to treat addictive behaviors like any other therapy issue. In my early years as a family therapist, I often encountered individuals who had spent years in psychotherapy, never confronting their runaway addictions. The addicted man would speak to his therapist each week about all manner of interesting issues—childhood wounds, marital tensions, new areas of growth in his personality—all the while driving his family to the brink of despair with his drinking, drugging, or other compulsive behaviors. Many believed that one could cure such behaviors using traditional therapy techniques that addressed the patient's underlying emotional dynamics. But the evolving expertise in addictions recovery has convinced most mental health professionals that they cannot cure addictive behaviors with five days a week on the couch, any more than by simply throwing antidepressant medication at them. Only after the shame cycle has stopped, after the addictive pattern itself has been broken, and after the person has moved into "sobriety" can the pain of covert depression be addressed.

This double-edged approach, stopping the addictive cycle and dealing with the emergent depression, calls for the "dual diagnosis" of both depression and addiction. Covertly depressed men who self-medicate with substances have the greatest chance of a correct diagnosis and of receiving effective treatment for both aspects of their disorder.

Less fortunate are those covertly depressed men who turn for self-medication not to substances but to people, as in a love addiction, or to actions, particularly violence. In such cases, most mental health professionals would not correctly diagnose either the addictive behavior or the underlying depression that fuels it. Covertly depressed men who turn to persons or to activities to medicate their shame are generally labeled as having *personality disorders*. Many of the men who appear in this book would be classed as having personality disorders in conventional psychiatric thinking.

The term *personality disorder* does not denote a disease at all but rather a variety of serious problems in one's basic character, an insufficient development of the psyche itself. A neurotic disorder, by contrast, involves conflicts between different parts of the psyche, such as the classic Freudian conflict between our uncivilized sexual drives and the superego, the seat of moral principle. Neuroses involve psychic conflicts; personality disorders involve structural damage. Personality disordered people are described as impulsive, unable to regulate feelings, having poor judgment or undeveloped consciences.

In their level of seriousness, difficulty of treatment, and degree of impairment, personality disorders are viewed by psychiatry as occupying a domain between neurotics, like those who inhabit Woody Allen movies, and outright psychotics, like the protagonist in *Taxi Driver* or those who suffer from schizophrenia. Personality disordered people are thought to be better off than psychotics because they do not actually lose touch with reality. However, they are thought to be more "primitive" than neurotics in their development because they tend to locate their difficulties outside themselves. They show little insight or capacity for emotional responsibility. They blame the world for their problems and often engage in vociferous struggles with their environment, as did my father. They are all, in one form or another, antisocial.

The problem with this well-established psychiatric tradition is that it ignores the effects of gender. In our society, women are raised to pull pain into themselves—they tend to blame themselves, feel bad. Men are socialized to externalize distress; they tend not to consider themselves defective so much as unfairly treated; they tend not to be sensitive to their part in relational difficulties and not to be as in touch with their own feelings and needs. In psychology, measures have been devised for calculating these tendencies in direction, called internalizing/externalizing scales. Women rate high in internalizing, men in externalizing. Internalizing has been found to have a high correlation with overt depression. When researchers compared the high rates of externalization in men with their low rates of depression they speculated that men's capacity to externalize might somehow protect them from the disease. But while the capacity to externalize pain protects some men from *feeling* depressed, it does not stop them from *being* depressed; it just helps them to disconnect further from their own experience. The capacity to externalize helps men escape overt depression, only to drive them toward covert depression.

In the value system of traditional psychiatry, pain that is internal, lucidly experienced, and able to be spoken about is seen as less disturbed than pain that is externalized and unconsciously "acted out." The withdrawn depressed girl in the back of the classroom is seen as somehow less troubled than the acting-out, disruptive boy in the front row. Because psychotherapy since Freud has been "the talking cure," it relies on the patient's insight into his or her problems and feelings as its chief therapeutic agent. One difficulty with such a methodology is that it is much more in keeping with the traditional skills of women than with those of men. Men do not have readily at hand the same level of insight into their emotional lives as women, because our culture works hard to dislocate them from those aspects of themselves. Men are less used to voicing emotional issues, because we teach them that it is unmanly to do so. Even a cursory look at gender socialization in our culture indicates that a man would be far more likely to act out distress than to talk about it, while a woman would have the skills, the community, and the ease to discuss her problems. Having forcefully pushed our boys and men away from the exercise and development of these psychological skills, we add insult to injury when we turn around and label them more disturbed and less evolved than women who have been encouraged to keep them.

Overt depression, prevalent in women, can be viewed as internalized oppression, as the psychological experience of victimization. Covert depression, prevalent in men, can be viewed as internalized disconnection—the experience of victimization warded off through grandiosity, perhaps through victimizing. Morally, one might place an unequal judgment on these related disorders. Self-laceration may seem more evolved than attack, masochism preferable to sadism. Certainly, to the innocent victims of an offender, implosion is preferable to explosion. But from a purely psychological perspective, we must understand that internalized pain and externalized pain are two faces of the same experience. We may find externalized pain more difficult, or even repugnant, but that does not make it a different condition, merely the same condition expressed in the ways men have been taught to express it.

We know this about male children. We know that the disruptive boy is no less depressed than the overly compliant little girl. "Acting out" behaviors are often the very symptoms we look for in making a diagnosis of depression in boys. And yet, for reasons that I have never seen explained, as a profession we have decided that when the boy hits the magic age of eighteen he is no longer depressed; he has crossed the Rubicon into the land of the personality disordered. This is not reason. This is moral judgment. This is the psychiatric equivalent of transferring a kid from "juvie" court to go stand for his crimes "like a real man."

That is not to say that covertly depressed men are not fully responsible for their offending behaviors. But it is clear that the stable ratio of women in therapy and men in prison has something to teach us about the ways in which each sex is taught by our culture to handle pain. Men make up close to 93 percent of the prison population, leading one "Men's Movement" leader to quip that the largest men's gathering in the United States is San Quentin.

In national figures on mental disorders, women outnumber men by two to one among those diagnosed exclusively as depressed. The lifetime incidence of a major depressive episode in women is 21.3 percent of the total population, while in men, the disorder strikes only 12.7 percent. But if we factor into the equation "personality disorders" and chemical dependency, the totals even right back out again. Antisocial personality in women runs at 1.2 percent of the total population, while in men it is 5.8 percent. Drug dependency in women runs at 5.9 percent of the total population, while in men it is 9.2 percent. And alcoholism in women runs at 8.2 percent of the total population, while in men it is 20.1 percent. When the incidence of these disorders is added to the incidence of depression, it balances the level of pathology in each sex (see chart).

LIFETIME INCIDENTS OF MENTAL DISORDERS
(as percentage of the population)

	Men	Women	Both
AFFECTIVE DISORDERS			
Major depressive episode	12.7	21.3	17.1
Manic episode	1.6	1.7	6.4
Dysthymia ("mild depression")	4.8	8.0	6.4
ANXIETY DISORDERS			
Panic disorder	2.0	5.0	3.5
Agoraphobia	3.5	7.0	5.3
Social phobia	11.1	15.5	13.3
Simple phobia	6.7	15.7	11.3
Generalized anxiety	3.6	6.6	5.1
SUBSTANCE ABUSE DISORDERS			
Alcohol abuse	12.5	6.4	9.4
Alcohol dependence	20.1	8.2	14.1
Drug abuse	5.4	3.5	4.4
Drug dependence	9.2	5.9	7.5
OTHER DISORDERS			
Antisocial personality	5.8	1.2	3.5
Nonaffective psychosis	0.6	0.6	0.7
TOTALS	48.7	47.3	48.0

It is time to conceptualize depression in men as a wide-ranging spectrum, with many variations and differences. Overtly depressed men like William Styron occupy one place along that spectrum. Covertly depressed men like David, Jimmy, and Damien occupy another. The common denominator linking them all is violence. All of these men are violent toward themselves, as

Styron was to the point of near suicide, or violent toward others, as David was to Chad and Damien was to Diane. And the origins of so much violence can be traced to the ordinary, everyday violence our boys are immersed in as a central part of their socialization. To understand depression in men, we must come to terms with the conditions that create it, the ways in which, in the name of masculinity and often with the best of intentions, we betray and deform our sons.

CHAPTER FOUR

A Band Around the Heart: Trauma and Biology

For the covertly depressed man, what lies at the center of the defense or addiction is the disowned overt depression he has run from. And in the center of the overt depression lies trauma. For some men the underlying injuries are blatant and extreme. For others, they are seemingly mild, even ordinary. And yet, for both, the damage in their capacity to sustain connection to themselves and others may be severe. No matter if the injuries have been quiet or loud, depressed men carry inside a hurt, bewildered boy whom they scarcely know how to care for. The moment of contact with that disavowed pain is the first step toward restoration.

"A lot has happened this week," Michael lets us know, before I even have time to close the door behind him and sit down in my chair. He has come a few minutes late to Wednesday night men's group, a gathering of eight men that I have facilitated for close to three years. Old members sometimes leave this group. New members arrive. A core of four have remained. I invited Michael to join us about four weeks ago and his entry has been edgy.

"I need to talk," Michael repeats. About forty-five, he is small and wiry, with an anxious, pointed face and dark, curly hair. His large, cornflower blue eyes bear down on me, searching, hungry. When I resist the impulse to turn away, the eyes meeting mine are opaque. There is no doorway into them. Even without other clues, those greedy, unreceptive eyes would give Michael away. The other men in the group instinctively draw back from him, perhaps without knowing it or wondering why. But I know why. Michael is intrusive and walled off at the same time. He pushes past other people's boundaries but then doesn't accept what they offer. His need to control, this combination of urgency and rejection, is difficult to live with, and his wife, Virginia, decided a few weeks earlier that she no longer wished to try.

I had seen them as a couple only twice before Ginny broke the news to him in my office one morning. When he heard it, Michael just doubled over in his chair and sat motionless with his head in his hands.

"Michael?" I asked. "Mike?"

He didn't cry. He didn't yell. Even when Virginia told him that she had been sleeping with another man for over a year, and that she was leaving to move in with him, Mike remained calm. They had a quiet discussion about what to say to the kids and agreed to see me later on in the week. Mike reassured both of us that he was fine. No surprise, really. He'd sort of known all along. Yes, he would call me if he needed to talk.

Michael did telephone early the following morning. He called to tell me about the handgun he'd purchased just after our last session. He spoke in whispers because the kids were still sleeping upstairs and he didn't want to disturb them. Mike and I, two avowed Massachusetts liberals, shared our sense of dismay that one could obtain a pistol so quickly even in staid old Boston. He told me the details of obtaining the gun. I asked whom he intended to use it on. At that, Michael grew cagey, ironic. "If I had any balls," he told me. "I'd use it on that homewrecker."

"Homewrecker," I thought. Such an out-of-step, Hollywood word. A word from another generation.

"But then again," Michael continued, "if I had any balls, I wouldn't be in this mess to begin with, would I?" I didn't respond. "Being the schmuck that I am, I'll no doubt take it out on myself if I use it on anyone."

"Are you thinking about doing that?" I asked him.

"I'm thinking about it, sure. Thinking about it."

"Where's the gun now?"

"I'm holding it," he told me. "Looking right at it. You know," he confided, "I really like the feel of it in my hand. Heft. It has heft."

"Michael, you're gonna scare the shit out of your kids if they walk downstairs and see you like this."

"I know," he sighed, petulant. "To tell you the truth, that's why I called. To tell you the truth, I think it may be the *only* reason I called."

"How about you put the gun away in a drawer?" I said.

"Fine," he replied, without a hint of struggle, as if he'd been waiting for me to tell him to. I could hear the drawer open and close. "You know, I never even bought bullets for it," he said.

"Probably wise," I answered.

We arranged for Michael to go with his brother to a local emergency room. His sister-in-law took the kids and his brother took away the gun. The emergency room psychiatrist evaluated Michael and decided to hospitalize him for a few days in order to start him on medication and check for suicide potential. Michael cooperated and was quickly released. The immediate storm had passed. As thoughts of suicide receded, overt depression settled in on Michael like a tough case of walking pneumonia. He couldn't sleep. He couldn't eat. He couldn't concentrate enough to work or even to drive without getting into an accident.

Like a lot of men, Michael, while appearing independent, had staved off his covert depression with his relationship. Along with the trauma of his wife's news and his grief for his marriage, Michael was in the acute phase of withdrawal from love addiction. His defense against underlying depression had just walked out with another man.

Antidepressant medication helped Michael once it "kicked in." I also allowed him to transfer some of his dependency from Ginny to me, meeting with him two or three times a week to help see him through the crisis. While I wanted him to survive it, I was in no hurry to take the crisis away. Working with covertly depressed men has taught me to respect crisis as a potential ally. It had taken Michael forty-five years to come unglued. While I wanted to help put him back together, I didn't want simply to return to the old status quo. If he was going to suffer the pain of this tumult, then at least he could make good use of it. In six weeks' time, Michael had "stabilized" enough for our real work to begin. I suspected that the combined support, wisdom, and confrontation of other men might help him along, and so I invited him to join us.

"I have a *lot* to tell you," Michael repeats, ignoring the other group members, impatient that I have taken so long to sit down. The other men shift in their chairs. Most are veterans of this process. They have some recovery on board. They know how to wait. Michael leans forward on the very edge of his seat, his clasped hands dangling between his spread legs, as if he were leaning over the side of a boat. He has pulled his chair to only a few inches away from mine and shifts his weight to get even closer.

"Michael," I say after backing my chair into the wall. "One of us is going to have to move or I'm going to suffer from short air supply."

"Huh?"

"Move your chair back," I request.

Annoyed, Michael pulls his chair back a full half inch and begins launching into his story.

"Further," I tell him.

Two inches.

"Here." I get up from my chair, ask him to rise, and place his chair at a distance I feel more comfortable with. "Sit down and lean back," I tell him. "If you got any closer, you'd spill off the seat."

"Okay," he says, breathlessly. "Now, where was I—"

"How do you feel, right now?" I interrupt.

I watch his jaw clamp and the tips of his ears turn red with anger. "Fine," he tells me. "Fine. I'm fine. I just want to get started."

"We already have."

"I don't really see—"

"Why your needs shouldn't take precedence over mine?" I ask.

Cornered, he wails. "I want *help!*"

I sit down again. Take a breath. "I'm giving it to you," I answer. "This is it."

"Michael, what is all this about, do you figure? This getting right up into my face business? All this urgency about getting things started? What do you think's going on for you in a moment like that?"

"I don't know," he says.

"Well, this is therapy, think about it," I tell him.

He shakes his head.

"What did you feel?"

"When?"

"Now."

"Frustrated," he moans.

"Frustrated," I think. One of those favorite male words for feeling, like "interesting." "Doc, I was frustrated when the plane went down and it was interesting when my leg got crushed."

"Can I help?" I ask.

"Sure."

"Okay, here's what you're feeling. I imagine that you feel pissed. Obstructed. Unlistened to. Uncared about. Like I was going to do what I wanted no matter what your needs were. . . ."

Hearing me, Michael almost begins to smile. "I can see this one coming from down the block," he says.

"I imagine," I conclude, "that you felt controlled."

"How did I know?" he says. He smiles, and so do some of the others.

"Well?" I ask. "A little control struggle here, do you think?"

"You mean, 'control,' as in that force by which I managed to push away my wife and ruin my family? The force I wake up to and lie down with each day? *That* force?"

"Michael."

"Yes?"

"You are what we call, in the technical language of modern psychiatry, 'a quick study.'"

"Thank you," he sighs.

"Yes," I say, softly. "That force. The one that's trying to destroy you."

Michael looks up at me with his blue, dead eyes and begins to cry—or, as he later put it, liquid leaked from his eye sockets. "I'm sick of this," he laments. "I'm really so fucking sick of this."

I hand Michael a box of tissues. He shakes his head and wipes his face with his sleeve.

Even though Michael was hard to comfort, even though it was difficult for me to feel touched by him, the grief he experienced at that moment was real. It was pain about the pattern he was caught in and its cost. Underneath that, however, I suspected there were deeper and earlier wounds. Michael was raised by upper-class German Jewish parents whom he would have described, before this crisis, as "Fine. Just fine." But as Michael learned to probe a bit deeper, his parents emerged as more than just fine. They were perfect. They lived in a perfect little house that was perfectly decorated. They enjoyed perfect health, perfect friends, and a perfect marriage. But nothing was more perfect than Michael himself—a "straight A" student, a Harvard undergraduate, a young entrepreneur with his own business, a lovely wife, two beautiful kids. And a year's worth of cuckoldry that he didn't even notice. It wasn't that Virginia was such an accomplished liar. She had all but left her journal open for his bedtime reading. Michael never bothered to wonder where his wife had gone for whole evenings at a time, because he was so busy leading his perfect life that nothing as messy as marital dissatisfaction ever dared cross his mind, even when his wife began flying into occasional violent rages. In such altered states, Ginny hurled dishes against walls, terrifying the children. A few times, Michael succeeded in calming her down only after he called her mother to drive over and help him contain her. My wife, family therapist Belinda Berman, has a fine saying that I often remember: "Beware of 'nice' men with 'bitchy' women." In Mike's marriage, as in his childhood, underneath the dust-free tables, the flower arrangements, and tasteful collections, lay wellsprings of emotional violence. In many ways, Virginia's eruptions served the marriage like a blessed storm, releasing tensions too suffocating to endure.

Michael was blissfully unaware of the impact he had on others. He moved Virginia around, nicely, politely, as if she were another art piece he had to sweep under. He moved her with that same implacable urgency he had leveled at me when I hadn't jumped quickly enough for him. Being on the receiving end of Michael's impatience, I knew something about the quality of the force he projected, which escaped him. I knew how mean it was. In small, nuanced ways, Michael was an effective tormentor. Sooner or later, any woman in her right mind would find herself unwilling to stay with him.

With the group's permission, Michael comes to sit next to me as he has seen others do. He closes his eyes and breathes deeply, allowing me to guide him into light trance.

"What are you feeling, now, as you sit there?" I ask.

"Nervous," he says.

"Nervous? Okay, and where is that in your body? What is the physical sensation connected to that?"

"It's here"—he points to his stomach—"like, all tied up in knots."

"It's tight? Constricted?"

"It's like a band," he says. "A band around my chest, my heart," and he begins to weep.

"You're feeling some pain?" I ask.

He nods again. He is having trouble catching his breath. "And fear," he says. "A lot of fear."

"In that band?" I ask.

"And here," Michael points to his throat. "I can't breathe," he says, starting to gasp. The other men lean forward, a little alarmed.

"Keep breathing," I tell him. "Deep breaths, nice and slow." He is still in trouble. It looks as though he may be at the beginning of an anxiety attack. "Okay," I say. "So, you start to feel some pain, keep breathing, Mike. Some pain comes up and some tears and then your throat constricts and there's fear?"

He nods, unable to speak.

"Right, so, a part of you starts to feel some of the pain and then another part starts to fight it?"

He nods again.

"Okay. That's fine, keep breathing. Listen, you don't have to perform for anyone here. If you cry, that's okay. If you don't cry. Whatever. . . . Can you hear me?"

He nods, settles down. His breathing returns to normal.

I begin to question Michael about his family. I ask him to look up at each parent in his mind's eye and describe them as they looked to him as a child. Initially, his recollections are vague. Then he begins to talk about his mother's rage. As the images coming to him take on more weight, more detail, Michael finds it increasingly difficult to talk.

"How old are you now?" I inquire.

"Seven," he answers. "Eight."

"What do you look like?"

"I can't breathe," he says.

"Take your time," I say. "When you're ready, say what you look like."

Michael begins to remember the yelling—dishes thrown, epithets hurled. As the memories crowd in, anxiety crackles around him like an electric field. Finally, Michael begins to remember it all.

"What do you see?" I ask him.

"I'm running," he answers slowly, concentrating. "She's chasing me."

"What does she look like?"

He shakes his head.

"Look at her."

"I don't want to."

"You're afraid?"

He nods.

"Try," I urge. "What do you see?"

"She's drooling," he says. "Jesus." His eyes squeeze hard and he turns away.

"Drooling?" I ask. "She's, like, foaming at the mouth?"

He nods.

"What's that like?"

"Its ugly," he says. "Frightening."

"Go on."

"There's a knife. . . . My God."

"Go on, Mike."

"She used to do this!" he cries out abruptly "She used to do this to all of us."

"Say it."

Eyes still closed, he shakes his head. "She's saying that she's going to kill me. If she catches me, she'll . . ." Michael begins to cry, strangled gasps.

"Breathe," I tell him, bending him forward. "Put some noise into it. Go 'Boo-hoo.' Don't choke it off."

A flood of sobbing breaks over him. "Good," I say. "Good, Mike. Let it release."

The sobbing stops abruptly and Michael begins hyperventilating.

"Breathe," I tell him. "Can you talk?"

He shakes his head, gasping, trembling. To the other men, I know, it must look as though he's heading into convulsions. I hold him tightly, one hand on his shoulder, the other pressing up against his knee. I begin talking him through it. "This is called a body memory," I tell him. "It looks frightening. It sometimes happens when you reexperience an old trauma. You're in it. A dissociated memory is breaking into consciousness. Keep breathing. Keep focused on my voice, Mike, like a beacon. Can you hear me?"

He nods.

"Good. This will wash over you. Concentrate on your breathing. Send breath to that little eight-year-old inside you. Breathe, Michael. Good." It takes a long, frightening ten minutes. I talk, he listens. "You're remembering something?"

He nods.

"Good, we'll get to it. Just focus now on your breath." Finally, the racking begins to subside. Like a storm passing, slower, gentler, the gasping and the trembling recede. "You did it," I tell him. "You made it through." Michael first smiles and then begins to cry—clean, uncomplicated tears.

"What have you remembered?" I ask him.

"When I would cry," he answers in the tiny voice of a vulnerable child. "When she would be like that. When I would cry, she would put her hand over my mouth and hold my nose."

"You mean she would block the air?"

He nods.

"She would smother you?"

He nods.

"Until what?" I ask. "How would it end?"

He shrugs. "I don't know. I think I'd pass out."

"I see." I tell him. "So, when you started to reconnect with that boy inside, when you started to feel the pain, you reexperienced the smothering."

"I was choking," he says, almost apologetically.

"I know," I say. "I know you were."

A few minutes later, Michael shares with the rest of us an image that comes to him, of the little eight-year-old. He has run out of the house, into the woods. He sits on a huge rock, the same one every time, waiting for dark and his father's return and safety. He tells himself stories, he makes up little plays. Mostly, what Michael remembers is the cold, since he would often run off with no jacket.

As the men give Mike feedback, Billy expresses the thought that had been uppermost in my own mind. "I'll say this," he tells Mike. "I have a lot more respect than I did when I walked in here tonight about why you need so damn much control."

Carl leans forward to catch Michael's eye. "Welcome to the group," he tells him. "I'm glad that you're here."

"So much for the perfect family," offers Tom.

"I knew that was bullshit," Michael begins, but I cut him off.

"Just listen," I tell him. "Let these men nurture you. Just take it in."

For a brief moment, Michael closes his eyes. He sighs, and then wills himself to lean back in his chair. That moment is his first conscious act of recovery.

*   *   *

"The mass of men lead lives of quiet desperation." Others, not so quiet. Michael's story is bold and dramatic; others are far more subtle. But the dynamics of depression in men remain the same. Helping a covertly depressed man like Michael requires peeling back the layers of the disorder. First, the addiction must fail, as it did in Mike's case when Virginia left him. The defense against the depression must either give out or else create so much trouble that the man is sent to me by those around him. He is sent by the wife who can no longer abide him, or by the employer who can not make him produce, or, in the most extreme cases, by the courts.

If the compensatory moves can be stopped, the underlying depression will stream up to the surface. Sometimes, this transition is so violent that the first priority is simply surviving it. If the man has been self-medicating with drugs or alcohol, as is often the case, he may also be in acute substance withdrawal. Hospitalization may be required. Twelve-step programs are often a help. With or without substance abuse, once the defenses of covert depression stop, unleashed pain often sweeps over the man with the intensity of a force long denied.

Since Freud's first formulation of depression as a kind of mourning, most psychological theories about the disorder have focused on the role of early childhood injury and loss. Psychiatrist Rene Spitz coined the term *hospitalism* when he studied the relationship between depression and early deprivation. Spitz studied infants housed in large orphanages with little emotional nurture, who showed signs of severe "failure to thrive syndrome." They were listless, made poor contact, had little interest in their environment, and were prone to illness. Many were so apathetic that they would not eat. A few came close to death. Although these infants were adequately fed and medically cared for, they were not emotionally stimulated or loved. Whereas such an extreme lack of nurture produces immediate results, less extreme forms of loss or failures in nurture may lay the foundations for later depressions. British child analyst John Bolby detailed case after case of childhood vulnerabilities resulting from even relatively minor disruptions in parental contact. In a classic documentary, Bolby's colleagues filmed a seventeen-month-old boy's reaction to his parents' two-week absence. The documentary follows the boy as he moves through the stages of traumatization: denial, protest, and despair. In the course of two weeks, this initially robust toddler moves from apparent calm to angry regression and then to apathy, as he curls up in a corner of the playroom. The documentary's final moment shows the parents' return. While the boy runs into his mother's arms, the camera closes in on his face, frozen in an expression of hostile mistrust. This extraordinary film exposes the kind of slight childhood fissures that later on, under sufficient stress, may crack open.

When compared to the experience of children in Sarajevo, Somalia, or even inner-city ghettos, the wound of a happy, affluent family's two-week absence seems barely the slightest of hurts. Children are enormously resilient, one hears, and life is full of difficulties one must master. Indeed, a child's capacity to survive extraordinary circumstances can seem, at times, nothing short of miraculous. But the vaunted resilience of our children should not blunt our sensitivity to the effects of childhood deprivation. Children will get by, often enough, but at what cost? By most measures, Michael had handily survived his childhood traumas. He was married, successful, the father of two children. But closer inspection reveals the wholesale maneuvers to which he resorted in order to keep his little ship afloat—the controlling, urgent behaviors, the disconnection he felt between himself and his own feelings. Childhood injury in boys creates both the wounds and the defenses against the wounds that are the foundation for adult depression.

Focusing on the importance of childhood experience does not stand in opposition to an increased understanding of the role biology plays in depression. Advances in physiological research finally seem at the point of concluding the age-old debate about "nature verses nurture." When I first trained twenty years ago, an enormous amount of attention was paid to distinguishing between two types of depression, one biological, the other not. This distinction had several names: major versus minor depression, biological versus neurotic, endogenous verses exogenous. The remnants of this old distinction still survive today in the DSM IV diagnoses "major depression" and "dysthymia." Traditionally, "major depression," often seen as "real depression," was thought to derive from a chemical imbalance. Considered to be a genetic disorder, it demanded medical intervention in the form of drugs or electroconvulsive therapy. The less serious disorder, "minor" or "neurotic" depression, was a reaction to life's stresses and was treated with "talking therapy."

Though the distinction between major and minor depression (now called dysthymia) still exists in the official nomenclature, in practical terms it has all but disappeared. The only real contrast between the two disorders is that major depression is more acute and severe than minor depression. It is simpler and more effective to think of them as one condition occurring along a spectrum of severity. Many patients who suffer the eruption of an acute severe depressive episode also have a chronic baseline of mild depression. Studies following patients with both disorders have shown that while "major" depression may be more severe in the short term, dysthymia may have devastating long-term effects. Patients suffering from dysthymia over the course of their lifetime prove harder to treat and have a higher recidivism rate. In addition, the overall economic and quality-of-life costs to these patients turns out to be, if anything, greater than it is for those who contend with depression in its more dramatic form. The relief afforded by Prozac and similar drugs to millions of people suffering from dysthymia further challenges the idea that "minor" depressions are not "biological." Prozac is no more effective than earlier antidepressants when treating classic "major" depression. Where it shines is in the relief of the "minor" conditions that earlier medications did not help much. The distinction between major and minor depressions, biology and character, seems to be breaking down.

*　　　*　　　*

Close to a year after Michael's first inclusion in our men's group, he was ready to invite his parents to a week of family therapy. With extraordinary care and courage, Mike, aided by his two sisters, confronted his mother about her periodic bouts of irrationality. After initial protests, Anna admitted what everyone in the family had known for years—that for a decade she had been addicted to prescription drugs. Anna sincerely did not recall her wild brutalization of her children, now openly discussed for the first time, but she did remember frequent blackouts from the drugs. Two months after that family session, Michael flew with his mother and father to Hazeldon hospital in Minnesota, where Anna fully "detoxed" for the first time in thirty-two years. At Hazeldon, the staff gave her a dual diagnosis of addiction and depression, the closest current psychiatric label to covert depression. They also noted a history of both depression and addiction throughout Anna and her husband's family.

Was Michael's covert depression genetic or environmental? From nature or nurture? Inherited or transmitted through trauma? The answer from all but those in the most extreme camps would be, both. For several decades, researchers in epidemiology, the science of tracking the course of disease, have been able to demonstrate that major depression runs genetically in families. By taking close family histories, and by studying identical twins raised in different settings, investigators have shown that there is a strong genetic component to major depression, independent of one's environment. Studies about the genetic basis of minor depression, however, proved far less convincing. Dissatisfied with these results, epidemiologist George Winokur tried factoring into his studies not merely dysthymia per se but a conglomerate of dysthymia, alcoholism, and "antisocial personality." He called this mix *Depression Spectrum Disease*. In all but a few aspects, Winokur's Depression Spectrum Disease is another name for covert depression. Winokur found that as soon as one broadened the scope of depression to include these addictive or violent behaviors, the resulting brew, Depression Spectrum Disease, could easily be shown to have a genetic basis. Winokur also considered gender distinctions in his research. In several studies, he and his colleagues found evidence of a genetic link between depression and alcoholism, with the former linked to women, the later to men. Winokur deduced from epidemiology what I have concluded from clinical data, that addictions and depression may not be distinct disorders but variants of the same disorder expressed differently along gender lines. Where I differ slightly from Winokur's conclusion is in his equating covert depression with minor depression. Anyone who has struggled with a severe addiction would not agree that his disorder is minor. Covert depression keeps a core depression at bay. One seldom finds major depression and the defenses of covert depression operating at the same time, for the simple reason that the defenses work, at least partially, to keep the depression looking minor. Once the defenses fail or the person stops self-medicating, the overt depression that emerges can look very much like major depression. This was the case for Michael, when his relationship to Virginia no longer soothed him, and for Damien Corleis, when he backed away from sex addiction to his wife. Both of these men were either hospitalized or near to it. The same can be said for William Styron, who was flooded with an utterly deliberating depression once he stopped drinking.

If the research is clear that both forms of depression, overt and covert, almost certainly have a biological basis, then one might wonder why we should concern ourselves with issues of childhood trauma at all. If the disease is simply inherited like other genetic disorders, an exclusive focus on medical rather than psychological issues would seem appropriate. While some researchers do take that position, others passionately counter it. The controversy concerning the question of nature and nurture, therapy or drugs, has been so hotly disputed that even in the midst of his own life-threatening struggle, William Styron could not resist tweaking his helpers about the absurdity of their argument. He writes: "The intense and sometimes comically strident factionalism that exists in present day psychiatry—the schism between the believers in psychotherapy and the adherents of psychopharmacology—resembles the medical quarrels of the eighteenth century (to bleed or not to bleed) and almost defines the inexplicable nature of the disorder."

The relationship between biology and psychology has never been as simple as the debate about it would imply. Both sides of the "nature/nurture" argument are wrong. The problem stems from framing the debate as if the influence of biology goes only one way—up, from our bodies to our minds. New research shows that the relationship between brain and mind runs in both directions. It has long been accepted that changes in our biochemistry, caused by illness, medication, or intoxicants, can effect our psychological states. But what has been less appreciated, until recently, is that changes affecting our psychological states may alter our biochemistries as well, even the very structures of our brains. Under certain circumstances these alterations can be permanent.

At the State University of New York at Stony Brook, Fritz Henn and Emmeline Edwards looked at the effect of environment on laboratory rats in a series of experiments that were as elegant as they were compelling. First, Henn and Edwards induced depression in a group of perfectly normal rats by giving them small electric shocks from which they could not escape. After an initial stage of protest, the rats eventually "gave up." They became despondent, isolated, and had trouble eating and sleeping. In other words, they displayed many of the "vegetative" (biological) symptoms that people do when plagued with "major" depression. The researchers next found that the brains of these rats had been altered. One part of the rats' brains had grown more than normally sensitive to a certain neurotransmitter, while another part was now less than normally sensitive to it.

Henn and Edwards gave these "depressed" rats the same antidepressants used by people. In about two weeks, the usual amount of time it takes for the medication to begin working, the rats' depressions cleared up. No longer helpless, they quickly learned to press a lever inside the cage and stop the shock. At about the same time, their brain abnormalities returned to normal. The emotional experience of helplessness changed the physiology of these rats and, conversely, a physiological change, medication, cleared up their emotional distress.

Henn and his colleagues followed up on this experiment by taking a different group of rats and stressing the new group into a state of depression. The same brain abnormality resulted, but this time, the researchers "treated" their little patients without medication. With a technique that mimicked psychotherapy, the researchers taught the rats how to escape their helplessness. A medical student knit the rats tiny sweaters with sleeves that fit over their front paws. A long string was left trailing from the rats' sleeves. By pulling the string, as on a marionette, researchers could coax the rats into pressing a lever, teaching them how to end their shock. As the rats learned to gain control over their circumstances, much as psychotherapy patients learn how to gain control over theirs, the rats' depressions subsided, and so did their brain abnormalities. Environmental factors produced changes in the brain that were reversed with equal success by altering the rats' neurochemistry and by affecting their learning. The relationship between physiology and psychology, body and mind, appears to be a reciprocal one. The wounded eight-year-old that Michael visualized and began to nurture that evening in men's group may exist not only in Michael's mind but also in his neurology.

A substantial and growing body of research teaches us that early childhood trauma and loss will have, as one researcher stated it, "lifelong psychobiological consequences." Primate infants who are separated from their mothers have been shown to have abnormal changes in levels of the brain neurotransmitter serotonin, a chemical whose imbalance has long been associated with depression, and which is affected by Prozac. Adrenal enzymes also change with maternal separation, as do blood cortisol levels, heart rate, body temperature, and sleep. Researcher Bessel van der Kolk notes that: "These changes are not transient or mild, and their persistence suggests that long-term neurobiological alterations underlie the psychological effects of early separation." In several experiments monkeys who suffered early isolation apparently adjusted well under normal circumstances, but proved to be markedly more vulnerable to both physical illness and severe depression when placed in a challenging situation, or faced again with loss. Antidepressant medications ameliorate or even reverse both the physiological signs and the behavioral changes that accompany early maternal separation in monkeys, leading some biologists to speculate that early maternal deprivation in monkeys might prove a good working model for depression in humans. These observations have implications for our understanding of addictions as well. If early maternal separation produces upset in monkeys, opioids, like morphine, relieve it. In fact, no substance has been shown to be more effective in alleviating such distress. Monkeys that had been isolated in youth display increased sensitivity to amphetamines and opioids, as well as increased alcohol consumption, when compared to normally raised controls. And these changes accelerate when the monkeys are put under stress.

Research on the biology of trauma is beginning to teach us that even apparently mild childhood injuries can produce lasting physiological change. But the harmful effects of trauma often go unrecognized. As a culture historically dominated by male values, we have always tended, and still tend, to deny vulnerability, and consequently, to deny the existence of trauma. Sigmund Freud was the first psychotherapist on record to document patients' reports of childhood trauma and sexual abuse. In one of the most famous mistakes of the twentieth century, Freud decided that his female patients, often daughters of friends and colleagues, were lying. Freud states flatly that his mind would not accept the idea that the decent men he knew could do the things these young women reported. Consequently, he did what most of us have done throughout history when faced with trauma survivors: he disbelieved and blamed them.

The issue of trauma did not surface again until tens of thousands of "shell-shocked" soldiers forced us to consider the topic once more during World War I. At first, we tried to deny the reality of psychological injury, blaming physical injury instead. The term *shell shock* derives from the mistaken theory that the distress occurs as a result of a concussion from explosives. When it became clear that our soldiers were not physically but emotionally overwhelmed, the typical response took over. We blamed them. The public rhetoric shifted from the language of medicine to the language of moral weakness. Shell-shocked soldiers lacked "fiber." They were frail malingerers or, more bluntly, cowards. The new medical specialty of psychiatry, brought out of relative obscurity into the mainstream because of the need to treat these combat veterans, dressed up essentially the same sentiments in technical garb, offering the picture of the "neurotically susceptible" "infantile" male. Not until the grassroots movement of Vietnam veterans forced the medical establishment to stop blaming the victim, did we as a culture acknowledge for the first time that any man, no matter how "well adjusted," could be overwhelmed if subjected to enough stress. The new diagnosis of *post traumatic stress disorder* was born.

As with depression, we tend to give credence to only the most extreme forms of trauma. We are no longer surprised, as we might have been a generation ago, to learn that virtually all of the men interred in notoriously cruel Japanese prisoner of war camps during World War II still have psychological symptoms close to fifty years later. We now grasp the lasting effects of such public, catastrophic injury—political captivity, torture, earthquakes, floods— just as we grasp the long-term effects of severe and blatant child abuse. But we are still reluctant to accept trauma or abuse in its subtler forms. And yet disqualifying the pain of subtler hurts ignores the fact that the most obvious injuries are not necessarily the ones that do the most harm. The flagrancy of childhood trauma does not always directly correlate with the extent of later damage.

The occasional brutal attacks Michael remembers irresistibly command our attention. But the compelling image of that boy chased with knives obscures the reality that on the other three hundred and sixty-odd days of the year Michael lived in a perfectionistic, constricted, mind-numbing atmosphere. Which of these two environmental forces, one deep and dramatic, the other ordinary and chronic, did him most harm? There is no simple answer.

*   *   *

Compared to what we usually think of as dramatic trauma, the kinds of injuries most boys sustain as an accepted part of growing up male tend to seem relatively mild. But I believe that the more we learn about the effects of childhood trauma, the more plausible the existence of such damage becomes. While it is true that children can be remarkably flexible, the research on the biology of trauma reminds us that, when compared to adults, they are nevertheless still delicate. And relatively delicate injury may harm. Stereotypically when we think of trauma, we think of the public catastrophic events that can overwhelm an adult, what some trauma experts called "Type I" trauma. But what most distinguishes childhood trauma from occurrences like combat stress is simply that the injury occurs to children. "Be kind to me, Lord," reads the epigram for the National Children's Defense Fund, "My boat is so small and the sea is so wide." A child's personality and his neurology—the little boat he must navigate in—are still developing. Relatively mild childhood injury can have long-lasting effects because it occurs while the very structures of the personality, body, and brain are being formed—or malformed. A growing body of evidence indicates that a heightened state of arousal—the body's inherent "fight or flight" reaction to stress—in small children may have permanent physiological consequences. Stressed children have a harder time modulating feelings, negotiating conflict, and "settling down" than other children, and this seems particularly true for males who appear, if anything, even more sensitive than females to injury or deprivation.

When a child is injured by his own caregiver, as is overwhelmingly often the case, danger is delivered to the child by the very persons he depends and relies on for protection. This tragic dilemma sets up an excruciating bind that lies at the heart of the child's trauma experience—the desperate need to reestablish a loving connection to his or her own abuser. When Michael sat shivering alone on his rock in the woods, the thing he remembered fantasizing about most was the theme of magic rescue. He, the brave prince, would swoop down upon the evil castle with ray guns of love and rescue the frozen princess. At forty-five years old, it had not occurred to him, until I pointed it out, that the frozen princess he so wished to liberate was his own addicted mother.

Finally, unlike adult trauma, childhood damage may not result merely from violation. Most of the animal research does not concern early assault so much as early deprivation. In working with traumatized men, I make a distinction between *active* versus *passive* injury. *Active trauma* is usually a boundary violation of some kind, a clearly toxic interaction. *Passive trauma*, on the other hand, is a form of physical or emotional neglect. Rather than a violent presence, passive trauma may be defined as a violent lack—the absence of nurture and responsibilities normally expected of a caregiver; the absence of connection. In an instance of active trauma, a boy might come home with a badly scraped knee and torn, bloody pants only to have his father scream at him for ruining his clothes. In an instance of passive trauma, a boy would show up with a badly scraped knee, and the father would promise to be there in a moment only to stay on a business call for another ten minutes while the boy waits beside him, bleeding. When we think of childhood trauma, we tend to think first of active trauma, although it is extreme neglect that causes the majority of the cases of children being taken from their homes. While there are no reliable estimates of the prevalence of even extreme passive trauma, most domestic violence experts estimate it occurs at least twice as frequently as active abuse. Richard Gelles, a pioneer of violence research, estimates that one in eleven children—4 to 5 million each year—suffers some form of extreme neglect. Just as with active abuse, however, issues of neglect do not need to be extreme to cause harm. And, just as with active trauma, passive trauma may be psychological as well as physical. Good parenting requires three elements: nurturing, limit setting, and guidance. A parent who is too absorbed to supply any one of these neglects the legitimate needs of the child. My client Ryan brought that point home to me one Wednesday night group.

*   *   *

When it is his turn, Ryan "checks in" with the tale of a "small road-side epiphany." Coming home from a party, Lilly, his wife, expressed anger and hurt at the way Ryan, affectionate in private, would frequently "disown and shun" her at public gatherings.

"She told me it felt as if I wanted to act like I didn't know her," Ryan tells us. "In the past, I would have gotten defensive and probably started a fight, but this time I was so . . . I don't know, so stunned. Because I knew she was right, you see. I pulled over on the side of the road and shut off the car." With a few years of therapy behind him, Ryan allowed himself to recognize not only the truth of Lilly's account and the pain it caused her, but also his own feelings and remembered associations. Ryan's parents rarely demonstrated physical affection for one another and, while they had shown physical nurture to him as a young boy and still did to his sister, they stopped displaying such affection for him at the age of six or seven.

Sitting on the side of the road, Ryan recalled a vivid memory of himself as a boy of seven or eight, crying hysterically in the middle of the kitchen asking for a "pickup," while his family bustled around him preparing dinner as if he simply wasn't there. "It was as though my parents made a decision one day to stop, although I'm sure they didn't because they didn't talk about things like that. I don't think my father touched me again, except maybe once or twice every few years he would totally lose it and throw me against a wall. I think that was it."

I lead Ryan through a quick guided imagery exercise, asking him to close his eyes and see himself lifting his own infant son in the air and laughing together, a scene he had described many times to the group. I ask him to note the joy, the sheer pleasure in each of their faces. Then I ask him to imagine himself as a child being touched with such joy by his own father. Ryan begins to cry, softly, silently. "That was your birthright," I tell him. "His thrill to be with you. You deserved that." Beside Ryan, Tom also begins to cry quietly. When I ask what triggered his feelings, he recalls that on the afternoon of his MBA graduation, his father hugged him and said he loved him for the first time in his life. "I was twenty-six years old," he muses. "Even a BA wasn't enough to get it out of him. I had to earn a fucking *graduate* degree." Tom smiles ruefully, tears still in his eyes. "If I'm still in this damn group when I have a child, I swear I am going to tell that precious creature I care about him or her at least once a day, do you hear me? At *least* once a day. If I don't, you can drag me out of the house and knock some goddamn sense into me."

Categorizing such neglect as trauma does not trivialize the nature of trauma. I think not touching a child for decades at a time is a form of injury. I think withholding any expression of love until a young boy is a grown man is a form of emotional violence. And I believe that the violence men level against themselves and others is bred from just such circumstances. Ryan first came to therapy after a year of alcohol abuse and several instances of hitting his fiancée. He lost the relationship but, with my help, entered treatment for his drinking and underlying depression. When Tom was referred to me for a consultation, he was suicidally depressed and on the verge of an emergency hospitalization. These men are not whining. Their injuries are not shallow. Minimizing their distress is not merely wrong; it is dangerous.

And yet, as a father of sons myself, inculcated as much as anyone else by the mores of masculinity, I know firsthand how easily we slip into the passive traumatization of boys.

Justin, my five-year old son, is very proud to have me, rather than his mother, attending his ice skating lesson. This is his eighth week and the first and only time this season I can free my schedule in the middle of a working day to be there.

Skating has been hard for him. Very athletic, Justin is used to sports coming easily and unused to having to work at something. He dislikes doing things badly, even from the start, and his mother has had to push him to keep him on the ice. I thought he had conquered his fears and shame. But now he appears to have regressed again, perhaps because I am there instead of Mom. He skates over to me and says he wants out of the lesson. His feet hurt, he complains. His shoes don't feel right. Thoroughly embarrassed in front of the other parents, I stand firm, nicely but clearly insisting that he "Go back out and try." Finally, he just sits down on the ice at the side of the rink and cries. Begrudgingly, I go and gather him up. Imagine how I felt when I pulled off his skates and found two nickel-sized blisters, one on each heel. In my rush to get him dressed on time, I had put his skates on the wrong feet.

Parents are human, myself included, and may this be the worst thing that ever happens to Justin. But nevertheless, one needs to ask, I needed to ask, "Would I have been as firm and unsympathetic to a daughter?" I honestly think not. When I ignored Justin as he sank lower and lower into despair, I abandoned him. Not lurid and awful, it was nevertheless the kind of abandonment that boys experience frequently. Studies indicate that from the moment of birth, boys are spoken to less than girls, comforted less, nurtured less. Passive trauma in boys is rarely extreme; it is however, pervasive.

The band Michael erected around his heart might well have been a necessary reaction to the extraordinary, unacknowledged threat to his life. This would fit the classic definition of Type I trauma, the kind so out of the bounds of the ordinary that it shatters our basic assumptions about life and safety. And yet Michael's band around the heart might just as equally have been the result of the persistent erosion of connection to self that characterized much of his ordinary life, and much of the ordinary life of many boys in our culture. This is Type II trauma, chronic and persistent, which occurs when childhood structures first form. Both types of trauma probably left their signature in Michael's body, his neurochemistry, perhaps even the structure of his brain, exacerbating what may have already been an inherited vulnerability to depression.

Six months have passed since I first met Michael and Virginia—four months since he came into the group, and two since he flew with his mother to her first treatment. He shows me a letter she has written to him:

> I look back in horror, as the recognition of what I have done can no longer be held back, not even from myself. I don't know how I will ever forgive myself. I don't dare even think about asking for

you or your sisters' forgiveness. It's like waking up from a bad dream, except that it's infinitely worse because the dream is real and the damage is real and here I am with thirty-two years beneath me, like an abyss. It is so vast, the size of it, I can hardly take it in or fully comprehend it. And of course, as I'm sure you imagine, I want desperately to run. So, what else is new?

In the midst of all this, one of my few consolations is that you have taken the steps you must in order to save yourself. You always were a brave boy! I don't know if I can be as brave by half, but I will try. I don't know what else I could possibly offer you now. Be well. You are in my prayers.

In Wednesday night group, Michael informs us that there are signs his mother has taken up drugs once again, but he is not despondent. Recovery often plays itself out in ragged chapters. Later, Michael shares a moment he had with his two daughters. He was dropping the girls off at their mother's new apartment. He bent down on the sidewalk by his car to give them a hug and he started to cry.

"Why are you crying, Daddy?" asked five-year-old Elene.

"Because," he told her, "now you are going to be with Mommy for a few days and I'm sad to miss you."

She had reached up to wipe away his tears. "Don't be sad, Daddy. Even when I'm with Mom, I still love you."

"I know that," he said, hugging her. "I know you do. But you know, it's really okay if Daddy cries. Its okay if people get sad and it's okay if they cry." Michael told the group that he had thought, as he watched his daughters dawdle their way up the path to their mother, that if he had learned to cry twenty years ago, he might not have been standing there watching them go.

I tell Michael I think his feet are firmly planted upon the dark path, the path that leads all the way down before it breaks into resplendent sunlight. "In the middle of the journey of our lives," Dante said beginning his voyage, "I found myself upon a dark path."

Michael suffered in an untreated depressed and addicted family, a situation someone of either sex might have been in. And yet his story rings unmistakably as a boy's story. The heroic, denying, covertly dependent defenses he erected between himself and his own experience, while possible for a women, strike one as familiarly male; strike one, in fact, as only slight exaggerations of much of what we have come to define as male. Michael's story is completely his own. The band around his heart, however, is a shared condition.

CHAPTER FIVE

Perpetrating Masculinity

Before they had attended school a week they saw what goats they had been not to remain on the island; but it was too late now, and soon they settled down to being as ordinary as you or me. . . . It is sad to have to say that the power to fly gradually left them.

—J. M. BARRIE,
Peter Pan

In a country in which 135,000 children take handguns to school each day, in which every fourteen hours a child under the age of five is murdered, and homicide has replaced automobile accidents as the leading cause of death in children under the age of one, few boys escape a firsthand acquaintance with active trauma. Once issues of race and class are considered, the picture grows even bleaker. There are more college-aged black men in prison than in school. And the leading cause of death in black men between eighteen and twenty-five—one young man in four—is murder. More than the childhood diseases we spend millions combating, more than accident or natural disaster, violence is the number one killer of boys and young men. By far most violent acts, both inside and outside the home, are committed by males. In our culture, almost without exception, boyhood involves being both the recipient and the sometime perpetrator of active trauma. Such boyhood injury operates like a fault line in troubled men, coloring their emotional lives, ready, given the right circumstance, to emerge anew. The

113

wounded boy they think they have long left behind acts like a reservoir of hurt and shame. Precisely to the degree to which that boy is not consciously felt and confronted, a man's hidden depression will permeate his actions.

When thirty-six-year-old Dave and his wife, Judy, first came to see me, they had been arguing furiously about ten-year-old Brian. Dave thought his son had a serious weight problem and Judy wanted Dave to stop haranguing the boy. Brian, a chubby but by no means obese child, felt a mixture of anger and shame. When I encounter a parent pressing hard on a boy, my working hypothesis is that the parent's own buttons are being pushed. My strategy then is to explore with the parent, in the boy's presence, the nature of that button. After some gentle prodding in such a session, Dave shared with his son for the first time his own experience of being "a fat boy," much heavier than Brian. He retold the story of a ten-year-old's terror as each day he was taunted and beaten by a group of older boys on his way home from school.

"How often did this happen?" I ask Dave.

"Every day," he answers, as though it were a vaguely stupid question.

"How long did it go on for?" I follow up.

Again, a look of impatience. "For the whole school year. Maybe into the next year as well."

"Let me get this straight. You were beaten up every day for a year, a year and a half?"

"A year and a few months," Dave corrects.

"Didn't your parents complain?"

"Of course they did. Bitterly."

"Well?"

And now Dave smiles, a wise, caustic smile. "Yes, well. You see that was the worst part of it. I would look up, you see. Look up at the school windows. The cheeky bastards would gang up on me right there in the yard, in plain view. And I would see them."

"See who?"

"My teachers," Dave said. "I could see their faces up in the window. They watched."

"They watched." It is hard to describe the raw wave of bitterness and helpless anger that radiated out of this man, close to three decades later, when he spoke those two words. It was clear that Dave's sense of betrayal had become a stable component of his emotional life, certainly of his parenting. The pain of that ten-year-old outcast now fueled Dave's aggressive stance toward his son. I told Dave that I viewed his preoccupation with Brian's weight as a misguided attempt at protection. Dave needed to find a way to be concerned about Brian without crossing over the line to intrusiveness. The danger lay in Dave's becoming so intent on protecting his son from the kind of abuse from which he had suffered that he would end up, ironically, doing him harm. This is a common dynamic between father and son. And the key to finding the balance between the extremes of neglect or intrusion was to resurface Dave's hidden depression. Once he acknowledged his own boyhood embarrassment and pain, Dave was able to grant Brian an experience that was Brian's and not his. Dave's job was difficult because of the reservoir of fear he still carried, and the bitterness reawakened by his son's situation. Dave knew how cruel life could be for a fat boy. Without the hard lines of a "real" boy's body, Dave's round softness had rendered him "like a girl." He had been deposited outside the circle. He had been fair game.

If Dave became the object of violence by virtue of his weight, Gerry, an overtly depressed man in his late twenties, drew violence to him by virtue of seeming "a geek." An MIT graduate, Gerry looks exactly like what he is—a terrifically smart, incredibly rigid engineer. One senses that he emerged from the womb with slide rule in hand. In the expensive and highly regarded New England prep school he had attended, Gerry's difference from the other boys was celebrated by an annual Get Gerry Day. Once a year, for four years, Gerry was hounded, like an animal. No matter where he tried to hide, he was caught, bound, gagged, and taken to a large recreation room. A group of boys wound duct tape around him from his feet all the way up to his head, until he looked like a silver mummy. They punched two airholes by his nose and deposited him, unable to move, upon a pool table, where he stayed until nighttime, "mostly, trying not to pee on myself." Throughout the school, boys wore little duct tape ribbons in honor of Gerry Day. "Gerry jokes" abounded. A student called upon in class might respond by clamping his lips as though gagged, saying, "Hmm! Hmm! Hmmm!" This was considered hysterically funny. Each year, the administration sent out the requisite memo chastising the boys. And each year they turned a blind eye until the torture was over. Boys will be boys, was their attitude, one supposes. Raised by two strict, punitive parents, Gerry is not a warm or likable man. I have little doubt he was not a particularly likable boy. Like Dave's weight, Gerry's "geeky" manner rendered him somehow not fully male. And that gave the boys license to do with him what they liked. At twenty-six, Gerry was hospitalized for psychotic depression. Among other delusions, he was convinced that the smell of urine leaked through the pores of his skin.

Gerry's and Dave's experiences of "schoolyard politics," while extreme in severity, are by no means uncommon in boys' lives. Studies of the earliest forms of violence, childhood bullying, confirm that boys in our society are more overtly aggressive than girls. While boys actually do not bully more than girls, they bully differently. Girls tend toward "indirect bullying": ridicule, name calling, spreading mean rumors. Boys engage in such behaviors as well, but they are much more likely to use straightforward brute force. Girls' aggression tends to be verbal. Boys hit, kick, and bite. While girls rarely bully boys, boys bully both boys and girls—anyone perceived as weak. But boys' most frequent and most ferocious attacks are reserved for other males. For most boys active trauma is an integral part of life.

One reason we are numb to the psychological damage that can result from boys' violence is that we have been lulled into viewing it as normal, as if it were an inevitable aspect of their development. Active trauma so saturates boy culture that many of us take it as "natural."

The idea that the violence permeating boy culture is biologically predetermined, that male bodies are simply "hardwired" for aggression, is currently enjoying a resurgence of popularity. While it might be tempting to make sweeping generalizations about masculinity and violence, evolutionary biologists and anthropologists have had to thread through a mare's nest of complexity in order to define aggression at all. Most researchers now distinguish several different kinds of aggression, such as fear-induced aggression, parental aggression, territorial aggression, instrumental aggression, and angry aggression, each with its own set of motives, emotions, and characteristic behaviors. A simplistic rationale of playground abuse as inherent, or biological—"Boys will be boys," or, more sophisticatedly, "Primates will be primates"—does an equal disservice to the intricacies of both humans and apes.

Evolutionary biologists teach us that "dominance aggression"— the kind of aggression apparent in the "alpha" gorilla who rears up to his full height, snarling and beating his chest—is distinguished from other forms of aggression precisely by the absence of violence. Dominance aggression is in almost all cases limited to an aggressive *display.* The animals demonstrate to one another what their fighting potential looks like. They size one another up, then the weaker animal, correctly assessing the potential outcome, yields to the stronger in ritual gestures of submission. The stronger animal accepts the deal and desists, often actively communicating his welcome and protection of the submissive. The evolutionary value of dominance aggression is obvious; it serves to give order to the troop while avoiding violence.

Freud once wrote: "The first man to hurl an epithet instead of a stick was the creator of civilization." As usual, Freud proved himself a genius at psychology and a bad anthropologist. In fact, the first "man" to use symbolic gestures in place of true violence was a gorilla. It is unfair of us to blame male "instincts" for our brutality. It is one thing to claim that boys may have a physiological push toward more activity than girls, or even toward more "rough and tumble play." It is quite another thing to say that boys' genes render them inherently violent. The unabashed kicking, hitting, and biting found in our playgrounds and the senseless cruelty that was turned upon Gerry or Dave would be an anathema to most apes. While some theorists may search for the arcane roots of male violence in our hairy ancestors or our DNA, it seems simpler, if more troubling, to confront a more obvious explanation—violence is inculcated in our boys through exposure to violence. Not all victims become perpetrators, but virtually all perpetrators have been schooled in the training ground of their own abuse.

If active injury in boys is pervasive and flagrant, passive injury is most often pervasive and subtle, as subtle as a father's refusal to check the skates of his crying son, as subtle as a birthday card. Diane, a forty-one-year old meteorologist, told me during one session about her six-year-old son Ben's birthday. She described Ben as a "typical" rough and tumble boy, a "boy boy," who loved hockey and baseball and anything that kicked, sliced, or jumped out at you. For his birthday, Diane gave Ben a new pair of hockey skates and a card she'd thought was cute. The card showed a boy in a dog's suit, with a big, mischievous grin. Inside a poem read:

> Son,
> We've seen you when
> you were sleeping
> Or kicking back
> Or howling
> We've seen you ready for a fight
> really growling.
> We've seen you when you were quiet
> And so wild
> No one could tame you.
> But we've never ever seen you
> When we weren't proud to claim you.
> HAPPY BIRTHDAY!

The whole family grouped around Ben and read the card aloud, joking and teasing. Mom ruffled his hair. The excitement of his new skates overshadowed the dark expression that passed over Ben's face as he listened. But his thoughtful mother noticed it. That night, as she put Ben to bed, Diane said "You know, when we read you that card we weren't laughing at you, we were laughing with you."

Ben turned away, his face suffused with blood and emotion. "I *hate* that card!" he said.

"But why, honey?" Diane tried.

Ben exploded. "I hate it!" He threw off the covers and ran to his bureau to get it, took one look, and threw it contemptuously into the hall. "It's *embarrassing!*"

"Why?" Diane asked.

"It just *is*. Get it *out!*"

Despite herself, Diane found her own feelings getting hurt. "All right, Ben, if you don't like it, you can just say so. You don't need to have a fit."

"Just get it *out*," her son repeated.

"Stressed out," Diane told me she'd thought to herself. "Hyped up from the party. Let's get him to bed and be done with it." Which is what she did. After a day spent preparing for, entertaining, and then cleaning up after fourteen six-year-olds, she was due for a break herself.

But evidently Ben was not quite ready to let things drop. The next morning at breakfast Diane found the birthday card lying on the kitchen table. Sometime during the night Ben had retrieved it, taken out his biggest, blackest marker, and proceeded to make giant Xs over all the words that offended him. And there were many. Out went "howling," then "fight," then "growling," then "no one could tame you." In the end, all that remained visible were the words "son," "quiet," and "Happy Birthday."

"This really bothered you, didn't it, Ben?" said Diane. He nodded, a little sheepish. "What was it you didn't like about all the words you crossed out?"

Then, Diane confessed, her little six-year-old leveled her, as only kids can, with clear, direct simplicity. "I'm not a *dog*, Mother," Ben told her. "I don't act like that, so don't call me those things." After a pause, he added, "They're *mean*."

Diane flushed with what is often called "appropriate shame." Ben was right. The words describing him and his behavior were mean. Ben did not howl, growl, kick, or bite, and he did not find it cute to be told that he did.

Had little Ben been victimized by a greeting card? Well, actually, yes, if only in a very small way. The card was a perfect instance of "masculine" role inscription, presenting boys as consumed by anger and aggression and implying by its tone that such behavior is not merely tolerable but somehow a source of pride. Even without the introductory "son," no girl in the world would have received such sentiments. Diane could not have been a more sensitive, thoughtful parent, and yet she had consented to a stereotyped vision of her son. In a tiny, relatively innocuous moment, Diane had perpetrated masculinity just as I had done with Justin, when I had insisted that he "tough it out" on the skating rink. Like me, she imposed a vision, tuning out the real needs and real experiences of her son. These slight instances of abandonment, in which we withdraw from that part of the boy that does not conform to our expectations, accumulate to great effect.

Understanding that innumerable small acts of passive trauma are driven by images of masculinity requires of us an act of conscious deliberation. Like fish trying to get a good look at the water they swim in, we find it hard to keep in focus the passive injuries we inflict on boys, because they are both so subtle and so common. Parents, teachers, and peers prod boys into role compliance, failing to respond to their unique needs, simply in the way they define boys' experience, just as the description in Ben's birthday card attempted to define Ben. Such subtle shaping, much of it out of the realm of conscious intent, permeates the lives of girls and boys. It is the essence of the socialization of gender. In the traditional setup, girls are encouraged to fully develop connection and relationship, but are discouraged from fully developing and exercising their public, assertive selves. Boys are encouraged to develop the skills of public, assertive action but discouraged from fully developing and exercising their relational, emotional selves.

Sociologist Barrie Thorne spent a year observing boys and girls in two American elementary schools. At first Thorne's observations confirmed the usual stereotypes: Girls are related. Boys are hierarchical. Girls' principal concern was with their attachments to one another. Boys' principal concerns were with winning and rules. When Thorne began her observations there seemed little ambiguity. But as time passed and her observations deepened, the anthropologist began finding so many incidents at odds with her expectations, so many exceptions and "crossovers," that she finally abandoned the "different cultures" framework she herself had championed for many years. Thorne writes frankly about how great a struggle it was for her, even with a trained ethnographer's eye, to begin allowing herself to see the boys as relational. The way we see a child will often shape the behaviors we evoke from him. In a well-known study, two educators placed children of average intelligence with teachers who were told that their new pupils were exceptionally bright. This "pseudo-gifted" group uniformly wound up with better grades and better scholastic performances than a matched group of controls. As with intelligence, so too with behaviors—malleable kids live up, or down, to our expectations. Sugar and spice and everything nice is what we expect little girls to be made of. As Ben reminds us, boys may not fare quite as well. By not attending to boys' relational needs—the need for connection, for nurture, support, the expression of vulnerability—we teach them, through passive injury, that those needs are not quite legitimate.

We begin sending boys the message that they have fewer emotional needs than girls in the very first moments of life. One research team studied parents' responses to newborns in the first twenty-four hours after delivery. The researchers selected newborns that matched in weight, length, alertness, and strength, so that there were no significant differences between boys and girls. Nevertheless, both mothers and fathers perceived newborn sons as: "more alert, stronger, larger featured, more coordinated, and firmer." They saw baby daughters as "less attentive, weaker, finer featured, less coordinated, softer, smaller, more fragile and prettier." In a classic study in the field of gender research, John and Sandra Cundry videotaped the reactions of a nine-month-old infant to various stimuli: a teddy bear, a jack-in-the-box, a buzzer, and a doll. They played the ten-minute tape for 204 male and female adults who were asked to interpret what they had seen. Some were told the baby was male, others in the group were told it was female. The adult subjects saw the crying "girl" baby as frightened, but when they thought they were watching a boy, they described "him" as angry. "If you think your child is *angry*," the authors ask, "would you treat 'him' differently than if you think 'she' is *afraid*? . . . It would seem reasonable to assume that a child who is thought to be afraid is held and cuddled more than a child who is thought to be angry."

Such research on parental response teaches us that we see what we expect to see—and we react to what we see. Researcher Jeanne Block used extensive cross-cultural data to suggest a number of important differences in the ways parents treat boys and girls. Block found that both mothers and fathers stressed achievement and competition in their sons, encouraged boys to control their emotions, emphasized independence, and developed a tendency to punish boys. Fathers in particular were stricter with boys, and mothers revealed concern that their sons conform to external standards. Both parents characterized their relationship to their daughters as warmer and physically closer than with their sons. They expressed greater confidence in girls' truthfulness and encouraged girls' introspection. At the same time, mothers were appreciably more restrictive with girls, monitoring them more closely than their sons. Researcher Beverly Fagot confirmed many of Block's observations in a study that examined parents' responses to stereotypical versus unconventional play in their children. Fagot found that parents gave significantly more favorable responses when their children conformed to "same-sex preferred" behavior and actively discouraged "cross-sex preferred" behavior. Girls, for example, elicited negative responses from their parents when engaged in large motor activities—running, jumping, throwing—and positive responses when they asked for help. Boys were encouraged to play by themselves and discouraged from staying close to the parent. Boys were praised for independent accomplishments and tacitly dissuaded from helping the parents with chores. One of the most interesting findings is that these parents, all of whom demonstrated significant force in shaping their children's conformity, saw themselves unequivocally as treating their sons and daughters alike. The discrepancy between the parents' own report of even-handed treatment of both sexes and the parents' actual behavior was vast. With remarkable understatement, Fagot concludes: "These data suggest that parents are not fully aware of the methods they use to socialize their young children."

For decades, feminist scholars and social researchers have patiently built up a body of evidence showing the psychological damage done by the coercive enforcement of gender roles in girls. But what about the damage to the psychological development of boys? If traditional socialization takes aim at girls' voices, it takes aim at boys' hearts.

Little boys and little girls start off with similar psychological profiles. They are equally emotional, expressive, and dependent, equally desirous of physical affection. At the youngest ages, both boys and girls are more like a stereotypical girl. If any differences exist, little boys are, in fact, slightly more sensitive and expressive than little girls. They cry more easily, seem more easily frustrated, appear more upset when a caregiver leaves the room. Until the age of four or five, both boys and girls rest comfortably in what one researcher has called "the expressive-affiliative mode." Studies indicate that girls are permitted to remain in that mode while boys are subtly—or forcibly—pushed out of it.

Australian anthropologist Bob Connell argues that bland-sounding sociological terms like "gender role acquisition" do not convey the emotional experience of those who are the ones being pushed. In his yearlong study of elementary-school boys, Connel encountered a profound impetus not referenced in earlier research— violence. The conventional view of socialization portrays boys as only too willing to "learn" the male role. All of the emphasis has been on those unfortunate few who lacked fathers or other "male role models" to mimic. No one thought to question the assumption that boys' squeeze into manhood was anything but eager. The results of his field study convinced Connel that the usual picture of boys hungrily digesting "the masculine role" only works "by playing down conflict and ignoring violence." Not all boys march off so willingly into manhood. Whether by active violation or passive nonresponsiveness, the rituals by which boys are taught to conform are often unpleasant. Connel writes: " 'Agencies of socialization' cannot produce mechanical effects in a growing person. What they do is invite the child to participate in social practice on given terms. The invitation may be, and often is, coercive—accompanied by heavy pressure to accept and no mention of an alternative." "Mama's boy," "faggot," "pussy," "wimp"—no boy I know of has escaped the experience of such ridicule. No man I have treated has fully eluded the taste of the lash one receives if one dares not accept masculinity's "invitation."

James remembers riding home with his dad from his music lesson. He is seven or eight. His father asks if he likes his new music teacher. James not only likes him; he's thrilled. "I'm real sweet on him, Dad," he tells me he replied. His father punches James hard in the arm, as if in fun. "Do not say 'you're sweet' on a man, James. Girls say that."

"You hurt me," James protested.

"I meant to."

"But, why?"

"That's just spice, James. That's so you'll remember. Now, do not whine about it. You'll be sounding just like a girl again."

In our session, James recalls his confusion as he looked out the window of the moving car, fighting back tears he felt ashamed of, and yet at the same time feeling the comfort and warmth of his father's hand on his shoulder.

Some boys grow up in flagrantly abusive environments. For

them, the active trauma of overt coercion may be a daily occurrence. We know statistically that most of the violence in families is perpetrated by men. We know that across a wide spectrum of strictness, fathers tend to be tougher than mothers and both are tougher on boys than on girls. In many homes, violent fathers pass on active trauma to their sons as if toughness were a gift, a necessary initiation. In the novel *The Prince of Tides*, the protagonist's father becomes intent on teaching his son about manhood when the boy cries because his older sister has hit him.

> "Tom, I'm ashamed of you, boy. . . . Crying when a little girl hits you. Boys never cry. Never. No matter what."
>
> "He's sensitive, Henry," my mother said, stroking my hair. "So, hush."
>
> "Oh, sensitive," my father teased. "Well, I wouldn't want to say anything that might hurt someone so sensitive. Now you'd never catch Luke crying like a baby over something like that. I've whipped Luke with a belt and never saw a tear. Luke was a man from the day he was born."

Believing it a part of his paternal responsibility, my father was no stranger to the manly value of whipping his boys into line. He whipped my brother and me if we dared to rebel. And, conversely, he whipped us if we showed too much vulnerability. Mostly, he whipped us as a proper man should, to keep us corralled and teach us our lessons. For my father, as was true of many men of his generation, pain was a form of pedagogy.

When I think back on the violence, it is the suddenness that I remember—the swat on the back of my head as he passed, the slap across my face if I "gave lip."

To this day, as I fall asleep, I will sometimes start, hearing in my mind the harsh call of my name, feeling the quick thrill of terror rush through my body, now close to forty years later. I remember the crash of the door swinging open, jarring me from sleep, and my father, silhouetted against the hall light, panting, his face flushed with rage, pulling me out of bed by the hair ("Oww, Dad. DAD!"), and dragging me off with no words, too disgusted for words, to the offending messy towel or capless toothpaste. "How many TIMES must I tell you?" my father would shake his head sorrowfully, bewildered, as his huge hand, disembodied, crashed down on me.

What I remember most is the belt. A thick black belt about three inches wide. I remember the slow way my father eased it out of the loops of his baggy gray work pants, tilting his head to the side as he folded it, carefully, thoughtfully.

Five, maybe six years old, I would lean over, with my pants down, bare, bent over my father's knee, bent over the bed, bent over to grab my own ankles. I had tried to run when I was quite young but the consequences of such disobedience had been demonstrated clearly enough.

With each stroke of the belt, my father intoned a word or short phrase as if he were trying to beat a message in through my skin. "Don't you EVER . . . talk BACK . . . to your MOTHER . . . like THAT . . . aGAIN. Not EVER . . . DO . . . YOU . . . under-STAND . . . me, BOY?" ("Yes.") "Yes WHAT?" ("Yes, sir.")

And then eventually enough blows would have fallen and the ritual would be over. I was allowed to go to my bed, or sometimes, I was forced to stand at attention in the center of the living room, with my pants still down, my hands clasped behind me, until my legs shook.

I remember, from the earliest age, teaching myself how to disas-sociate, consciously schooling myself in the art of leaving my own body to hover somewhere close to the ceiling. Looking back, I can recall it all clearly from an aerial view, my father's face suffused with blood, purple with exertion, his eyebrows drawn in concen-tration. The boy bent over, his pants at the ankles, like an embar-rassed spectator, turning away. The whiteness of the boy's skin.

Mostly, my father's aim was good, but at times anger would get the better of him and he would grow sloppy. Then the belt would land on the small of my back or the backs of my knees. That would bring me down from the ceiling in a hurry. Most often, though, after the first few blows, the pain would mean nothing to me at all, until the numbness and disassociation wore off a few hours later. Then, I would have trouble sitting, or sometimes even lying, just as my father had threatened I would. "I'm going to beat you so you won't sit down for a week." And, though I did sit down for fear and shame, I would often secretly wish that I hadn't.

"What are you making faces about?"

"Nothing, Dad."

"A little tender?"

"No, Dad."

There were no broken bones, no scars—some bruises, a few welts here and there, but nothing anyone would notice. Physical abuse? If you had said these words to my father, if you had said them to me, we would have laughed in your face. This wasn't abuse. This wasn't even a beating. My father knew what a real beating felt like. And he was right about that. What he dished out to his son was nothing compared to what he himself had received. And so the chain goes, across generations, link to link. Whether he knew it or not, my father was doing more than meting out punishment for imagined infractions. He was teaching me, just as he had been taught, what it means to be a man.

"I do not take shit from women," the father in *The Prince of Tides* tells his wife. "You're a woman and nothing but a goddamn woman and you keep your goddamn mouth shut when I'm disciplining one of the boys. I do not interfere with you and Savannah because I do not give a shit how you raise her. But it's important to raise a boy up right. Because there's nothing worse on earth than a boy who ain't been brought up right." For more boys than one might care to imagine, being "brought up right," means active trauma. But even boys who begin in a nonviolent atmosphere may find the enforcement of the masculine role ratcheting up if they dare try stepping outside of it. A young naval ensign, Kevin Manheim, broke the "do not ask, do not tell" code of today's military by informing the men of his unit that he was a practicing homosexual. Some of those men responded to Manheim's break with the traditional masculine role by stomping him to death.

In the movie *Dead Poets Society* an adolescent boy, Neil Perry, inspired by a gifted teacher, breaks from the masculine mold to discover himself as an artist and actor—directions that run counter to the wishes of his constricted, controlling father. The young man is only a few days away from playing Ariel, Shakespeare's fey sprite, when his father forbids it. Unwilling to wreck the performance that he and his classmates had worked so hard for and, what's more important, unwilling to turn his back on the realization of his own gifts, Neil disobeys his father for the first time in his life. He delivers a brilliant performance. Neil's father retaliates swiftly and thoroughly. He removes his son from his beloved school, separates him from his friends and the teacher he admires, and enlists him in a military academy. This boy, however, does not go gently into his father's night; he answers retaliation with retaliation. Dressed in the makeup and costume of Ariel—in clear defiance of the "hypermasculine" stance of his father—Neil commits suicide. His death is a lethal protest against the enforced betrayal of his own inner being. The suicide is at once an enactment of and a resistance to what one child abuse expert calls "soul murder." His story is an extreme form of the drama of repudiation and conformity which can be observed every day in our classrooms and playgrounds.

Some boys lose their "souls" in great chunks, others find it chipped away in small bits, through the most ordinary interactions, like my three-year-old son. Alexander has a gift and a great appetite for imaginative play. He likes Dracula, killer karate, and "monstees." But his unalloyed passion is reserved for Barbies and for dressing up. There is a simpler explanation than genes or nascent sexual preferences for Alexander's behavior. My son spends most of his days in a day care setting where he is the only boy. All day long he plays with his best friends, five three-year-old girls, and his penchant for dress-up and dolls doubtless has much to do with the current culture at their homes. To remove him from this setting and from the day care provider he has grown to love in the name of protecting his masculinity would be understandable and well within the range of "normal" action. But it would also be passively abusive.

Even within the supposedly enlightened atmosphere of a college community, the amount of stir my son's dresses has caused among our friends has surprised my wife and me. "Experts" we have known for years, psychologists who lecture around the country, have offered unsolicited advice about our "problem." People have expressed great concern about Alexander's impending "gender confusion."

Helen, Alexander's day care provider, gave us characteristically blunt advice, not about how to handle our son so much as how to handle our friends. "If it was Alexandra and not Alexander," she told us, "and if your daughter showed up in a hard hat and a tool belt instead of a dress, those same people bugging you now would be cheering you on. You just tell them not to worry about it."

My little son is not confused. He couldn't be clearer in his love for dressing up as all sorts of things—as Dracula, a cowboy, a lion. No one has felt the need to make sure Alexander understands he is not really a vampire or a cat. Our friends' uneasiness stems from our culture's discomfort with femininity in boys, not from Alexander's discomfort. He has none. But he is learning.

One day Alexander's big brother, Justin, had some boys over to play. Alexander ran excitedly upstairs to change into his favorite dog-eared dress and grab his magic-fairy wand, then dashed down to the kitchen to display his regalia. The boys looked up, startled, and stared blankly. Not a word passed between them, but the moment was molten. Alexander turned heel and fled back upstairs. "That's beautiful, A," Justin weakly called after him. But it was too little, too late. Off went the dress, back on went the pants. Without a fuss, Alexander rejoined the group and they went together to the basement for woodworking on some sword or gun. The dress has not been worn again.

In that moment, I witnessed a pure instance of cultural transmission through passive trauma. Alexander rushed downstairs innocently expecting appreciation and delight. The stares of the older boys contained an emotion, shame, and a message: *You are not to do that.* Since these were nice boys, the message was devoid of outright ridicule and, even so, I felt my face burn in sympathy with Alexander when the discrepancy between the reaction he wanted and the reaction he got washed over him like a wave of humiliation—when he began learning, at three, what it takes to be a boy.

For most boys, the achievement of masculine identity is not an acquisition so much as a disavowal. When researchers asked girls and women to define what it means to be feminine, the girls answered with positive language: to be compassionate, to be connected, to care about others. Boys and men, on the other hand, when asked to describe masculinity, predominantly responded with double negatives. Boys and men did not talk about being strong so much as about not being weak. They do not list independence so much as not being dependent. They did not speak about being close to their fathers so much as about pulling away from their mothers. In short, being a man generally means not being a woman. As a result, boys' acquisition of gender is a negative achievement. Their developing sense of their own masculinity is not, as in most other forms of identity development, a steady movement toward something valued so much as a repulsion from something devalued. Masculine identity development turns out to be not a process of development at all but rather a process of elimination, a successive unfolding of loss. Along with whatever genetic proclivities one might inherit, it is this loss that lays the foundation for depression later in men's lives.

Just as girls are pressured to yield that half of their human potential consonant with assertive action, just as they have been systematically discouraged from developing and celebrating the self-concepts and skills that belong to the public world, so are boys pressured to yield attributes of dependency, expressiveness, affiliation—all the self-concepts and skills that belong to the relational, emotive world. These wholesale excisions are equally damaging to the healthy development of both girls and boys. The price for traditional socialization of girls is oppression, as Lyn Brown and Carol Gilligan put it, "the tyranny of the kind and nice." The price of traditional socialization for boys is disconnection—from themselves, from their mothers, from those around them.

*   *   *

Guiding these pressures directed toward boys, and motivating characters as diverse as my academic friends who were concerned about Alexander's dress, and the savage father in *The Prince of Tides*, is a myth. It is a myth about how boys develop, what they need to be "turned into" men, and what the consequences are if they fail. This myth has been believed by most in this culture for a long time, from Sigmund Freud to Robert Bly, from conservative sociologists like Talcott Parsons to progressive feminists like Nancy Chodorow and Carol Gilligan. It is one of the unquestioned assumptions of our society. The myth I speak of is the idea that boys must be turned into men to begin with, that boys, unlike girls, must *achieve* masculinity. Boys must repudiate their connection to mother and to all things feminine. They must "dis-identify" with mother and "identify" with father in order to develop a "stable internal masculine identity." If they fail, if their "masculine identity" is weak or unstable, dread consequences may result. Over the decades, sociologists and psychologists have blamed unstable masculine identity formation on everything from juvenile gangs to homosexuality, drug addiction, and even murder.

Each of the misguided assumptions embedded in this myth is easily disputed. First, why must we distinguish between the gender development of boys and girls to begin with? As anthropologist Barrie Thorne points out, a woman's basic femininity is never questioned in our culture. There may be questions raised about what kind of woman she is—flirtatious, tough, even "butch"—but it is rarely in doubt that she remains a woman, feels herself to be a woman, is not driven by anxiety about her own femininity. But for boys and men, masculine identity is perceived as precious and perilous, though not a shred of evidence has emerged to indicate the existence of this supposed precarious internal structure, masculine identity. Studies indicate that both boys and girls have a clear sense of which sex they are from about the age of two, and that this knowledge is extremely solid and unambiguous in all but the most severely disturbed children, those who are brain damaged, psychotic, or autistic. Some sociologists now distinguish between such a basic knowledge of one's own sex, which they call "sex role identity" from knowledge of what it *means* to be a boy or a girl, which they call "gender role identity." It is at this point that things grow murky. In order to be well adjusted, boys and men need to have internalized a clear, stable sense of what it means to be male. Confusion about what "maleness" means can result in severe psychological difficulties and "antisocial" behaviors. Now, do I, for one, possess such a clear, unchanging set of beliefs about masculinity? I confess that I, though solidly middle-aged, with two marriages, two children, and close to twenty years of practice behind me, do not. In these changing times, I know of few men who do. More current research has begun to suggest that it is not truly adaptive to possess some hypothesized internal repository of unchanging images and expectations in our changing world. Rigid notions about masculinity, far from being a necessary component of good psychological adjustment, may be a negative factor. "Androgyny," the fluid capacity to access many qualities, has been shown to correlate with psychological well-being. But even calling a man who can be empathic or a woman who can be assertive "androgynous" presupposes that some human qualities are inherently male, others female. A more accurate judgment is that the fluid capacity to access many different kinds of strengths and characteristics seems to be good for humans of both sexes.

Boys do not need to be turned into males. They are males. Boys do not need to develop their masculinity. They are masculine, no less than girls are feminine. Once we understand that "masculine identity" is not about an internal structure but rather a socially accepted definition of what it means to be male, then the processes by which we impose those definitions on boys sharpens in clarity. Like the myth of the Procrustean bed, like circumcision, the oldest and most common rite of passage throughout the world, boys "become" men by lopping off, or having lopped off, the most sensitive parts of their psychic and, in some cases, physical selves. The passage from boyhood to manhood is about ritual wounding. It is about giving up those parts of the self that do not fit within the confines of the role. It is about pain and the withstanding of pain.

In his autobiography, Nelson Mandela recalls his transition to manhood through the tribal rite of circumcision. He speaks with characteristic simplicity and directness:

> Suddenly, I heard the first boy cry out, *"Ndiyindoda!"* (I am a man!), which we were trained to say in the moment of circumcision. Seconds later, I heard Justice's strangled voice pronounce the same phrase. . . . Before I knew it, the old man was kneeling in front of me. I looked directly into his eyes. He was pale, and though the day was cold, his face was shining with perspiration. . . . Without a word, he took my foreskin, pulled it forward, and then in a single motion, brought down his assegai. I felt as if fire was shooting through my veins; the pain was so intense that I buried my chin into my chest. Many seconds seemed to pass before I remembered the cry, and then I recovered and called out, *"Ndiyindoda!"*
>
> . . . . I felt ashamed because the other boys seemed much stronger and braver than I had been: they had called out more promptly than I had. I was distressed that I had been disabled . . . and I did my best to hide my agony. A boy may cry; a man conceals his pain.

The process Mandela recalls as a single transformational event, occurs in Western culture without much ceremony each day in the lives of our sons. Their "masculinization" through wounding and the concealment of pain are mundane occurrences. It is no longer a formally accepted part of Western culture to physically injure sons in the name of masculinity. Psychological injury, however, is another matter.

These emotional amputations can be effected through active or passive injury, in transactions severe or seemingly mild. They can occur with extraordinary drama, as for Michael and his mother, or for my father and me. They can appear as mundane as dinner non-conversation in a middle-class family, as banal as the scene described one afternoon by my client Janie. Janie and her sons sit at the dining room table. Janie's husband, Robert, who is fatigued and somewhat depressed, joins them after a long day at the office followed by a hectic commute home. Janie wants to talk to Robert and the boys about their days and hers. Robert wants to "relax," that is, to be left alone. After a few abortive efforts, Janie gives up and, rather than confront Robert, compensates for his lack of interest with redoubled efforts toward the kids. The boys, particularly the oldest, pick up Dad's cue and freeze out their mother with monosyllabic responses. Janie, reluctant to "smother," willing to give her men "their space," eventually, amiably withdraws. She putters about the kitchen and cleans up while Robert listens to the news and the boys go off to sports or video games or homework. This transaction is seamless. There occurs, in this family, hardly a ripple of overt discontent. And yet, as Janie and I work together to deconstruct this simple, everyday scene, it begins to seem nothing short of chilling. What have Janie's sons learned about what it means to be a man?

They have learned not to expect their father to attend to them or to be expressive about much of anything. They have come to expect him to be psychologically unavailable. They have also learned that he is not accountable in his emotional absence, that Mother does not have the power either to engage him or to confront him. In other words, Father's neglect and Mother's ineffectiveness at countering it teach the boys that, in this family at least, men's participation is not a responsibility but rather a voluntary and discretionary act. Third, they learn that Mother, and perhaps women in general, need not be taken too seriously. Finally, they learn that not just Mother but the values she manifests in the family—connection, expressivity—are to be devalued and ignored. The subtext message is, "engage in 'feminine' values and activities and risk a similar devaluation yourself." The paradox for the boys is that the only way to connect with their father is to echo his disconnection. Conversely, being too much like Mother threatens further disengagement or perhaps, even active reprisal. In this moment, and thousands of other ordinary moments, these boys are learning to accept psychological neglect, to discount nurture, and to turn the vice of such abandonment into a manly virtue.

Janie brought first Robert and then the boys into therapy. She refused to stand by while a level of isolation many would not even recognize as problematic grew steadily in her family. Yet even

Janie, an exceptionally strong, capable woman, did not enter my door with such clarity of purpose. She was referred to me with a growing problem of anxiety and depression. In her mind, initially, she was the family's problem. In short order, however, it became apparent to us both that the family was her problem, not the other way around. Thus, rather than trying to change Jamie, we tried changing the context around her. It took a bit of effort to convince Robert to "buy in," as he put it, to our analysis. But, once she grasped the reasons for her discomfort, Janie would not back down. She insisted on greater levels of communication not just between her and Robert but also, with Robert's help, between them all. Nowadays, at their table, Robert has come out from behind his newspaper and the boys have come out from behind one-word answers. Everyone seems happier for the change.

Janie is an unusual woman. Faced with the encroachment of the force of disconnection in her family, she found the resources to stand up and meet it head-on, first in her marriage and then in their parenting. She took such strong action for her own sake—her family was becoming lonely for her to live in. But, more than for herself, she struggled for increased connection for the sake of her sons. More and more, parents of both sexes are trying to value and hold on to the relational connection with their sons as well as their daughters. Despite these good efforts, traditional forms of both active and passive trauma are still very much alive in our culture. Both inside and outside our homes, the old roles have far from disappeared as an influence in the lives of most boys.

CHAPTER SIX

The Loss
of the Relational

Sister, mother
And spirit of the river, spirit of the sea,
Suffer me not to be separated

And let my cry come unto Thee.
—T. S. ELIOT,
"Ash Wednesday"

The trauma inherent in boys' socialization can be grouped into three domains—diminished connection to the mother, diminished connection to aspects of the self, and diminished connection to others. Taken together, these severances comprise what I call *the loss of the relational*—that wound in boys' lives that sets up their vulnerability to depression as men. Of the three dislocations—to mother, self, and others—the earliest and prototypical loss, for many boys, is the attenuation of closeness to their mother.

The idea that boys must rupture an effeminizing connection to mother is one of the oldest, least questioned, and most deeply rooted myths of patriarchy. Freud himself sounded the clarion call close to a century ago, when he wrote: "[The boy's] relationship of the mother is the first and most intense. Therefore, it must be destroyed."

Thirty-eight-year-old Ann Buchet knew what it felt like to be on the receiving end of the impulse Freud voiced with such passion. "I remember the first time Bill did it," Ann told me one session. "Timmy couldn't have been more than seven. He was lying in my lap, just resting, and Bill simply walked over and took Timmy's hand and said, 'Come here,' and whisked him off. I didn't realize what he was doing, at first. I thought he was just taking him somewhere. But then it became obvious.

"So, I said to him, 'Bill, what are you doing?' and he got very angry with me. He said, 'He's too old. You have to learn to let go of him.' And I said, 'He's just a child.' And he bent right over me, very close, very upset and told me, 'You will *not maul* that boy!' " In her lap, Ann's hands clench and unclench. "I knew, of course," she continues, "that he was talking about his relationship with his own mother. But I honestly didn't know what to say. I still don't know what to say."

"So," I asked, "Have you obeyed? Have you left Timmy alone?" Ann grins mischievously. "I *sneak*," she confessed.

Ann's smile is so impish. Her solution has such a familiar feel, it seems mean-spirited to break with her light-hearted tone. Yet this simple transaction speaks volumes about mothers and sons inside the modern family. And most of what it has to tell is not good news. Bill was attempting to ensure that his son was not babied, coddled, drained by the "regressive" pull of his mother. He was acting like "a good father," in accordance with the prevailing myth that teaches that boys must be helped to gain distance from their "enmeshing" mothers. For many decades, in both our popular imagination and in psychological theory, helping the boy sever his "psychological umbilical cord" was viewed as one of the father's main functions. The underlying assumption is that mothers and sons, left to their own devices, would maintain some sort of fusion that would "sissify" the boy. In Conroy's *The Prince of Tides,* Henry, the brutal father, addresses his children as he is about to depart for the war in Korea:

> "I'm going to miss my babies," my father said. . . . "I'm going to
> write you letters every single week and seal each one with a million

kisses. Except for you boys. You boys don't want anything to do with kisses, do you?"

"No, Daddy," Luke and I answered simultaneously.

"I'm raising you boys to be fighters. Right! I'm not raising you to be lovers," he said, cuffing our heads roughly. "Tell me you won't let your mother turn you into lovers when I'm away. She's too soft on you. Don't let her put you in dresses and take you to teas."

Conventional theory long held that mothers, left unchecked, would, at least psychologically, "put their sons into dresses." Boys without strong "father figures" to help them ward off their mothers were in grave peril of either succumbing to the mother's feminizing influence, becoming homosexual or ineffective (the two were equated), or else of "overcompensating" by becoming "hypermasculine"—caricaturing bravado in order to hide their hidden insecurities. The "hypermasculine" theory was the favored explanation for boys' destructive behaviors—from juvenile delinquency, to gangs, to drug addiction. The root of boys' difficulties lay in an unnaturally close connection to the mother, unmitigated by an absent or ineffectual male. This formula—too much mother and too little father—has been a mainstay in our thinking about "problem" boys for generations.

James Dean put his stamp on a whole generation in the film *Rebel Without a Cause*. This cautionary tale of troubled youth does not, despite its title, shy away from positing a cause for Dean's angst. In an oft-quoted scene, the hero tries to engage his father in conversation. The father is shown earnestly trying to comprehend his son but he is distracted because he's nervous about getting the floors washed before his domineering wife returns home. "Son," says the father. "I just don't understand." The camera pulls back to show him on his knees, scrub brush in hand, wearing his wife's frilly apron. The visual message is clear: "Beware debased fathers who stoop to do housework!" Dad has been castrated, the film suggests, and his son needs a desperate infusion of "balls" (common parlance for "a stable masculine identity"). Enraged at his father, young Dean slams out of his house. In the next scene he is drag racing other boys. With a truly haunted look on his face, Dean drives like a madman, hurtling himself into danger. Left on his own to cut the maternal tie, Dean is on a dangerous, reckless quest for "balls."

Despite Freud's talk about castrating fathers, it is the emasculating mother who looms larger than life in our culture's imagination. The assumption in all this is that women in general and mothers in particular can "feminize" a male, robbing him of his masculinity. It takes other men—fathers, mentors, the tribe—to loosen the apron strings. Manly men, Iron Johns, must flank and encircle, protecting their own.

The fear of the feminizing mother is still very much with us today. In a recent article on fathers appearing in *Esquire* magazine, for example, journalist Michael Segell reiterates the decades-old explanation for homosexuality without question or criticism.

> As a result of [a weak] father's abdication of power to his mother, a toddler is unable to identify—is often prevented from identifying—with his father and to separate from his mother. The boy's and his mother's boundaries become blurred, and the boy persists in his feminine identification with her, which causes him great guilt and anxiety. When it's time for him to latch on to his father for his primary identification, his mother again refuses to let go, and, with only an ineffectual male figure to turn to, the boy's hunger for a male role model, for a male rescuer, becomes eroticised. *When he finally manages to flee his mother,* he flees all women—safe, finally, in the land of men.

This "scientific" explanation of the cause of homosexuality has about as much empirical support as the theory of the four humors. It harks back to the days when psychiatry listed homosexuality as a disease, and when therapists "treated" thousands of men—some volunteers, many brought by their families—for the "perversion" of being gay.

It is time to recognize that this myth is repulsive. Amid all the furor and dread, has anyone stopped to inquire—is this really what "women" want from their men? Do mothers, unrestrained by strong fathers, inevitably gravitate toward emasculation? These images of castrating mothers and sissy boys are grotesque, revealing our culture's irrational fear that holding the door open to "the feminine"—and to females—will "turn" our sons into castrates, or homosexuals, or, as Robert Bly would have it, "soft males."

Despite years of research, not a shred of evidence has been found to substantiate this fairy tale of fusional mothers or of fathers as the necessary objects of masculine identification. Recent studies indicate that boys raised by women, including single women and lesbian couples, do not suffer in their adjustment; they are not appreciably less "masculine"; they do not show signs of psychological impairment. What many boys without fathers inarguably do face is a precipitous drop in their socioeconomic status. When families dissolve, the average standard of living for mothers and children can fall as much as 60 percent, while that of the man usually rises. When we focus on the highly speculative psychological effects of fatherlessness we draw away from concrete political concerns, like the role of increased poverty. Again, there are as yet no data suggesting that boys without fathers to model masculinity are necessarily impaired. Those boys who do have fathers are happiest and most well adjusted with warm, loving fathers, fathers who score high in precisely "feminine" qualities. The key component of a boy's healthy relationship to his father is affection, not "masculinity." The boys who fare poorly in their psychological adjustment are not those without fathers, but those with abusive or neglectful fathers. Contrary to the traditional stereotype, a sweet man in an apron who helps out with the housework may be just the nurturant kind of father a boy most needs. The tragic irony is that a man like Bill or like the father in *The Prince of Tides* may become the worst father in the very act of trying to live up to traditional notions about what makes a good one.

When Bill Buchet unceremoniously rips his son away from Ann's physical nurture, he is motivated by a wish to help his son. Bill's behavior is fueled by a drive that is evident throughout our culture. That force manifests itself in the voice of a gym teacher who mocks Timmy, however good-naturedly, when he deserts a schoolyard game in favor of greeting his mother; or it might appear in Timmy's school chums who also ridicule him for leaving their game, though less good-naturedly. That force inhabits Timmy's mother when she doesn't quite know what to say to her son when he begins to cry in response to the teasing—whether she should support his tears, or his instinct to conceal them. Where is the line between nurture and coddling? How close to her is too close?

"Mother died today. Or, maybe, yesterday; I can't be sure." So read the opening lines of Albert Camus's *The Stranger*, a novel that has become the very emblem of alienation. Grief for the lost maternal begins this chronicle of extreme disconnection. With intuitive resonance, these first two lines announce the progress of the entire work. First there is the loss of the mother. Immediately following, there is dislocation in time and place.

While artists have concerned themselves with this issue for some time, psychology has just begun to focus on the role of maternal loss in boys' lives. Psychologist William Pollock suspects that beneath the undeniable "father wound," the emotional toll taken on boys by "absent fathers," there may be an even earlier "mother wound." This is not the wound of the stereotypical mother who will not let go, but the wound of the mother who, in compliance to society's fears and rules, lets go too early. When Ann Bouchet complies with Bill's mandate for Timmy, when Janie accepts her sons' withdrawal from emotional contact, they abandon their boys, yielding momentarily, not just to their particular family dynamic, but to obligations both older and deeper. In such moments of passive trauma, these mothers have allowed themselves to be silenced by the conventions of patriarchy. Furthermore, by diminished connection to the mother I do not mean merely the connection through nurture. At least as damaging to the boy is the mother's diminished authority.

The traditional idea that only men know how to raise sons undermines not just a mother's instinct to care, but also her capacity to guide and to set limits. The stereotype that mothers nurture while fathers discipline is overdrawn. While studies indicate that men are harsher to their children than women, they are not necessarily the family's main disciplinarian. The typical American father spends on average only eleven minutes a day with his children. And most of that brief amount of time is spent in play. While in certain circumstances fathers may be brought in like heavy artillery to support mothers in unusual circumstances, by and large mothers, not fathers, handle the lion's share of discipline, for the simple reason that mothers handle most of the parenting functions. As devastating as the taboo of mothers' tenderness is for boys in our society, the undercutting of mothers' power is at least as destructive. When a boy rejects his mother's authority because she is "only a woman," when a mother shrinks from the full exercise of her parental rights and responsibilities, both play out the values of patriarchy. The mother's higher authority as a parent is counterbalanced by the son's higher status as a male. The psychiatric units I sometimes consult to are filled with such abandoned, grandiose young men. These boys suffer less from their relationship to the absent fathers who have disappeared from their lives than they suffer from their relationship to the overwhelmed mothers they must live with, mothers they have managed to bully into silence, much to their own detriment. Conventional psychiatry often reflects these same values when, rather than empowering the mother, it offers to replace her by a therapist (preferably male) or (male-run) institution. Traditionally oriented therapists may actively discourage family therapy, citing the need for the boy to have "a place of his own," in which to "work out separation." But the true meaning of psychological "separation" is maturity, and we humans stand a better chance of maturing when we do not disconnect from one another. Such literal thinking misses the point that boys must work out "separation" with the people they are "separating" from. There is no way they can work it out on their own. And the current notion that mentors—"male mothers" as Bly calls them—must help the boy "leave" begs the question of why he must "leave" at all. Traditional visions of masculinity, even in the very language of "separation," equate growing up with severance. But what maturity truly requires is the replacement of childish forms of closeness *with more adult forms of closeness,* not with dislocation.

There are virtually no images in this culture representing close, mature ties between males and their mothers. Almost all of the positive imagery concerning mothers and sons is limited to young boys. If the tie between mothers and older boys is referenced at all it is usually depicted as pathological. Most often, though, as the young boy grows older, the presence of the mother just disappears. As family therapist Olga Silverstein described in *The Courage to Raise Good Men*, in order to clear the decks for a boy's growth and adventure a good mother is supposed to get out of the way. Such is the message of countless tales of adopted, orphaned, motherless heroes. In the legend of the Holy Grail, for example, the boy Perceval, whose father has been killed in knightly combat, is hidden away by his protective mother. He grows up in an enchanted grotto, as a pastoral naïf, until a group of knights thunder by. Seeing the sun glint off their armor the boy mistakes them for gods. Instantly seduced, he runs off with them and poor Mom, seeing his dust, drops dead on the spot, never to be referred to again. In George Lucas's *Star Wars* trilogy, all three films track Luke Skywalker's quest and confrontation with his complex father. His mother, by contrast, is not once mentioned. As boys turn into young men, closeness not just to the mother but to both parents—indeed dependent closeness to anyone—is equated with childishness. Growing up becomes synonymous with moving out. Maturity and connection are set up as choices that exclude one another.

As devastating as the disconnection from the mother may be, it is merely the beachhead of a larger social mandate, the instruction to turn away, not just from the mother, but from intimacy itself, and from cultivating, or even grasping, the values and skills that sustain deep emotional connection. The diminished attachment to the mother is a particular manifestation of the disavowal of all things deemed feminine, including many of the most emotionally rich parts of the self. My son Alexander must forgo his dress and magic fairy wand; the adolescent in *Dead Poets Society* must give up that part of him that wishes to play Ariel. If the tie to the mother is the first disconnect on the road to manhood, the tie to oneself is the second. A boy's disavowal of the "feminine" in himself falls into two spheres: rejection of expressivity and rejection of vulnerability.

Alice Blake, a wry thirty-four-year-old businesswoman, leans forward and tells me about the "gender bombardment" she encounters in just one morning with her seven-year-old son. "Here's a two-hour slice called *Mom's Life with Small Boy*," she announces. Jeff starts off the day by declaring he's not wearing the powder blue shirt she just bought for him.

"They'll make fun of me, Mom," he protests.

"But it's *blue*," she replies. Jeff flings the shirt onto the floor, ending the discussion.

"Not blue enough," he declares.

Alice and Jeff then go off to his classroom where she drops in and helps out one morning a week. The students are decorating the stuffed animals they were asked to bring for sick or hospitalized children. "How come you didn't bring in one of your animals?" Alice asks Jeff privately. She knows better than to publicly ask a first grade boy about his stuffed animals. Jeff scans the room, looking, as Alice describes it, like a midget drug dealer on the lookout for feds. He "confesses" to having given all of his animals away to his older brother.

"Oh?" says Alice. "Then how come they're still all over your room?"

"Mom"—Jeff drops an arm around her shoulder—"they're on loan."

The teacher gathers the children in a circle and asks them to offer suggestions for what to write on cards to be attached to each animal. "Get better soon," says one. "Cuddle me," says another. "Hug me," says a third. "I hope you feel better," says a fourth. None of the suggestions came from the boys.

"So," Alice asks me, "when it comes time to write the cards, how many of the boys do you think chose 'Hug me,' or 'Cuddle me'?" The answer comes as no great surprise. "Zip," she says. While the girls selected from the entire range of greetings, every boy in the room picked the most emotionally constricted inscriptions possible: "Get better soon," or "I hope you feel better." Already they have herded themselves into an emotional corner. Even at age seven, they have learned to dampen their natural capacity for vivid emotional expression. They understand the rules of the game, rules that they will play by for the rest of their lives.

In our culture, expressiveness—even talking in an animated way with great emotional range—is reserved for women. Despite occasional rhetoric about increased communication, "the strong silent type" remains the ideal for men. Real men—men like Clint Eastwood or Arnold Schwarzenegger—are laconic bullet biters. They say things like "Make my day" or "I'll be back." This impassive quality of traditional masculinity blends into the demeanor of depression. But the loss cuts a lot deeper than mere matters of style. Many boys are taught to be so proficient at burying their exuberance that they manage to bury it even from themselves. Recent research indicates that in this society most males have difficulty not just in expressing, but even in identifying their feelings. The psychiatric term for this impairment is *alexithymia* and psychologist Ron Levant estimates that close to *eighty percent* of men in our society have a mild to severe form of it.

The relationship between emotional numbing and overt depression is well documented. In fact, lack of feeling is one of the two main criteria for a diagnosis of overt depression. Less well known is the relationship between alexithymia and the addictive defenses used in covert depression. Addictive behaviors are commonly seen as sedating and medicating pain. For several decades, however, researchers like Edward Khantzian have hypothesized that certain addictions, such as cocaine or alcohol, work to "self-medicate" a person not by sedating him but rather by "revving him up" or "enlivening" dead feelings. These substance abusers are "sensation seekers"—people whose ordinary psychic states are muffled and muted. We know that a great many men in our culture have dampened emotional experience. We know that male drug takers and alcoholics outnumber females by well over two to one. A connection between masculine socialization, alexithymia, covert depression, and substance abuse seems obvious.

The intensification of muted feelings can be achieved not just by using drugs but also by using action, by throwing oneself into crisis situations. Risk taking, gambling, infatuation, and rage all trigger our bodies' "fight or flight" response, releasing both endorphins, the body's opioids, and adrenal secretions, the body's natural stimulants. The body's capacity to release internal medicators when under stress has led researcher Bessel van der Kolk to write about what he calls "addiction to trauma." Noting the high prevalence of crisis in the lives of people who have histories of trauma, he hypothesizes that some may seek intensity to "self-medicate" internal pain not by reaching for an external stimulant, but by throwing themselves into extreme states of physiological hyperarousal. Trauma survivors may develop dependency on the release of their body's own "drugs." Van der Kolk's research points the way toward an understanding of the physiological basis for those defenses used in covert depression that rely on behaviors rather than substances.

While both traumatized men and women may seek increased intensity, their behavior is not equally dangerous. Studies indicate that from boyhood through adolescence and manhood, traumatized males display a distinct proclivity toward "externalizing" distress by inflicting it.

The most profound expression of this impulse to enliven through violence that I have encountered is in male prisoners who are kept in solitary confinement to protect other inmates. Alone, these brutal men frequently turn to self-mutilation—carving names in their arms, biting themselves, swallowing razor blades. They evoke the men in Dante's lowest rung of hell, frozen up to their necks in ice, gnawing on one another's heads. These men uniformly describe the self-mutilation as bringing a sense of relief. It may be that at a most elemental level these prisoners are describing release from the torment of feeling nothing at all. They embody extreme patterns of emotional deadening that, in much milder forms, play an important role in most covert depression. Similarly, the emotional numbing common in both overt and covert depression may itself be an extreme form of the way in which society truncates the capacity of many men and boys to feel.

*   *   *

Just as notions of traditional masculinity view the strong expression of emotion as unmanly, so too they prohibit most expressions of vulnerability. Stereotypically, being a man means being strong, being "on top of it." There is little room for faltering, confusion, or weakness. The shame attached to vulnerability is one of the reasons why so many overtly depressed men don't want to talk about it, why they don't admit the disorder or get the help that could change their lives, and why people surrounding overtly depressed men shy away from confronting them about their condition. It is also one of the powerful dynamics underlying covert depression, since a covertly depressed man is one who finds the vulnerability of depression unacceptable even to himself.

In the same way that the injunction against vulnerability blocks men from resolving depression, it also impedes many men's capacity to heal from the active and passive trauma that contributed to setting up the disorder. Research teaches us that the capacity to reach out to others for help in dealing with fear and pain is the best single remedy for emotional injury. Whether the person is struggling with the effects of combat, rape, or childhood injury, the best predictor of trauma resolution is good social support. But the pressure for men to minimize pain eclipses their desire for help. First, boys are wounded. Then they are taught to foster "self-reliance," eroding their willingness to reach for the healing salve of community. Unacknowledged vulnerabilities seldom cooperate and stay buried, however; they tend to rise up to exact their own toll.

Frank Riorden was a staunch self-made scrapper from East Boston, who had risen through the ranks in the textile business from millworker to become owner of a textile manufacturing plant worth millions. He had struggled with the Boston Brahmin "old boy network," with labor unions, and even with organized crime. And he had about as much patience for my "psychodrivel" as he had for lessons in etiquette. Now in his early sixties, after a lifetime of hard work, in glorious good health, with more money than he knew what to do with, Frank found himself with six wonderful children, three grandchildren, and a beautiful wife—all of whom thoroughly despised him. For many years, Frank's business had taken him "on the road" between 50 and 80 percent of his time, and this proved a dangerous place for a guy who was wealthy and good-looking and "just didn't like spending time alone." Frank filled his travels with a succession of young women, all of whom he treated well, most of whom he genuinely cared for. Frank believed that, in comparison to his heartless exploitative colleagues, he was a sexually sensitive guy.

Frank's world split open on the day his wife, Dana, and his oldest son, Steve, desperately tried to reach him on the road to tell him that a lump that looked like cancer had been discovered in Dana's breast. While Dana was in the hospital for what began as exploratory surgery and wound up as a radical mastectomy, Frank was partying with a flight attendant in Rio de Janeiro. Steve finally tracked his father down two days later. Without therapy this family might have taken two to three generations to heal fully from the trauma of those few days. As it was, it took six months of therapy before Steven would even agree to sit in the same room with his father.

Frank confessed to me in an individual session that in the fancy hotel rooms with those young, adoring, and uncomplicated women, he had felt able to "let down," as he was unable to do anywhere else in his life. He was comfortable talking to his companions about worries and fears—his loneliness, his age—in ways he couldn't imagine doing with people in his "real life." As mistresses from time immemorial have understood, men like Frank are not drawn by the promise of sex alone but by the promise of sex and comfort. Unlike many chronic philanderers, Frank did not blame his wife for the way he had split sexual and emotional nurturance off from his marriage. In fact, Dana could be both nurturant and sexually passionate. The difficulty lay not in her capacity to give but in Frank's willingness to receive. It no more occurred to him to "burden Dana with my troubles," as he put it, than to "blow my own head off." Early on in his marriage Frank had adopted a

Superman stance. Strong, secure, in charge, he was the tree every-one else could lean upon. It took three months of what I call "jack-hammer therapy,"—like boring through asphalt with a pneumatic drill—before Frank finally "got" that there might be a connection between the total denial of his own humanity within his family and his occasional jaunts to exotic locales with twenty-year-olds.

As for the idea of covert depression, Frank sneered at the thought that his tough background—he had a "hard-drinking," blue-collar dad who "beat the snot" out of him and his brothers on a weekly basis—had anything to do with his drivenness, with unacknowledged pain he might still carry inside, or with a reluctance to get too close to anyone he really knew. His childhood, he objected, wasn't much different from that of the other boys in his neighborhood. I told Frank that I wholeheartedly believed this to be true, and yet I wondered just how well those other boys were now doing in their careers and in their family lives.

Frank was typical of many of the covertly depressed men I see, in that he would have rocketed out of my office if I didn't have high-powered leverage. Frank tolerated therapy because I had something he wanted—his wife and kids. There was no benefit in trying to "form a trusting alliance" with him by being sympa-thetic, as most therapists are taught to do. Frank was seeing me because his wife had made it clear that "getting it together" in ther-apy was his only hope of winning her back. He was what I call a "life-mandated referral"—there under duress.

With my encouragement, Frank agreed to call Henry, a man I had worked with years ago who was also in his sixties. Like Frank, Henry had struggled with covert depression—along with a history of cocaine abuse and womanizing. Henry, who had about eight years of therapy and twelve-step work under his belt, managed to drag Frank to ten minutes of an Adult Children of Alcoholics meet-ing, but it didn't much suit Frank. He later explained, "If the fate of my marriage depends on my sitting in some church basement next to some grown man holding a teddy bear on his lap, then the hell with my marriage!" Even though Frank never set foot in a twelve-step meeting again, he surprised both of us by finding coffee with

Henry "halfway tolerable." Henry soon added a couple of friends and Frank found himself talking to this group of seasoned men his own age or older in ways he had never spoken before to anyone but his mistresses. Frank had always been well liked from a distance, with dozens of warm acquaintances and no real friends. Over time, he slowly experimented with opening up, first to Henry and his companions, then to his own wife.

I considered Frank a workaholic, but he felt pathologized by that label. In his own eyes, he had done what it takes to become a self-made millionaire. I considered Frank's relationship to sex addictive, but Frank thought this hopelessly naive. Every businessman he knew had "a little action on the side now and then." I saw Frank as covertly depressed, still carrying injuries from childhood. He saw me as a "bleeding heart liberal" who wouldn't rest until I'd turned him into Alan Alda or some other version of a "sensitive nineties sniveler." Frank had a ready answer for all of my concerns, but the fact remained that this "normal" man had spent his life working most of the time, cheating on his wife, and barely communicating with anyone about anything beyond mundane logistics. He adored his two daughters and criticized his four sons, but only from a distance. Hearing Frank and Dana's description of the extreme emotional disengagement that had existed between them for so many years, I immediately suspected some form of addiction. Humans can rarely tolerate such levels of detachment for long; it is just too lonely. In a marriage as consistently distant as theirs, there is usually a "third leg of the triangle"—booze, work, an affair—that augments an insufferably empty relationship. Many covertly depressed men, unwilling to face the vulnerability of their own hidden pain, and unable to be intimate with their own hearts, cannot face intimacy with anyone else. Where had Frank learned to need so much distance? Where had he learned to mistrust vulnerability and turn for succor outside his family? What was he so afraid of?

One of the things Frank finally shared with Dana and me was his fear of growing old, alone and despised by his children, as, in fact, his father had.

"There's an old saying in family therapy," I told him. "They say it takes three generations to heal from trauma. Your dad never made it and you're in the middle. Let's see what bringing in your children can do."

Bringing Frank, his six kids, and his estranged wife into one room was no small feat. The family flew into Boston from different parts of the country and stayed in various homes or hotel rooms during the week of our work together. Steven, the youngest boy, and the child most obviously hurt by his father's actions, was reluctant to join us at first. It was part of our contract that they were to meet in the days between sessions to spend time together and talk about whatever came to them in the wake of the previous day's work. As is often the case, these informal sessions without me proved as useful as the work done in my office.

I began by eliciting from the Riorden family information in order to silhouette their current crisis against the backdrop of their own history, the burden of unfinished business passed along from parent to child. One way to help a family heal from actions as hurtful as Frank's is to place them in context. The point is not to excuse the man's behavior but to understand it.

As the family story slowly unfolded, I learned that the force that obstructed Frank's connection to himself and his family was the ghost of his older brother, James. James died of complications of pneumonia when he was eight and Frank was six. The family had been visiting relatives in Canada, when little James caught a bad chest cold. A physical exam suggested bronchitis, but James's high fever concerned the doctor, who advised an overnight stay in the hospital. Frank's father, Peter, was restless and anxious to get home. It had been a long visit with his in-laws; he needed to report back to work the next day, and he didn't trust doctors much anyway. "Let him sweat it out," Peter said as they bundled the boy up for the long train ride back to Boston.

James fell into a coma somewhere in northern Pennsylvania. He never recovered. Neither did his parents. Allyssa, Frank's mother, retired into a martyred cloud of chronic depression that left no doubt that she blamed both herself and her spouse for the death of their son. Peter, who once had held aspirations of upward mobility, dropped into factory work like a penitent, medicating his guilt and unspoken rage with alcohol and ritualized attacks on the sons who seemed to affront him by remaining alive. Particularly repugnant to him was Frank, the next oldest boy. Peter outlived his wife, as well as his son. He died at the age of eighty-four, estranged from his family, in a roominghouse in South Boston. He had become, by most accounts, a lonely, mean man the family was relieved to be without.

In our final four-hour session of intense family therapy, I thought it was time to see if Frank could move into some of the vulnerability he had spent most of his life denying. I asked him to participate in a role-played enactment of a typical scene with his father. At first Frank refused, but gradually, with a lot of support and guidance, he slowly warmed to the task. In the scene Frank constructed, he is nine or ten years old. His mother is in bed early, as was her habit. His father comes in late, not drunk enough to be falling down, sloppy, but drunk enough to slur his words and drunk enough to be cruel. Perhaps because Frank is not ready to show it, perhaps because it is not the most painful of his injuries, Frank does not dramatize a scene of physical abuse. In the vignette Peter does not hit the boy, but he does mock him. Peter sneers at Frank for his interest in science. He ridicules him for his hard work at school, for "putting on airs," for "useless ambitions," and, most hurtfully, for his closeness to his mother—"as if it were dirty," Frank tells us, "something to be ashamed of." Frank reports all this sheepishly, not looking at anyone, his voice without emotion.

"Show me," I tell Frank. "Show me what it looked like."

We clear away my office furniture and set up the scene. "The living room couch was over here," Frank indicates. "There was a big desk here along the wall. . . ."

Gradually, I enroll Frank as his father—what Peter looked like, what he wore, how he stood, how he sounded as he said those terrible things. At first Frank, role-playing his father, is stiff, timid. But he cannot accurately portray Peter that way, and soon the force of the role begins to grab hold of him. As the family looks on, Frank and I go over it once, twice, a third time. Each time Frank, playing Peter, grows louder and meaner. "Go on and run to her," he is saying to the imaginary boy. "You little sniveler. You've always been a conniving little sniveler and you know it. Go run under your mother's covers if you don't like hearing what I'm telling you. If you can't stand listening to what a man has to say."

Across the room, thirty-six-year-old Steven looks pale. When I ask him if he would be willing to take over the role of his grandfather, Steven shakes his head. He looks upset. Later, Steven will tell us that hearing the contempt in his "grandfather's" tone hit too close to home for him, was too much like his own tone at times, particularly now, toward his philandering father. But at that moment I speak to him, Steven does not say all that. He only shares that he is reluctant to role-play Peter, but that, if we are patient with him, he will attempt it. Steven walks slowly to where "Peter" had stood, and I watch his posture transform as he steps into the role. Steven draws himself up so that he towers over his father and, without warmup, begins screaming at him, picking up the role without missing a beat. Frank, playing himself as a boy, crouches, thoroughly uncomfortable both in and out of the role. It is an excruciating scene for all of us.

"Go on, you little sniveler," Steven, as Peter, shouts.

"How did you answer?" I ask the nine-year-old Frank.

"I didn't," Frank tells me.

"You just stood there and took it?" I say.

"Yes, for a time."

"For a time?" I ask, but Frank just looks down at the floor. He seems on the verge of tears, but desperate not to cry in front of us.

I put my hand on his shoulder. "And what would you have *liked* to have said?" I ask him.

"What do you mean?"

I direct Steven, as Peter, to start up the tirade, which he does with considerably more noise than Frank had put into it. "You think you're so smart," Steven-as-Peter was shouting, pointing his finger, his face scrunched up in disgust. "You're still wet behind the ears. You know that? Who do you think you are?"

"Look at him," I direct Frank. "Look at your father. What do you *really* want to say to him, now?"

"Fuck off," Frank offers, half joking.

"Go ahead," I urge. "Say it."

"Fuck off," Frank says meekly, barely enrolled.

"Don't you talk to me that way," springs back Steven, who is thoroughly engaged and visibly angry.

"Fuck you, Dad," Frank repeats.

"Louder," I instruct.

"Fuck you, Dad."

"Louder, Again!"

"Who do you think you are?" Steven-as-Peter approaches Frank. "You don't ever—"

"Fuck you, I said!" Frank shouts, uncoiling to meet him. "Fuck you, asshole!"

I put my hand on Frank's shoulder, supporting and restraining him. "Tell him!" I say.

"Who do I think I am?" Frank answers, "Well, who do you think you are, asshole?"

"Don't you dare—" Peter tries, but Frank shouts him down.

"Shut up, you! Shut your mouth! Shut your mouth!" Frank balls his fists, fights back tears. "Just shut your fucking mouth, do you hear me? I can't stand it, do you hear?"

Silence falls over us. It hovers, jittery and jagged. Steven steps back, but I push him into place again with my hand against his shoulder blades.

"Is that it?" I ask Frank softly. "Is that how it was?"

Across the room, Dana cries softly. Frank nods, shaken.

"Now, this is what I want you to do," I tell Frank, standing close, almost whispering in his ear. "I want you to fix it. I want you to redo this scene, only this time, bring into it whatever has to happen to heal it."

"You want me to . . ."

"I want you to make it right," I straighten up. "Take it right from the last line, 'Shut up!' " I say. This time, I ask Steven to play Frank, while Frank portrays Peter—but not Peter as he really was, Peter as he should have been, as Frank would have wished him to be.

Peter begins by apologizing to his son. "I'm sorry," he says. "I have no reason to behave this way toward you." He then begins to talk haltingly about his own pain, his guilt over James's death, his collapse into the working-class life he despises, about his feeling trapped and relentlessly judged in his marriage. Underneath the brutality, Frank-as-Peter now unleashes a flood of hurt, depression, and regret.

"Well done," I tell Frank. "Now I want you to go back to playing yourself as that boy. Come back here, crouch down again. I want you to imagine, even if just for a few minutes, what it might have felt like to have heard words like these from your father when you were a boy."

"But I never would have," he protests.

"I know that. Hear them now."

Frank leaves the role of Peter and crouches again, assuming the position of the nine-year-old boy. I ask Steven once more to role-play his grandfather. When Steven answers this time, there is no hesitation. Role-playing Peter, he bends down and lifts up Frank's face, cupping Frank's chin in his hand. "Listen to me," Steven says. "Forgive me, and let me forgive you. We can't go on living like this anymore. Full of shit and blame. It's done. It's over. Let's make the most out of what we have left."

"Say that again," I instruct Steven.

"Let's make the most out of what we have left," he says once again. He has begun to cry.

"Tell him you love him," I say, softly.

In role, Steven lifts his father into his arms. "I love you," he tells Frank. "I'm very proud of you . . . son."

Frank reaches up to Steven, who holds on tight. "I love you, too," he answers.

*   *   *

Frank Riorden carried his father's pain and guilt like an albatross around his neck. That generational transmission, coupled with his own childhood trauma, formed the core of a covert depression he managed by cutting off from his own vulnerability. This defensive maneuver cost him a capacity for true intimacy with anyone, particularly himself. Without the slightest conscious recognition, Frank constructed his life to be a negative template of his hated father's. As Peter was resigned, Frank was driven; as Peter failed, Frank succeeded; as Peter felt overwhelming guilt, Frank felt none; as Peter was trapped in an unhappy marriage, Frank never fully entered into his. The one thing both men shared was an unwillingness to deal with vulnerability and a willingness to leverage their family rather than face their own experience. Pride goeth before a fall, the proverb advises.

There is a story told by the Roman Stoic Cato about a young thief. One day, after stealing a fox, the youth was stopped and interrogated by a constable. He hid the fox under his cloak and calmly answered his interrogator's questions while the fox gnawed away his side. For both Peter and his son, invulnerability, commonly called male pride, was like the fox they hugged to themselves. Peter, spiteful of his accusing wife and compelled to "be strong" for the family, never once openly showed the remorse that surely ate away at his soul. He went to his grave without healing and without forgiveness. Frank poured his energies into being everything his father was not. And yet, in unconscious loyalty, Frank in his own marriage was no more vulnerable than Peter had been in his, and not much happier, either.

Frank Riorden began to divest himself of his father's pain and shame that afternoon in my office. In its place he attended to mending the wreckage he had made of his life. As frightening as it was—and, for the first time, he could admit that it was frightening—Frank fully committed to the marriage he had only gone through the motions of being in for thirty-eight years. He never did break down and cry or launch into the kind of deep emotional work some of the men I treat do. Nevertheless, he did manage to turn around and face the pain of a depression he had run from for most of his life. He passed through his fear and mistrust enough to sit still and rest inside his own family. The most courageous act of this shielded man was the surrender of his armor.

When a man like Frank Riorden positions himself in the world as though he were invulnerable, the trauma of his relational losses further perpetuates itself. The losses repeat like a time-released capsule, as the boy learns to reject help and comfort over and over again throughout his childhood, and, indeed, throughout his lifetime. By internalizing the value of invulnerability and the devaluation of dependency, boys like Frank learn to reject comfort and connection in an ongoing manner.

A reverse of the usual stereotype, Frank had suffered from too little mother and too much toxic father. Raised in such an abusive environment, defending against a depression he was loath to admit, Frank desperately needed comfort from somewhere. Yet he could tolerate receiving it only in situations in which he retained almost total control, as with his young women. The cultivation of a stance of invulnerability robs men of a wisdom known to most women in this culture—that people actually connect better when they expose their weakness. Linguist Deborah Tannen, analyzing women's "rapport talk" versus men's "report talk," found that a vital component of conversation between women was what she called "trouble talk"—inviting the listener in by opening up one's own points of vulnerability. Finally, to the degree to which a man learns to "be strong" and to devalue weakness, his compassion toward frailty not just in himself but also in those around him may be limited or condescending. In this and many other ways, the loss of expressivity and the loss of vulnerability inevitably lead to diminished connection with others.

Just as for many depressed women recovery is inextricably linked to shedding the traces of oppression and finding empowerment, for many depressed men, recovery is linked to opposing the force of disconnection, and reentering the world of relationship—to the "feminine," to themselves, and to others. Frank, by remembering himself as a boy and by surfacing the unfinished conversation with his ruined father, reached out in one moment to that father, to his long-dead brother, to his wife, and to his son Steven. I sometimes tell the depressed men I work with that recovery requires *dragging them back into the relational*—often kicking and screaming, initially. A man cannot recover from either overt or covert depression and remain emotionally numb at the same time; he cannot be related and walled off simultaneously; he cannot be intimate with others before establishing intimate terms with his own heart.

My work with depressed men has led me to turn the conventional thinking about sons and their fathers on its head. If we give credence to the research detailing the centrality of affection in father-son relations and the relative irrelevance of the father's "masculinity," it becomes clear that boys don't hunger for fathers who will model traditional mores of masculinity. They hunger for fathers who will rescue them from it. They need fathers who have themselves emerged from the gauntlet of their own socialization with some degree of emotional intactness. Sons don't want their father's "balls"; they want their hearts. And, for many, the heart of a father is a difficult item to come by. Oftentimes, the lost boy the depressed son must recover is the one not he but his father has disavowed.

CHAPTER SEVEN

Collateral Damage

What serveth a man if he gain the whole world and
lose his immortal soul?

—NEW TESTAMENT, MARK 8:36

The final steps in the process of molding boys are practices
that reinforce the boy's grandiosity, his male privilege, his
"better than" position. Relational impoverishment creates
the insecure base for the feelings of shame, worthlessness, emptiness that haunt many men and, at their most extreme, blossom
into overt depression. When we reinforce a boy's grandiosity, we
invite him to escape such pain by flights into addiction or the illusion of dominance.

To understand the role of grandiosity in boys' lives, we must
appreciate that in the halving process by which we create polarized
gender distinctions, each sex makes a kind of deal. And there are
costs and benefits to each side of the bargain. Traditionally, girls and
women are encouraged to maintain connection—to the emotional
parts of themselves and to others. But in order to preserve their
attachments, girls must learn to silence and subjugate themselves.
They must learn to appear, as David Halberstam bluntly stated it,
"pretty, polite, not too smart." While these traditional roles may be
in the process of changing, adolescent girls still struggle with the
conflict between performance and affiliation. If a girl is too smart
and assertive, she places in jeopardy her relationships both to boys
and to other girls who may feel competitive with her. Studies like
those of Peggy Ornstein or Lyn Brown and Carol Gilligan indicate

that mixed classrooms seem to teach young women how to defer. Boys are called on more than girls. Girls speak less in mixed groups than in all-girl settings. They interrupt less, apologize more, and use more disclaimers when they talk. These findings have led several women's educators to suggest, with some regret, that girls and young women may perform better academically in same-sex settings. Boys seem largely unaffected by switching from same-sex to mixed classrooms, leaving the impression that boys will do pretty much what they want to with whomever happens to be there. These are some of the advantages boys come to expect. Some of the benefits of the male side of the bargain.

In patriarchal cultures throughout the world, female initiation rituals reinforce women's deference to men. When women are wounded, the manner of their wounding usually plays out the theme of bondage. Rape can be seen not just as a sexual act but as an act of aggression and possession. The feet of girls in Imperial China were broken and tightly bandaged to make them appear more delicate. Genital mutilation dampens a woman's sexual appetite, rendering her safer, less threatening. Common in all of these acts is a demarcation of women as property.

Boys' initiation rites, by contrast, are not about captivity. They are about pain and the boy's capacity to bear it. A provider, hunter, warrior must be tough. What toughness requires is the capacity to separate from one's own experience; to ignore fear and pain, in the service of doing what needs be done, despite severe hardships. Boys' initiations culminate the toughening process that begins early in childhood. They frequently mock and shame the boy. The ritual wounds are often physical, sometimes sexual. Boys in the New Guinea Highlands are terrorized into performing self-inflicted nosebleeds. The boys force sharp, long grass up their nostrils, provoking copious bleeding, which is greeted with war cries from the grown men. After being taken from their mothers and publicly beaten, Sambian boys are forced to practice fellatio on the older men, who think ingested semen will make their boys strong. Tewa boys are removed from their mothers, ritually washed, and then "beaten mercilessly by the Katchinas (their fathers in disguise)." Amhara boys engage in whipping contexts in which "faces are lacerated, ears torn open, and red and bleeding welts appear. Any sign of weakness is greeted with taunts and mockery." Such traditional rites of passage, currently romanticized by some in the Men's Movement, leave many boys maimed or dead. But if the child survives, his wounds did not cripple him, as a girl's wounds do; rather, they transform him. It is the boy's capacity to detach from his own painful experience that proves him worthy of membership in the community of men. Girls' wounds keep them penned; boys' wounds exalt.

In modern culture, the pattern of the wound that transforms has moved largely from the physical realm to the psychological. Boys learn to forgo much of the emotional and relational richness that is their birthright, gaining in its place the unfettered development of public assertive action. Males enjoy the privilege of assumed superiority. The forces in our society that whisper to boys and men that they are "better than" are ubiquitous. Decades of feminist analysis has documented countless ways in which, beginning with Adam and Eve, men are held up as the standard, women as the deficient counterpart. In contemporary children's lore—the stories we tell them, the books they read, the television and movies they digest—the boy is almost always the pivotal character. Males are bigger, stronger, more daring, and more interesting. From *Star Trek* to *Sesame Street,* male characters take center stage. Women are commonly relegated to the role of damsel in distress, such as Princess Leia in *Star Wars.* The rare assertive female character, like *Sesame Street*'s Miss Piggy, is often presented ambivalently—as comic, or as an object of ridicule.

The traditional view of girls and women as dependent, emotional, unable to care for themselves, and boys and men as strong, rational, the saviors of delicate damsels is rehearsed in hundreds upon hundreds of ways, saturating the socialization of children. Boys and men are the heroes who sacrifice self, who brave danger "to serve and protect." Boys are Peter Pan rescuing Wendy from Captain Hook; they are the Nutcracker who transforms into a handsome prince and rescues Clara from the frightening Mouse

King; they are Prince Philip fighting Maleficent to save Sleeping Beauty. The theme of the powerful disconnected male proving his worth through the violent rescue of the dependent female is a drama endlessly replayed in our culture.

It is this pervasive social influence which belies our attempts to raise our children differently than we were. Many, myself included, have made great efforts to keep their sons and daughters out of the traditional mold. Many encourage their sons to cry when they are upset, encourage their daughters to climb trees. But signs of boys' superiority still permeate our childrens' lives; images of the traditional roles are everywhere. Even if we do not allow our boys to watch *The Mighty Morphin' Power Rangers* or play with GI Joe, are we really going to forbid the male rescue dramas, *Peter Pan, Sleeping Beauty, The Nutcracker?* Will they never hear of Robin Hood saving Maid Marion or of Lancelot's great feats for Guinevere? How much of Western civilization should we be willing to lop off for the sake of political correctness? And while there may be a particular, rather rarefied segment of the population that carefully screens the effects of such cultural influences on their daughters and sons, the majority of parents do not.

Statistically, the average American child watches twenty-eight hours of television a week, not counting rented movies or video games. Some evidence suggests that in working-class and poor families that number may be as much as double. By the time a boy is eighteen he has watched on average *twenty-six thousand* television murders, almost all of them committed by men. Some of them are bad men who kill for bad reasons; many are good men who kill off the bad. Over 235 studies on the relationship between television and violence have been conducted, spawning close to 3,000 articles and books, including reports from the National Institute of Mental Health and the Office of the Surgeon General. There is a wide-ranging consensus that watching television violence increases aggressive behavior, that much of the material in television programming is sexually stereotyped in the extreme, and that such stereotyping directly influences the attitudes and beliefs of the children who watch. An NIMH report found that 70 percent of the references to sex on television referred to either extramarital affairs or to prostitution. Men were rarely shown as interested in their families, and sex was commonly linked to violence. In 1980, psychologist Leon Efron reported the results of a longitudinal study he began in rural New York state in the late 1950s. In following 875 eight-year-old children, Efron found that "the single best predictor of how aggressive a young man would be when he was 19 years old was the violence of the television programs he preferred when he was 8 years old." While some may argue that the traditional roles affecting our sons may be changing, they are clearly not changing in television programming.

Educators Diane Levin and Nancy Carlsson-Paige voice specific concerns about the contrast between children's developmental needs and what they learn by watching television. They characterize the portrait of the world conveyed through kids' television as often frightening, and dominated by both gender and ethnic stereotyping. Problem solving is rarely demonstrated; community and diversity are practically nonexistent, and right prevails through might. They point out that young children should be shown a world in which individuals can act autonomously while still maintaining connection, in which they can be both relational and assertive. But on current programs

> The themes of separation and connection are presented to children as mutually exclusive. Autonomy is commonly equated with violence and hurt toward others and connection with helplessness and victimization. To be separate usually means to be male, strong, powerful, armed with weapons, unfeeling, and able to care for oneself. To be connected usually means to be female, weak, dependent, and constantly in need of rescue.

Adults may enjoy the sophisticated charm of plays against the masculine role like a pregnant Arnold Schwarzenegger in the film *Junior,* or "drag comedies" like *Tootsie* or *Mrs. Doubtfire,* but our children are still being saturated with the most extreme forms of traditional sex stereotyping. Girls relate—often to their own detriment. Boys rescue and fight—equally, though less obviously, to theirs.

These circumstances bring to mind a distinction first made by trauma expert Pia Mellody, which I have found helpful in work with depressed men—the distinction between *disempowering abuse* and *falsely empowering abuse. Disempowering abuse* is the kind of abuse one normally thinks of. It is characterized by a major caregiver shaming a child, placing him in a one-down, less-than, or helpless position. *False empowerment,* by contrast, lifts the child up to an inordinately powerful position, pumping up, or at the least not appropriately checking, the child's grandiosity. Mellody's insight is that both styles of inappropriate parenting lead to disorders of self-esteem. Disempowering abuse shames the child setting the stage for victimization later in life. False empowerment instills grandiosity in the child and sets the adult up to become offensive. The first is a disorder of too much shame, the second a disorder of too little. Disempowering abuse leads to overt depression, falsely empowering abuse leads to covert depression.

When girls and women in our society are injured, they tend to be subject to disempowering abuse; they are silenced, shamed, made to feel defective. A formulaic analysis might conclude that boys, by contrast, are predominantly subject to false empowerment, but the reality is not quite so simple. Perhaps the single most important discovery that has come from my work with men and their families is the realization that most boys and men have been subject to a preponderance of neither disempowering nor falsely empowering abuse, but to *alternations between the two.* This sudden switch from "one down" to "one up" and back again leaves boys and men in a perpetual state of anxiety about their status. No matter how "up" a man may be today, there is always tomorrow. There is always someone younger, faster, smarter crowding the wings. We raise boys to live in a world in which they are either winners or losers, grandiose or shame filled, or, in the most extreme cases, such as life in some prisons or combat situations, either perpetrators or victims, the rapist or the raped. "I'd rather be a hammer than a nail," Paul Simon sings. There isn't a man I have met who doesn't understand the chilling implications of that sentiment. If healthy self-esteem is the experience of oneself as essentially worth neither more nor less than others, there is precious little training for it in the current culture of boys.

If boys have any difficulty picking up the message about hierarchy and dominance at home or in the media, there is little subtlety about it in the gymnasium or on the athletic field. Sports are enormously important in the lives of most boys, both the sports in which they themselves participate and the sports heroes whom they adore from afar. Although competitive sports have many obvious benefits, there are few activities that inculcate boys with the mores and values of traditional masculinity as powerfully. For a great many boys, what begins as fun quickly becomes a high-stakes endeavor. As baseball legend Vince Lombardi once quipped, "Winning isn't everything; it's the *only* thing."

The sports arena is one of the last clear bastions of traditional masculine heroics left in our culture. The basketball court and hockey rink have replaced the tournament and jousting pavilions of yore. We still tend to link athletic prowess with moral goodness. The Larry Birds and Michael Jordans of our world stand in as modern-day Lancelots and Odysseuses. In the medieval *Song of Roland*, a prototypical account of knightly heroics, young Roland confronts a dreaded opponent in combat, takes a moment to pray that God will grant him strength, and, "*being virtuous and valorous,*" raises his sword and not only beats the enemy knight, but in one mighty stroke cleaves the man, his saddle, and his horse in two. Roland, like every medieval hero, did not prevail based on physical strength—no amount of human muscle could have accomplished such a feat. Rippling through Roland's arm was the power of *valor,* a word connoting both bravery and worth. In the medieval worlds, where outward occurrences were always imbued with spiritual significance, what a man could *do* was inextricably mixed to his inner being. Roland was strong because God was with him. When Lancelot vanquished all foes, it was as much a testament to his *courtesy,* his chivalry, his love for Guinevere, as it was a sign of his outward prowess. Hero tales from the *Aeneid* to *Star Wars* are filled with cautionary figures, like Faust, or like Darth Vader, who have placed their innate gifts into the service of unworthy masters. These are the fallen angels. The hero, by contrast, is both inherently strong and also imbued with force from above by virtue of his discipline and fidelity to principle. As Joseph Campbell reminds us, these heroes' feats, full of rectitude, are not performed for their individual glory, but almost always in the service of their community. Traditionally, heroes are righters of wrongs, defenders of the realm, knights of the Round Table, adventurers for the glory of the Paideia.

In modern culture, heroism has been stripped of virtually all of its spiritual significance. Removed from morality as well as from human community, heroism in our society has become a secular, individual achievement. Most often, it simply means winning big, whether on the baseball diamond or in the stock exchange. In the same way that we used to speak of a man's *valor,* meaning both his worth and his bravery, we now speak of his *value,* meaning both his worth and the weight of his assets. We now celebrate corporate raiders, not buccaneers. But the old stirrings still speak to us, no matter how degraded their form. Both in our own lives and in the spectacles around us, we still search for higher meaning in achievement. We still equate performance with virtue.

The ideology of sports for boys contains the promise of enhanced self-esteem, of valorous deeds and increased value. Organized competitive sports and deliberate forms of masculinization like the Boy Scouts and the armed services are supposed to "build boys up," both physically and psychologically. Unfortunately, most of the evidence points to the opposite effect. While there may be lip service paid to good teamwork, both in the media and the sports boys play at school, most of the attention is given to the few star performers. As a number of sociologists have pointed out, a tremendous discrepancy exists between the experience of those few extraordinary boys and that of the vast majority of young players. Despite dreams of glory, a boy's chances to make the big leagues are minuscule. The statistical chance, for example, of a boy's growing up to become a professional football player is estimated at one in twelve thousand, about on a par with winning a state lottery. Sociologist Michael Messner sums up the research: "The disjuncture between the ideology of success and the socially structured reality that most do not 'succeed' brings about widespread feelings of failure, lowered self-images, and problems with interpersonal relationships." Young athletes who "fail" often blame themselves, and some sociologists have argued that such problems in self-esteem are particularly damaging to young black athletes, who are "disproportionately channeled into sports and yet have no safety net" to catch them when they fall.

And what about those who win? Our conventional imagery would figure them as young heroes, Rolands in the height of their glory. But does that match up with boys' actual experiences? Contrast that idealized description with the real voice of Michael Oriard, who played for Notre Dame:

> On play after play I rammed my shoulders and forearm into the . . . headgear of the man trying to block me. I wanted him to feel an ache that night at ten o'clock and think, "That sonuvabitch Oriard." . . . I wanted to physically dominate . . . to feel contempt for their inability, and the satisfaction in knowing I was tougher than they were.

The golden sunlight drenching these young heroes is too often the light of naked dominance. And the cost they must pay for their glory is high. Just how tough does one have to be? Football star Dave Meggyesy answered the claim that athletics "builds boys" in the following way:

> Young men are having their bodies destroyed, not developed. As a matter of fact, few players can escape from college football without some form of permanent disability. During my four years I accumulated a broken wrist, separations of both shoulders, an ankle

that was torn up so badly that it broke the arch of my foot, three major brain concussions, and an arm that almost had to be amputated. . . . And I was one of the lucky ones.

A recent survey reveals that 78 percent of professional football players retire with permanent disabilities, and their average life expectancy is only fifty-six years. There are sports less physically damaging than football, certainly, but there are also sports that do even more harm, like boxing, the most unalloyed form of aggression as entertainment. An estimated 60 to 87 percent of boxers retire with chronic brain damage, an effect alarming enough to convince the American Medical Association to demand that the sport be abolished. Such are the means by which we seek to improve our sons' self-esteem.

Organized competitive sports as we know them today grew in the first few decades of the twentieth century, at a time when men were siphoned away from the family farms to work in the growing industrial centers, a time when the new women's movement questioned and threatened traditional roles. The advent of organized sports for boys parallels the growth of Boy Scouts of America and carried much the same avowed ideology. Sports, like scouting, were conceived of as places where boys could fall under the beneficial influence of men, removed from feminine rule. One wonders what the early architects of organized sports almost a century ago would think today as they listened to Dave Meggyesy's recitation of damaged body parts.

The lesson many young athletes learn is just a different incarnation of the lesson Frank Riorden learned, the lesson most boys learn in our culture—turn your back on your own needs and vulnerabilities and you become special. Refuse to shoulder that burden and you are less than a man.

In *Death of a Salesman*, Willy Loman drives home the connection between specialness and success again and again. In his disordered mind, he speaks to Biff, his athletic son, and an imaginary friend:

> Without a penny to his name, three great Universities are begging for him, and from there the sky's the limit, because it's not what you

do, Ben. It's who you know and the smile on your face! It's contacts, Ben, contacts! (*To Biff*) And that's why when you get out into that field today it's important. Because thousands of people will be watching you and loving you . . . And, Ben! when he walks into a business office his name will sound out like a bell and all the doors will open for him! I've seen it, Ben, I've seen it a thousand times!

The almost biblical hyperbole with which Loman stuffs his sons does not help them in the real world. Biff is a kleptomaniac. His younger brother, Happy, is a womanizer. Both have made nothing of their lives. Happy, a lowly store clerk, complains: "Sometimes I want to just rip my clothes off in the middle of the store and outbox that goddam merchandise manager. I mean I can outbox, outrun, and out-lift anybody in that store, and I have to take orders from those common, petty sons-of-bitches till I can't stand it anymore." With such an attitude, it is a small wonder why he is not getting ahead. Bulging with innappropriate false empowerment, Happy tries to drown the pain of his hidden shame in the exercise of sexual prowess. But it doesn't really solve his problem. He tells his brother: "I get [beautiful women] anytime I want, Biff. Whenever I feel disgusted. The only trouble is, it gets to be like bowling or something. I keep knocking them over and it doesn't mean anything."

Such are the rewards of false empowerment, when playing means winning and winning means dominating, when sex becomes "knocking them over," and other people become "common, petty sons-of-bitches." Glory, perhaps, for a moment. But warmth, richness, humanity? Not much. Nevertheless, if winning is lonely, losing is worse.

To fail in the agenda of grandiosity, of achieving specialness through dominance, is to lose one's masculinity and pronounce oneself that most hated thing—a sissy, a "wuss" (a word that combines "wimp" and "pussy"), a girl. Those who seek to push boys out of the affiliative, vulnerable mode often use the threat of such gender ridicule. Sociologist Gary Fine reports that in Little League, boys and coaches freely used expressions like "he's so gay," or "girl," or "wuss." When displeased with a particular student's performance, Indiana University coach Bobby Knight was known to put a box of sanitary napkins in the boy's locker as a way of letting the student and those around him know what the coach thought of the player's masculinity. It is almost impossible to imagine a woman coach treating a girl in a similar fashion, but all too easy to imagine such behavior between an admired role model and a vulnerable boy. Athlete Dave Meggyesy writes: "this sort of attack on a player's manhood is a coach's doomsday weapon. And it almost always works, for the players have wrapped up their identity in their masculinity, which is eternally precarious for it not only depends upon not exhibiting fear of any kind on the playing field, but it is also something that can be given or withdrawn by a coach at his pleasure."

Once we realize that the elusive "masculine identity" does not exist inside the boy's psyche, but rather that it is a social construct to which the boy must bend and comply, we can understand why it is impossible for most boys to feel secure about it. Being "man enough" isn't something one has definitively once and for all. It is something one is granted by the community of men whom we experience as watching, weighing, and judging. To "become" a man—an act that is supposed to be quintessentially independent—in fact means that a male reference group consents to call one a man. The construction of manhood turns out to be as social as a sewing circle. Masculinity, unlike femininity, is conferred. And since it is bestowed, it can also be taken away. That is why a mentoring figure like a coach can carry such authority for a boy.

For many boys, a favored coach is a surrogate parent and a figure of enormous moral importance. To the thirteen-, fourteen-, and fifteen-year-old boys at Camden Junior High, Coach Nevins was a luminous being. Beautifully built, funny, and smart, he talked to us as if we were already men. He cursed, spat, laid down the law, and broke a few rules when he wanted to. I remember how good it felt just to be with him, just to bask in his presence.

My classmate Eddie was as uncool as Coach Nevins was cool.

Stiff-jointed, dull, with acne all over his face and a bizarre penchant for reciting the numbers of buses on various bus lines, Eddie was not normal. In hindsight, I realize that Eddie was probably autistic, but no one thought in those terms back then. Coach Nevins hated Eddie. Eddie, who was always the last in line. Eddie, off dreaming instead of "falling in." Eddie, hanging comically from the ropes we all climbed. Afraid. Screaming. Unable to get down.

"Eddie, here, boy. Here's the planet Earth!" One day Coach Nevins hurled a huge medicine ball at Eddie's head while we watched, twenty or so of us, an entire class. Only this time an extraordinary thing happened. Instead of crashing down in a jumble, Eddie's arms instinctively reached up to snatch the heavy ball. He hurled it, twice as hard, smack into Coach Nevins's chest, winding him. Without pausing for a single word, the coach took three quick strides across the gym and punched Eddie hard in the gut.

We watched Eddie crumple, gasping. His body folded to the floor, where he rested his head, as if on a pillow, and cried. Instinctively, three or four of us stepped forward, angry. But Coach Nevins reeled on us. "Fuck around with that pansy and you fuck with me." We froze; Eddie panted. A long moment passed. We could hear a game of basketball on the far side of the partitioned gym, the solid resonance of the ball as it thudded, the spring of the backboard. Then Coach Nevins flashed his resplendent smile. He put his arms around Eddie, lifted him up, whispered to him, joked with him. We saw Eddie laugh, still shaky. Coach told us to get into our coats and run together, blocks at a time, an arduous exercise. Coach Nevins and Eddie ran side by side the whole while, talking and smiling. The coach's camaraderie was like soft, sticky cotton muffling our minds, sending a message to us and to Eddie himself that what had happened was nothing. This was how things were done between men. Only "a pansy" would take it to heart.

I remember running a long time as the autumn afternoon grew dark. I remember the cold on my face and hands. Like a lot of the boys, I imagine, although we didn't talk about it, I wanted to go to

Eddie and comfort him. I wanted to tell him not to be bought off so easily with a smile and a stupid joke or two. But I couldn't bring myself to do it. I was too afraid of being tainted by association with him. And I was confused by Coach Nevins, too lulled and charmed to act. Even though I felt bad for Eddie, I had already learned to despise him, despise his pimples and his ugliness, his weakness so close to those parts of myself that I had grown wise enough to conceal.

As a thirteen-year-old, my choice seemed either to join Coach Nevins and the rest of the boys in dominance or risk the ostracism of becoming like Eddie myself. I experienced myself as already having one foot in the hole Eddie lived in. I did not feel secure enough within the class to do what my heart commanded me. I realize now, at forty-four, that at that moment, probably every other boy in the class had feelings akin to my own. The need to save one's own insecure place in the circle of manhood by participating in oppression, or at the least in remaining silent, while the weak fail is one of the principal dilemmas for boys. Fear of losing membership in the clan of winners often costs boys their capacity for compassion. "Do it to her or we'll do it to you," threatens the sergeant, only a teen himself, to Private Ericksson, in the film *Casualties of War.* In his account of surviving Aucshwitz, Elie Wiesel remembers a moment when he witnessed a guard beating his beloved father with an iron bar. With great shame, Wiesel confesses that he was not angry at the guard, but at his own father for not being smart enough to have avoided it. "That," writes Wiesel, "was what concentration camp life had done to me."

While we both had our share of ill treatment, between my brother and me, I became more the active "troublemaker" in our family and my brother would grow furious with me for running afoul of Dad. Why couldn't I keep my head down and my mouth shut as he'd learned to do? At the time I hated him for betraying me. If he didn't stand up for me, then at least he could show enough grace to not take Dad's side. "Do it to him or we'll do it to you." I now believe such choices are an ineluctable part of boyhood. And the "Sophie's choice" of hammer or nail, victimizer or victim is not relegated to extreme instances. It is an inescapable part of the game we call "success." Boys learn that the game requires fierce loyalty to those on the inside of the circle. But the outsiders, those judged weak or lacking, one must be willing to betray. Most boys learn the precise nature and extent of the cruelty leveled against deviants, because they themselves experience both sides. They learn to betray the humanity in others—the fat boys, the effeminate boys, the Eddies of this world—as a way of protecting themselves, and in so doing they also learn to disconnect from their own compassionate hearts. This is the most fundamental damage of false empowerment.

In *1984*, George Orwell brilliantly analyzed the intentions and tactics of the totalitarian mind. The novel reads like a morality play between the forces of connection, as represented by the illegal lovers, Julia and Winston, and the state that tries to "break" them. After standing up to the most extraordinary pressure, intimidation, and torture, the protagonist does finally collapse. His torturers ferret out his deepest childhood fear—rats. They construct a cage in which hungry rats will be clamped onto his face. Finally, terrorized beyond all reason, Winston Smith screams out, "Don't do it to me. Do it to *her*. Do it to *her*." His captors remove the threat. They know they have won. Smith's will, his integrity has been broken. *Integrity* is an interesting word in this context. It means acting with principle and it also means wholeness, intactness. By forcing him to betray his human attachment, to disconnect from his lover, Smith's interrogators produced the intended result of a profound disconnection inside himself.

The paradox of the grandiose position is that it solidifies the very relational disconnections whose pain it seeks to soothe. Willy Loman's son Happy desperately needs to become competent in the world and to find intimacy. Instead, like Frank Riorden, he medicates his pain, not with the demands of a real relationship but with the grandiosity of sexual conquest. Such measures fail because they do not address the real hunger. In fact, by reaching for prowess instead of connection, Happy objectifies those who might provide solace and only succeeds in further isolating himself. How much nurture can one get from a bowling pin? Striving for specialness and objectifying others are processes that are intrinsically linked.

John McMurty, former Canadian football player, writes of the contrast between the ideology and the reality of sportsmanship: "the truly professional attitude is not to think of the opponent as a human being at all—he is a 'position' to be removed as efficiently as possible in order to benefit the team's corporate enterprise of gaining points." Michael Oriard states, "I could not have continued to maul someone I had come to *know*—even if only a little. But I did not know them." Nor could Oriard afford to know them. If he had, he would have lost the benefit of the powerful drug, grandiose dominance. He writes: "I loved to dominate my opponents physically in a public arena. Such dominance was a salve for the many wounds my adolescent ego received during my high school years." That misguided adolescent had no means of understanding that many of the wounds to his ego that he sought to salve sprang from the very disconnection from self and others that his dominance reinforced. In the same way that grandiosity demands a disconnection from the humanity of "the opponent," it requires a disconnection from one's own. Trauma pioneer Robert J. Lifton has called this process of self-alienation "doubling," the compartmentalization of self. Doubling is a psychological mechanism for denying or distorting reality, which is shared by both the perpetrator and his victim. When my father was carried away by his rage, both he and I dropped into different variations of trance. My father moved into the intoxication of dominance while I split off from my own body, hovering above the scene.

When boys are taught to objectify themselves and others, they learn to turn themselves into a kind of commodity to be weighed and judged, as they weigh and judge those around them. The ultimate expression of this capacity to turn humans, including oneself, into things is war. In *The Things They Carried*, writer Tim O'Brien remembers this process in Vietnam:

> It's easier to cope with a kicked bucket than a corpse; if it isn't human, it doesn't matter much if it's dead. And so a VC nurse, fried by napalm, was a crispy critter. A Vietnamese baby, which lay

nearby, was a roasted peanut. "Just a crunchie munchie," Rat Kiley said as he stepped over the body.

Just as foot soldiers turn the foreign enemy and civilians alike into objects, they themselves have been objectified by the men who dispatched them. Ron Kovac, Vietnam vet, paraplegic, author of *Born on the Fourth of July*, writes of himself, fittingly, in the third person:

> He had never been anything but a thing to them, a thing to put a uniform on and train to kill. . . . They were smooth talkers, men who wore suits and smiled and were polite, men who wore watches and sat behind desks sticking pins in maps. . . . They had never seen blood and guts and heads and arms. They had never picked up the shattered legs of children and watched the blood drip.

If we are to come to grips with the extent and the power of the pressures brought to bear on our sons, we must understand that masculine socialization, throughout history and in almost all cultures throughout the world, is inextricably bound up with war. The process of "masculinization" is one potent enough to take my sweet son Alexander, who loves makeup and dresses, whose favorite identity is a magic fairy, and deliver him, a decade or so later, into a state in which he will be prepared to kill and be killed. In *Boys Will Be Boys*, philosopher Myriam Miedzian summarizes:

> Boys are raised to be soldiers. They are prepared from the youngest age to view war as a thrilling adventure. Their play with war toys is great fun without pain. The books they read (and today the TV shows and films they see) focus on exciting violence. In schools all over the world, little boys learn that their country is the greatest in the world, and the highest honor that could befall them would be to defend it heroically someday. *The fact that empathy has traditionally been conditioned out of boys facilitates their obedience to leaders who order them to kill strangers.*

It is also the "conditioning out of empathy" that allows the leaders to send in the boys to begin with, cloaking the reality of war with metaphors like "necessary losses" and "collateral damage."

The tragic bind for boys and men in traditional socialization is that in order to demonstrate themselves worthy of human connection they must perform competitively, they must become winners, which intrinsically demands disconnection, the exact opposite of what they truly seek. How do you connect to someone by beating him? Is it likely that a young athlete like Michael Oriard, who reports growing to love publicly dominating others, enjoyed rich, nourishing forms of interpersonal intimacy? I think it a safe bet that he was a confused, lonely boy who felt at his best in those rare moments of approved violence played out before an adoring crowd. As Oriard himself grew to realize, this state of affairs was not heroic; it was grotesque. He was, himself, his own collateral damage.

Twenty-year-old Jason reported in therapy a small triumph he had enjoyed earlier that morning. Jason was cycling on a deserted road when he spotted another cyclist coming up behind him. This second cyclist was dressed in a fancy outfit with an enormously expensive bike. "But," Jason told me, "I put a little weight into it and totally blew him away." A look of sadness crossed over my face and Jason asked about it.

"It really is typical of the way you can sometimes relate," I told him. "Instead of 'blowing him away,' you might have found out who he was. You might have cultivated a partner for your workouts. Do you know what you were attempting to say when you left him in the dust like that?" I asked. "I think you meant to say, 'Hello.' I think grinding him into the dirt was your way of saying, 'Hi.'"

Jason told me later that this confrontation was the most important moment in our work together. Groomed in a fairly mean family, he was taught to introduce himself by metaphorically clipping someone in the jaw.

Trying to connect by going "one up" on someone seems an odd strategy. Yet this is exactly what men are doing when they joke and jostle for position at social gatherings. A woman friend of mine calls it "antlering behavior," like stags butting heads in good fun. Sometimes it works. Sometimes Robin Hood can meet Little John on the bridge, have a glorious fight, get trashed, and both jump up to become great pals. Here and there, I suppose, there are hearty Lawrencian wrestlers flinging each other around before roaring fires. But more often the reality between men is edged and unpleasant. We have grown accustomed to think of all this jockeying as being principally about power. But I believe that, underneath, it is really an attempt at connection. In the hierarchical world of boys and men, some degree of power is a necessary security; it ensures against the dread of either subordination or abandonment. Being one up means that you won't wind up as an Eddie. But power is not the driving force here; belonging is.

The problem for many boys and men lies in the paradox that one must dominate in order to belong. First you slay the dragon, or the other boy. Only then do you win the princess. First the male must renounce the emotive, affiliative mode. Only after the tournament has been won does he return to the relational wealth he himself turned his back on. Psychiatrist Steve Bergman calls this pattern the "Hi, Mom," syndrome, a name that came to him one day when he had seen a third young male Olympic winner wave to the camera and mouth, "Hi, Mom!" triumphantly. Why doesn't anyone say, "Hi, Dad!" Bergman wondered. It is because the connection to Dad had not been renounced to begin with and therefore it did not need to be won back.

This tripartite cycle—the boy's renunciation of mother and home, the challenging ordeal and the triumphant return—is such a pervasive design throughout our history that mythologist Joseph Campbell called it the "Ur Myth"—the prototype for all myths, the "Hero with a Thousand Masks." There are endless examples of this pattern. Moses, separated from his real mother, is found in a basket, only to become united with God. Orpheus descends to Hades and wins back Eurydice. Odysseus wanders and returns to Penelope. Dante plunges to the depths of hell to find Beatrice. All these men leave mother and home, succeed in perilous adventure, and then reunite with abundance and femininity in glory.

Each boy, like Faust, makes a deal with the devil gaining worlds of knowledge and power—the capacity to *do*—in exchange for his very (relational) soul. The boy's position in this culture is like that of the "special" child in disordered families. "Special" children function as extensions of self, for one or both parents. They find themselves in an ambiguous position. On the one hand, since they are entrusted with the psychological equilibrium of the parent, and since they become caretakers to their own caretakers, they enjoy inordinate power within the family. But that inordinate power is based, as for Faust, on forfeiting the most precious part of them, their souls, their deepest vulnerabilities and needs.

I call such a trade-off "conditional grandiosity." It lies at the core of the male experience. Boys and men are granted privilege and special status, but only on the condition that they turn their backs on vulnerability and connection to join in the fray. Those who resist, like unconventional men or gay men, are punished for it. Those who lose or who cannot compete, like boys and men with disabilities, or of the wrong class or color, are marginalized, rendered all but invisible. Having abandoned real affiliation, the stakes for boys and men are very high. An entrepreneur in my practice told me once that there is a phrase for a "player" whose fortunes have fallen. They say of such a one that he has "gone over the side without a ripple." The exclusion, isolation, of a failed winner is so great, it as if he had never existed at all.

Oppressed women sometimes find it difficult to grasp why privileged men feel so pressured. But boys and men live each day with a kind of fear that can only rarely be assuaged. Strait is the gate and narrow is the path. One false step and it's a long drop down. If a man is not a winner, he is a loser. And the cost of losing is more than just the game at hand; it is abandonment. A *New Yorker* cartoon shows a boss, flanked by underlings and sitting behind a large desk on some frozen embankment. Facing him stands a modern everyman in a business suit, with briefcase and hat. The hero stands facing the shore on a small chunk of ice that is drifting away, receding out toward the icy sea. As he's cut adrift on his little ice floe, the caption reads, "We're sorry to have to tell you this, Bob."

Since connection is experienced as conditional, since he must prove himself worthy of love, if a man does not succeed, he risks an abandonment he may feel he deserves. The bind is that in order to succeed, it is often at the cost of neglecting much of who he is and his relationship to those around him. In an increasingly materialistic world, winning, for men, means making money. The bumper sticker trumpets: HE WHO DIES WITH THE MOST TOYS WINS. Another *New Yorker* cartoon shows two well-heeled middle-aged men at a plush bar, where one confides to the other, "Money is life's report card." Trailing throughout Willy Loman's remembrances and dementia is the ghostly figure of Ben, who "went into the jungle empty-handed and emerged a year later a wealthy man." Loman feverishly asks the apparition, "What's the secret, Ben? Tell me, how is it done?" How does one make money, Loman wants to know, but underneath that, how does one gain recognition, how does one become the hammer instead of the nail? How does one get into the club? Traditional masculinity rests on such an insecure foundation of wonder, smugness, or dread, depending on one's position on the ladder. It instills in our sons not healthy but *performance-based esteem.*

Healthy self-esteem is an inherent, nonfluctuating sense of oneself as essentially worthwhile. Shame states, or failures in self-esteem, are experienced as a sense of not being enough and not mattering, as emptiness, fear, or impotence. This is why oppression is intrinsically shaming. A shame state can be triggered in anyone who is sufficiently disempowered. The discomfort of the shame state sets the stage for overt depression and is defended against by intoxication and grandiosity in covert depression. Shame hounds boys and men throughout most of their lives for two reasons. First, since the standard of masculinity against which most boys and men measure themselves is unrealistically narrow and perfectionist, virtually no one feels he sufficiently measures up. Second, since masculinity is conferred more than won, since it represents membership, not a state of being, it is always in danger of being revoked. One can always "go over the side without a ripple."

Healthy self-esteem is the capacity—rarely taught to either sex in our culture—to hold oneself in warm regard even when colliding with one's human shortcomings. Our capacity to stay rooted in a compassionate understanding of one another's flaws keeps us humane. When we lose touch with our own frailties we become judgmental and dangerous to others. Psychoanalysts and developmental psychologists have been clear that the capacity to esteem the self arises from a history of unconditional regard from one's caregivers. Our capacity to esteem the self is an internalization of, in one famous description, "the gleam in the mother's eye," as she gazes upon her child. But do we, in fact, offer our boys such unconditional regard? Perhaps we might as individual parents or teachers, but we most emphatically do not as a society. What we offer boys in our culture is highly conditional, performance-based esteem, not an essential sense of worth that comes from within. One cannot *earn* healthy self-esteem. One has it. Performance-based esteem augments an insufficient, internal sense of worth by the measuring of one's accomplishments against those of others and coming out on top. As a new acquaintance introduces himself to me at a function in our children's school, I note very quickly that he is younger and more fit-looking than I am. I wonder how much money he has, and whether he has earned it or has had it handed to him. Almost simultaneously, I note, however, that I am wittier, and warmer. I'm probably a more compassionate person. And so we weigh one another, sizing each other up, until the voice of maturity reminds me to stop such nonsense.

There is nothing wrong with a nuanced assessment of one's own or another's talents, limitations, gifts, and difficulties. Such discrimination becomes unhealthy when it puts one's own or another person's essential worth on the line. Mature people do not question their intrinsic value at a working lunch or a PTA meeting. But most men do, whether they want to admit it or not. Most men are not far behind Colonel Catcart in Joseph Heller's *Catch-22*, who carried with him a little notebook in which he noted that day's events in two separate rows. One column was headed "Feathers in my Cap," the other was headed "Black Eyes." At the end of each day, Colonel Catcart would tally up the reflection of his experience and give himself a report on his status as a human being.

One of the reasons, I believe, for the popularity of the film *Forrest Gump* is that the main character, by dint of his low IQ, does not judge himself or others by performance. The audience experiences his "innocence," his gift for acceptance, as warm and refreshing. A variation on the same theme is found in the film *Regarding Henry.* Harrison Ford, a quintessential "type A" personality, steps off the fast track after a bullet in the head causes brain damage. The film makes it clear that he is a better, if slower, person for it. Brain damage may represent a radical cure for unhealthy forms of masculinity, but one hopes less extreme measures may lead to change as well. In fact, sociologists have long noted that men spontaneously seem to become more "androgynous" when they hit middle and retirement age. Circumstances like disability or retirement can relieve some men of the burden of performance, allowing relational capacities and concerns to surface. The cultivation of these yearnings and skills need not have been discouraged to begin with, but, unfortunately, the lack of their full expression and development is a central part of most boys' lives in this culture no matter how "gender sensitive" or "nonsexist" their parents may be. Short of removing them as young Perceval's mother tried to do, to some remote grotto where there are no television, superheroes, Nintendo, or peers, our sons are bombarded with news about their role's requirements and privileges each and every day.

Performance-based esteem is the foundation for elevating intoxication, reliance on those substances or acts that give one a sense of dominion and grandiose power. It is a short step from Michael Oriard's thirst for public domination as a "salve" for his adolescent wounds to the dynamics of battering or other forms of dominance. And studies have shown a high correlation between athleticism in high school–and college-aged men and increased rates of "date rape," violence, and the destruction of property.

It is a rare man, however, a man who is truly on the extreme of Narcissistic disturbance, who performs solely for his own self-aggrandizement. The great majority of men feel at least as much burdened as enhanced by the need to perform. What motivates

them is not principally privilege and domination so much as love—
"coming through" in the eyes of one's boss, one's colleagues, one's
wife. "A well-liked man is a successful man," Willy Loman
instructs his boys over and over again. Loman tells Biff to win the
big game because "a thousand people will be rooting for you and
loving you." My work with men and their families has convinced
me that boys and men are fundamentally just as relational as girls
and women. They have been taught to turn their backs on many of
their relational needs and instead have been stuffed with the privilege of insensitivity. But there is nothing intrinsically "hardwired"
about it. Research indicates that when men are placed in empathy-
demanding situations, as single, custodial parents or caretakers of
the ill or the elderly, they are readily capable of becoming just as
nurturant and empathic as female counterparts. The human emotional palette is vast. It isn't that men have fewer relational needs
than women, but that they have been conditioned to filter those
needs through the screen of achievement.

But attempting to secure connection through performance is a
high-risk endeavor. In the competitive marketplace a man can be
digested and then thrown away. As Willy Loman learns all too
painfully, in *Death of a Salesman,* even if one succeeds, there are no
guarantees for the future. At Willy's funeral a friend defines him as
simply "a salesman," a man, "way out there in the blue, riding on a
smile and a shoeshine. And when they start not smiling back, that's
an earthquake. And then you get yourself a couple of spots on your
hat you're finished."

In the play's climactic scene, Loman's son Biff tries desperately
to resign from performance-based esteem, and make his father recognize how toxic the agenda of specialness has been.

> BIFF: I am not a leader of men, Willy, and neither are you. You
> were never anything but a hard working drummer who landed in
> the ash can like all the rest of them! I'm one dollar an hour, Willy! I
> tried seven states and couldn't raise it. A buck an hour! Do you
> gather my meaning? I'm not bringing home any prizes any more,
> and you're going to stop waiting for me to bring them home!

WILLY: You vengeful, spiteful mutt!

BIFF, *at the peak of his fury:* Pop, I'm nothing! I'm nothing, Pop. Can't you understand that? There's no spite in it anymore. I'm just what I am, that's all.

Biff's fury has spent itself and he breaks down, sobbing, holding on to Willy, who dumbly fumbles for Biff's face.

WILLY, *astonished:* What're you doing? What're you doing? *To Linda:* Why is he crying?

BIFF, *crying, broken:* Will you let me go, for Christ's sake? Will you take that phony dream and burn it before something happens?

The figure of Willy Loman is an American icon of overt male depression. His two sons, Happy and Biff, are spoon-fed a legacy of false empowerment and tacit shame that pushes both toward covert depression. At the play's end, Biff steps off the track of performance esteem and grandiosity and frees himself. Biff's younger brother, Happy, has learned nothing.

"Willy Loman did not die in vain," Happy tells Biff. "He had a good dream. It's the only dream you can have—to come out number one man. He fought it out here and this is where I'm going to win it for him." Biff looks at his brother with pity and leads their stricken mother away.

The Loman family was caught in a lethal encounter with the masculine dream. Willy gives up his very life to land insurance money in his son's pocket, saying, "That boy will be magnificent!" He never once understands that his son, like all children, has been magnificent all along. Performance-based esteem claims the life of one family member and severely damages the others.

In the film *Searching for Bobby Fischer,* based on the true story of Josh Waitzkin, the highest-ranking U.S. chess player under eighteen, a father wrestles with many of the same issues that defeated Willy Loman. This man, however, awakens from the dream.

Nine-year-old Josh, an ordinary boy in most respects, is a true child prodigy in chess. Through the camera's eye, we watch him watch the Afro-American men banter as they play in the park. We watch him take in the pieces and how they move for the first time. A few days later, we experience the thrill as he offhandedly demolishes his father by calling down moves from upstairs in his room while he plays with his toys, without even bothering to look at the board. Within this sweet, lovable little boy we encounter a force of genius, unexplainable, miraculous. In a world that values performance, here is a performer of magnitude.

Josh's mother brings him back to the park, where he plays with a tough black man who soon becomes his mentor. The father goes further by securing for him an embittered old master, Bruce Pacclan, played by Ben Kingsley looking for all the world like an aging Samuel Beckett, with about that much warmth. Pacclan takes over Josh's education, forbidding contact with the "crude" players in the park, and chiseling not just the boy's skill but his intensity, his aggression. In one scene, Pacclan puts a problem before his young student and when Josh has trouble with it, says, "Here, let me make it easier for you." Pacclan sweeps the pieces from the board in a grand, ferocious swipe. One sees the shock and fear cross Josh's face, and then he settles into the problem, which in fact is easier to grasp now that the board has been cleared. The teacher lures Josh with the promise of working toward a revered end. Pacclan lovingly produces a dog-eared certificate. "Careful, touching it!" he breathes. "It's *rare!*" The certificate deems the holder a "Grand Master."

"It takes *many* points to win this," Pacclan tells the boy, kindly.

"How do I get points?" Josh asks, and his teacher smiles.

"You have already begun!"

Passion, violence, and nurture are seamlessly fused in the scene. Pacclan is teaching his protégé not just about chess, but about being a winner, about being a man.

A troubling force begins to take hold of the adults surrounding this boy, however. In a humorous scene, Josh's first competition starts off with a very stern lecture on comportment by the tournament official. The camera draws back to reveal that he has been lecturing not the kids but their highly competitive parents. Eventually, two fathers break out in a fistfight, and the official leads all the parents to the basement and locks the door. In response to their parents' incarceration, the children, at first timidly and then with gusto, applaud.

Later, Josh's schoolteacher, a young woman, timidly voices her concern to Josh's parents that chess is beginning to consume him. What about museums, sports, hobbies? What about friends? The father, who had been shown as a warm, sensitive man up to this point, suddenly wheels on the teacher with contempt. "My son has a gift." He raises his voice, incensed. "He has a *gift*. He is better at this than I have been at anything. He is better at this than you will *ever* be at anything. Understand *that* and we have a basis to talk." He turns heel and walks out, leaving his wife behind, bewildered and helpless.

Before a big competition, Josh confesses to his father that he's frightened of losing. In an excruciating scene, the father repeatedly reassures his son that he's the "champ," that "it's the other boys who need to be afraid of you." Josh repeats his plea and his well-meaning father keeps missing the point. It is painfully clear that the boy needs his father to tell him that he will be loved whether he wins or loses. But the father does not respond. This scene, admirably delicate, is an excellent illustration of the subtlety of what is, in fact, quite damaging passive abuse. This father's vicarious performance esteem blinds him to his son's needs, and his son is visibly frightened by his father's inexplicable abandonment.

Josh, like Neil Perry in *Dead Poets Society,* dares an act of resistance. He deliberately loses his next tournament. The film shows his father pacing before him in the pouring rain, beside himself with anger. Josh's small frame huddles in a narrow doorway.

"You *could* have taken him." He paces, confused, furious. "I *know* you could. You deliberately threw that game. What is the *matter* with you?"

Josh listens to the diatribe, cold, wet, huddled into almost a fetal position. He finally looks up at his father and says, ever so softly, "Why are you so far away from me?"

"What?" the father asks.

"Why are you standing so far away from me?" Josh repeats, crying.

Finally the father holds him, but the look on his face does not soften. As he stares off in the distance, the father looks driven and frightened.

Josh's father is to Josh at that moment what Willy Loman was to Biff, what David Ingles was to Chad. Over the years, countless troubled Joshes and Chads have crossed into my office—slouching, "underachieving" boys whose parents are at their wits' end. I often frame them in my mind as little protesters, sit-down strikers refusing to march off into the state of alienation we call manhood. If the choice is between success and connection, many boys simply refuse to play. We usually call these boys delinquents.

If a boy's mandate is to separate from nurture, grow up, and learn to take care of himself, then competence out in the world equals relational abandonment. Josh threw the game because he needed to know that he would be cherished for who he was, independent of his gifts. Like Biff, he was attempting to say, "I'm just who I am." Other boys throw more than a chess game. They throw their grades or their health or even their safety. Fathers, or even school counselors, will often say of a boy's acting-out behavior, "We think he's just looking for attention." To which I say, "Right! For God's sake let's give him some! And let's try our best to make it the kind he most needs."

Josh Waitzkin begins to fade. Like an emotional consumptive, his spirit wanes. Pacclan discerns the change in his pupil and it enrages him. He taunts Josh, ridicules him, and finally decimates him.

"Do you want a Grand Master's certificate?" Pacclan sneers. "Take one." He reaches into his briefcase and pulls out the beloved document. "Take two. How many do you want?" Pacclan produces another certificate and slaps it on the table. "You want one, two, *more*?" He pulls out a whole sheaf of them, filmy Xerox copies, and flings them all on the table. The "rare" document that had so motivated Josh turns out to have been nothing but a cheap trick. With sadistic triumph, Pacclan enjoys the shock he produces in the boy. Josh's face does not even register the bewildered pain he surely feels. He is utterly overwhelmed. But his mother is not paralyzed. Her response to Pacclan's psychological violence consists of a single sentence.

"Get out of my house!"

Pacclan wheels on her as Josh's father wheeled on Josh's teacher, saying what men have said to mothers for a very long time: "It's a tough world out there. You cannot ask your son to face what he will face and then fail to equip him to handle it." The mother replies by swinging open the door for Pacclan to leave.

Josh's father agrees with Pacclan—his son must be toughened up. But Josh's mother, unlike Timmy's, or Chad's, or my own, is able to find the resources to protect her son, even though it requires putting her marriage on the line.

"Josh is a decent boy," she tells her husband. "And if you or anyone else tries to beat that decency out of him, I will leave you. I swear I will!"

Josh's mother refuses to buckle under the force of patriarchy. Only her rare confidence in standing up for relational values reverses the "soul murder" that has been taking place. The father is called back to his senses and, against all advice, both parents begin supporting Josh's childhood as a childhood, and not just a chess player's training camp.

In the film's climactic scene, Josh beats a robotlike archrival to win his first national championship. Just before winning, Josh offers the boy a tie game.

"I've got you beat in three moves," he says, extending his hand across the table. "Take the draw."

Josh's opponent, already schooled in arrogance, indignantly refuses.

"Please," Josh begs him. "Take the draw."

When Josh wins the game, he runs to his father. Visibly shaken, Josh repeats over and over again, "I tried to give him a way out, Dad. I tried to give him an out." His father squeezes him, tearfully, at last more proud of his son's decency than his achievement.

"I know you did, son," he tells him.

The grief Josh feels in that moment of "victory" comes from the very immediate experience of having decimated the self-esteem of his opponent. People who wonder how so many men can become inured to inflicting pain are blind to the reality that, in the competitive, hierarchical realm of achievement, one cannot win without inflicting pain. Winning means inflicting loss, by definition. Try as he might, Josh could not find a way of fully exercising his gifts without betraying the other boy.

There are no bad people in this story, no overt oppression, no beatings, no poverty, very little active abuse. And yet, if Josh's mother had not stood up to the forces that attempted to disempower her, her son would have collapsed as surely as Biff or Happy Loman—as surely, the film suggests, as the frighteningly eccentric chess prodigy of a preceding era, Bobby Fischer. Josh's story is so compelling because we intuitively grasp that, at a psychological level, it is nothing less than a struggle for emotional life or death.

In the film's final scene, Josh's father looks through a window affectionately as his son strolls through the yard with a young chess buddy. Josh's friend berates himself for his imperfect performance at their previous tournament.

"I shouldn't have brought out my queen so early," he bemoans.

Josh reassuringly drapes an arm around his young friend's shoulders. "I know," he soothes. "I've made the same mistake. But you know, you're a much better chess player than I was at your age."

The film closes with a shot of the two friends together. A message scrolls across the screen informing us that Josh has gone on to become the highest-ranked chess player for his age in the nation and that he also enjoys baseball, art, friends, and vacations. The healing moral of this story is clear—a boy can be a performer and a connected human being at the same time. Josh and his family, after some painful learning, narrowly avoided the usual course of emotional and relational amputation that accompanies specialness based upon performance.

There is nothing intrinsically wrong with vigorous competition; there is nothing wrong with boys working hard and playing hard.

Indeed, there is something wonderful in the feeling that comes from working up a sweat and going all out to defeat one's opponent on the tennis court or baseball court or hockey rink—so long as the passion falls short of placing the boy's or his opponent's self-worth on the line. The difference between the healthy enjoyment of achievement and competition and its unhealthy expression is analogous to the distinction between the recreational and the abusive use of intoxicants. A recreational drinker begins with a baseline feeling of relative contentment and the drug is used as an enhancement. The state he returns to after the drug has worn off is the satisfactory state he began with. The abusive drinker medicates a baseline experience that is painful or empty, and when the drug wears off, the underlying ill ease returns or worsens. Similarly, healthy joy in competition and achievement enhances an already invigorated boy. He does not rely on it to feel worthy, and he is not devastated on occasions of failure. In the same way that performance is not the boy's ticket to a sense of self-worth, it is also not a ticket to relational connection. Contrary to conventional ideas that link self-worth and self-reliance, in fact it is more acurate to link self-worth and relational connection. Unlike traditional mythic images of the lone, utterly self-sufficient hero, real boys and men need social connection just as much as do girls and women. A sense of self-worth always implies a secure sense of membership—a sense of mattering to someone, of being worthy of intimacy. In a healthy relationship to performance, achievement is a labor of love that exists within the context of secure connection, not an act of grandiosity that takes the place of connection.

Although the path of learning was painful for Josh and his family, he and they emerge intact. Other boys his age, with parents less willing or less able to resist traditional values, are not as fortunate. And for many men my age, raised a generation ago, the questions answered by Josh and his family would not even have been considered. The filtering of self-worth and relational needs through the screen of performance leaves these men and boys in a vulnerable position. Such men risk further alienation if they succeed and the threat of psychological breakdown if they fail.

CHAPTER EIGHT

Two Inner Children

B illy Jodein was a disheveled, wisecracking, overweight college freshman referred to me by his university health service in a last-ditch attempt to keep him in school. An acute episode of overt depression had taken its toll on Billy, leaving him barely enough energy to get out of bed in the morning, and little left over for study, friends, or sustained concentration. Although Billy's brash style might at first hide his condition, depression had gripped this young man, and it was about to toss him out of school and back home to his parents. For close to a month, Billy "just didn't have it" to get himself to many of his classes, let alone to the library. The few friends he had made were steadfast enough, although he was convinced he was boring to be around. When alone, he ached to be with other people. When with other people, he felt alienated and burdened—out of step—and he spent much of his time wishing they would just go away.

If Billy offered poor fellowship to others, he was far worse company to himself. When I ask him what he does all day, sitting for hours alone in his little dorm room, Billy answers with the warped bravado of his self-described "grunge sensibility."

"Mostly," he replies, smiling pleasantly, "I'd say I flay myself."

"You flay yourself?" I ask, willing to take on the role of straight man.

"Psychological self-immolation." Billy nods, a parody of sincerity. "Self-immolation is my favorite hobby."

"How is it?" I ask.

"Oh, it's *loads* of fun," he answers.

"I meant, how does it go?" I try again.

Billy spreads his hands. "That's just it," he tells me. "It doesn't go. It doesn't go anywhere. It just sits there, right on top of me. Right here on my chest. And it goddamn refuses to move."

Billy has managed to evade my question, and I suspect he is not yet ready to expose to me the dialogue that rages inside his head. But I have seen enough depressed men in my practice to guess what "flaying" himself signifies. At Billy's age, I myself was no stranger to such self-immolation. At sixteen, seventeen, I did not manage to sit still long enough to allow the voices inside my head to have their way with me. I ran from them. But even without giving in, I knew their essential message well enough: There was something wrong with me, something unlike other people—something frightening and bleak. I felt a perverse sense of blackness, sadness, a grim coldness at the center of things. I can recall this state of dead disconnection since early childhood.

As I write, a memory floats up to me. I am in Hebrew school, at eight or nine. I am tall for my age, an early developer. It is a dark winter afternoon, overwhelmingly dreary. If my experience at public school was bad, my experience at Hebrew school was worse. Ira Springle was my chief tormentor. Freckled, pudgy faced, Ira loved to taunt me, his face a mask of glee as he inflicted pain. Hebrew school felt so forlorn to me, I could hardly bear it— the children, clearly not wanting to be there; the teacher, incompetent, barely able to maintain order; the subject—God and suffering—confusing, painful. Looking back, I realize that the distress I felt in the classroom, the sense of meaninglessness and disconnection, was a displacement of my experience of chaos at home. But, at the time, I only knew that I hated being there and that, often, sitting in the back of the classroom, as far away from the others as possible, a profound languor poured over me, a blanket of muffled fatigue. I would, with great relief, drift off. Finally, one day, Mr. Seigal got mad.

"What the *hell's* the matter with you, Real?" he shouts from the front of the class, snapping me awake.

I blink up at him, disoriented in the jittery fluorescent light.

"What's your *problem? Sleeping sickness?*" he sneers.

The other kids smirk at me, excited.

"You been bit recently by a tsetse fly?" he taunts.

Ira sticks his face out at me from the aisle, grinning. "*Tsetse fly!*" He takes up the phrase. "*Tsetse fly!*" Ira bangs on his desktop, leading the chant, "*Tsetse fly! Tsetse fly!*" The class takes up the chorus, while Mr. Seigal looks on. "*Tsetse fly! Tsetse fly!*" Louder, in my ears.

Still half asleep, I just want the noise to stop. Without thinking, I cross to Ira's desk, pick it up, with him in it, and somehow throw it across the room. The class explodes into action, swirling around me, but I don't hear them. I stand in the middle of the classroom, oversized and disconsolate, sobbing for no reason at all.

Weeks later, Rabbi Wein thrusts his bespectacled face into mine as closely as Ira Springle used to do, but I don't much mind. Through his Coke bottle lenses, the rabbi's eyes are just about blind.

"So, why did you *do* it?" he asks me, sincerely trying to understand.

I shuffle about in my chair.

"Answer the rabbi!" My father clamps a firm, threatening hand on the back of my neck.

I look up into Rabbi Wein's milky eyes. I feel so sad—sad for him, sad for my parents to have to be there, sad for the mess I've made. I turn away from him, choking back tears that rise to my throat.

The rabbi looks at me even more closely, moves to put his arm around me. I flinch.

"Can you tell me, young man?" he asks again. "Terry?"

I drop my eyes to the floor. "I don't know," I manage.

The rabbi sent me back into the classroom with a few kind vagaries about "getting along." I was expelled from Hebrew school for aggressive behavior in the spring of the following year.

*   *   *

"Stupid, ugly, defective, coldhearted"—these are the phrases I would have flayed myself with if I could have put my inchoate feelings of self-hatred into words, if I had stopped "acting out" long enough to let them catch up to me.

By seventeen, I had already been suspended from school many times, cruised through my classes with a low D average, run drugs for local thugs, been arrested, and narrowly skirted commitment to the state mental hospital. Jazz was my passion. Jazz and drugs. I do not know if the drug-soaked "counterculture" of the sixties amplified or merely ratified my addictive career. Looking back, I draw the same distinction for myself that I now draw with adolescents and college-aged kids.

"A lot of kids your age drink and use drugs," I might say to a young man I am convinced is covertly depressed. "It's patently obvious that most of those kids will not go on to become addicts or alcoholics. But the difference is that those kids use booze and drugs to party; you use them to get hammered. You're not looking for a good time. You're looking for relief."

When I was seventeen and for the next dozen years, I cannot even claim to have been looking for relief. I was looking for oblivion. Other kids may have experimented with LSD, but Tommy Daimes and I injected it. Other kids may have been stoned now and again. But I spent a dozen years being straight now and again. Anything you could do straight, you could have more fun doing buzzed. Every day, all day long.

We called ourselves, with the innocent self-righteousness of those times, "psychonauts"—cosmic adventures. And, hey, if we died, we died. Psychonuts would have been more fitting. How crazy was I to try blue morphine with a man nicknamed "Lemon" for his chronic jaundice? How crazy was I to "drop" LSD and then spend my night cruising to nowhere in particular in a stolen car stuffed with delinquents, drugs, and, now and then, someone's gun?

"Mother's here!" Tommy Daimes yelled, flinging open the door of Zekial's basement apartment one evening. Three of my friends were with him. They were on a rescue mission, I later learned, for me. My buddy Zeke, a jazz singer, had introduced me to the joys of injected cocaine. That was a week earlier. I had been high ever since, not sleeping, barely eating. I felt myself hoisted over Tommy's broad shoulder. "The things I do," he muttered. "See ya, Zeke!" my friends called, while Zeke smiled, nodding pleasantly. Zeke was later shot in some drug deal. Lemon overdosed. Tommy has spent years in and out of mental institutions. The damage I did to my body has left permanent traces, which will probably shorten my life. And yet, while I emphatically hold myself responsible for the injury I brought to myself and to others, I do not really blame myself for running. Anyone in their right mind would have run from the gnawing blackness that dogged me.

I think I understood what Billy Jodein meant when he told me that he flayed himself.

In *A Season in Hell*, journalist Percy Knauth describes the way depression flayed him night after night:

> The nights were the worst. I started drinking more than usual, and often when I got to bed I was sodden with alcohol. I longed for sleeping pills, and rummaged everywhere to find some. . . . But pill or no pill, I never slept for more than three or four hours. Then I would awaken and lie there staring into the darkness while my mind began its endless circling. . . .
>
> In my own eyes I became worthless. In long night sessions, I reviewed my life and saw everything that I had done wrong. Not even the most trivial detail escaped this deadly scrutiny. I remembered arguments I had had with my children when they were very young. . . . I realized what a poor excuse for a father I had been. . . . I understood precisely why my . . . wife had left me for another man. . . . Even my work appeared to me to have been a fraud. . . .
>
> Next came despair. It was black as all the legions of darkness I had ever heard about, and it came at me screaming.

In an early session, I read Knauth's description to Billy. He turned his face away from me, struggling to hold back his tears.

"Lyric's a little different," Billy told me, "but the beat's similar enough."

"Thought so," I said gently, putting the book away.

There are many ways to describe the experience of depression, many aspects of the disorder one might choose to center on. My focus in treating depressed men has been primarily relational. *What kind of relationship does a depressed man have with others?* I ask, followed by: *What kind of relationship does he have with himself?* The answer to both of these questions is often: a bad one. Writers like Knauth or William Styron vividly describe the "pure psychical anguish" that patients like Billy endure. In the last twenty years, all manner of depressed men have passed through my doorway—young, old, successful, incompetent, kind, and angry. Each one of them has had one thing in common: his relationship to himself was a cruel one.

I tell Billy Jodein that I think of depression as an *auto-aggressive disease*, a disorder in which the self turns against the self. If we were able to take a psychic stethoscope and listen in to the unremitting conversation looping inside Billy's mind, we would hear harsh, perfectionist judgment matched with bitterness, mistrust, and hopelessness.

Billy comes by such harshness "honestly," as they say. Like most of the depressed men I have encountered, Billy had a history of sustained childhood injury. The bridge that links injury in childhood and depression in manhood is violence. Psychological violence lies at the core of the traditional socialization of boys in our culture. For many boys, that social wound is further aggravated by their unique family experiences. If "boy culture" exposes most young males to some degree of psychological injury, those growing up in especially difficult circumstances, particularly those also possessing genetic vulnerabilities, are most at risk for depression later in life. The violence they are exposed to as children takes up residence inside their minds as adults. Overtly depressed men like Billy are frozen, endlessly rehearsing repetitions of pain and despair. If overtly depressed men are paralyzed, men who are covertly depressed, as I was, cannot stand still. They run, desperately trying to outdistance shame by medicating their pain, pumping up their tenuous self-esteem, or, if all else fails, inflicting their torture on others. Overt depression is violence endured. Covert depression is violence deflected. In either case, understanding depression in men means coming to grips with men's violence. How has the door of the psyche been opened to such a dark visitation? By what mechanisms does violence in the boy's environment become internalized as a stable force inside his own mind? Although he is unaware of his knowledge, Billy Jodein knows how.

"Every night before he came home, I would watch my mother scurry around the house like a fat little hamster," Billy tells me during one session, crossing the legs of his artfully ripped blue jeans. With his acne-ridden face, spiky hair, and pudgy disorder, Bill thrusts himself out into the world, a pugnacious whirl of chaos, daring someone to try cleaning him up. This is our fourth session, and Billy has already threatened to stop coming. His demeanor makes it clear that he is in therapy to placate his school, his worried parents, and me, in that order.

"What do you mean, 'hamster?' " I ask.

Billy pushes up the glasses that threaten to slide down his nose—an abrupt, jabbing motion—and curls his lip in a sneer. "You know, like totally frenetic. Trying to get everything all straightened out before Dad got home. Every dish, every ashtray. I could see the fear in her eyes. I mean subtle, but definitely frantic, in her own controlled little way."

"Go on." I lean forward.

Bill takes a big swig of diet Coke and rests the wet can on a bare knee sticking up through his jeans. "I had this realization one day," he tells me. "This 'ah, hah!' experience, you know? And I told her. She was all running around and, like, I said, 'Hey, you know, Mom. I hope you understand that everything you're doing is *totally* useless.' "

"And?" I ask.

He shakes his head. "She hardly heard me," he says. "But I told her anyway. I said, " 'You *do* know that no matter what you do, he's still going to go off on you. If he feels like it. I mean, no matter what. No matter how nice the dinner is or whatever.' "

"Go off?" I ask.

"You know, flip out." Billy combs through thick, unruly hair with his chubby fingers.

"And how did she take it?" I ask.

"Could have saved my breath." He pulls on the Coke. "Believe me."

"Why?" I ask.

"Well, she heard me, I guess. I mean physically. Just sort of blinked at me and kept going." He grins to himself. "Just like one of those little Duracell guys, you know. *Just kept on tickin'.*"

Even though it is a pose, even though I know he is young, I find Billy's snide mannerisms annoying. "Is this funny?" I challenge him.

"Excuse me?" he bridles.

I take a breath, try to relax. "I was just wondering what you might be feeling if you weren't joking" I say, halfheartedly, suddenly tired.

Billy squints up at me for a moment, as if considering for the first time that I am in the room with him. He looks at my face longer, and more seriously, than I have been accustomed to.

"Long day?" he asks, not mockingly.

I look back at him. "Yes," I say. "To be honest. Why?"

He shrugs. "You looked kinda tired."

"Thanks, Billy," I tell him. "I appreciate that." And, after a pause, "Do you want to answer?"

"Your question?" He smiles.

I nod, waiting for some big revelation, but he only shrugs.

"Kinda useless, I guess. That's how I'd feel if I didn't make a joke out of it," he tells me.

I let it go. "And when your dad did get home?" I ask him.

"Yeah, so"—he looks down at his soda can—"why would it be different from every other night he came home?" he asks, with another reckless jab at his glasses. I worry he'll miss and poke his eye.

"Meaning, they argued?" I ask him.

"That's one way to put it," he answers.

"You have another—" I begin, but he cuts me off.

"No, you're right. They fight." He seems nervous.

"Describe it," I ask him.

"Like what? What would they say? The words?"

I nod.

"Aw, you know, just, *'Fuck you! I won't live like this anymore,'* and then, *'You're such an asshole! I can't believe you treat me like this!'* " He shakes his head. "Et cetera. Et cetera. Et cetera," he intones. "Believe me."

"And this would go on every night?" I ask.

"Most nights," he tells me.

"Where would you be?"

"Are you kidding?" he sits up. "Hey, I'm at a friend's. Really, 'Have a nice day!' " Under my gaze, Billy's ready smile dissipates. He sits back, deflated. "Or, maybe, up in my room," he says, sounding like a kid, "listening to music."

"Billy," I ask. "Are you feeling anything as you say this?"

"Now?" he asks, "Naw." Although I can see he is sad.

"And how would you feel back then?" I pursue.

"About their fighting?" He stalls.

I nod. "About anything. All of it."

"Not too much," he says, appearing more and more a little boy, kicking his feet in the chair. "Sorry for them, mostly, I guess. They were just so *pathetic.*"

"So, you're aware of feeling sadness for them," I tell him.

"Well, just that they're both such *jerks,*" he replies.

"Uh-huh. And what about you, Bill?" I lean toward him. "You were the kid listening to all of this night after night. The kid upstairs in his bedroom."

"What about it?" he says, sullen, pugnacious.

"You felt sad for them, but what about your feelings for your-self?" I ask.

"Yeah, I'm pretty used to it," he says, a tough guy.

"Oh, you are." I lean back.

"Hey," he says, "this has been going on a long time."

"Yeah," I say. "How long? How old were you when all this first started?" I ask him. "Give me the youngest age you can remember them bickering."

"It's been like this the whole time," he protests.

"Nine, ten, seven, eight?"

"Yeah, all of it," he says.

"And you think that little nine-year-old might not have had some feelings?" I ask him. "That seven-year-old boy?"

"It was a long time ago."

"You can't remember?" I press.

"No," said quickly, belligerently, then, "Why should I?"

"I'm just wondering what happened to them, that's all."

"My feelings?" he asks.

"Right," I say.

He flashes a supercilious smile. "Well, that's *assuming* I had them," he says.

"Billy." I lean forward and catch his eye. "I think you still have them."

"You know, *Terry*," Billy sneers, "not *everyone* needs to fit inside your neat little—"

I cut him off, speaking softly. "You finally manage to get out of that hellhole of a family and not five months into your freshman year you're so depressed you can't sleep, eat, or make it to class. But you sit here and tell me this is our last session, you have nothing to work on, and you don't have any feelings." His face flushes, but I keep going. He is either going to get on board or not. "You know, if you keep going on like this, Billy, I think you'll be headed right back home again. Is that what this is really about?" I ask. "Before the end of next semester, I'd guess." I lean back in my chair. "Believe me."

He turns on me, angry. "That was a low blow, mister!"

Even though it is in anger, I can feel his connection. "You need help, Billy," I tell him, flatly.

" '*You need help, man. Hey. You really need help,*' " Billy mocks me, furious, turning his face to the wall. But his eyes fill with tears, despite himself. We sit, quiet awhile, not looking at one another. A few minutes pass. "I'm a *loser,*" Billy says at last, the apathetic veneer collapsing. He sounds small, frightened. "A big fucking loser!"

"You're a boy," I answer. "A sad boy trying to deal with it all."

Billy stays quiet awhile, still not looking at me. A few minutes later he says, still in his child's voice, "You want to hear the sickest thing?"

"Okay, sure," I say gently.

"I swear," he begins to cry softly, "this is so fucking *ill.*"

"Go on," I tell him.

"The sickest thing is . . . I think I miss them." He stifles his tears. "If you really want to know the truth. I mean, how is *that?*" He twists further away in his chair. "I think that, really, what this whole thing is, is I'm homesick is all. I finally get the fuck out of there and then I fall apart 'cause I'm homesick. Jesus!" Billy buries his face in his hands and, for a brief moment, fully gives in to his tears.

I hand him a tissue. "Go on and cry, Billy," I say. "There's a lot to be sad about. You have a right to be sad."

"I *hate* this!" he gasps. "Breaking down."

"You're not breaking down. You're crying. Breaking down happens to people who don't cry."

Billy blows his nose, loudly, a couple of times. He squints up at me with his belligerent, acne-ridden face. "Do you know what the *fuck* you're talking about?" he asks, collecting a mound of tissues on his lap.

"Here." I hold up the wastepaper basket, like a hoop, for him to throw his wet tissues into. "Take a shot."

Billy Jodein's case provides great insight into how trauma metamorphoses into depression. The first clue of his condition is an absence rather than a presence—an absence of feeling for himself. Billy tells me that he felt the pathos of his bickering parents but did not feel, and still does not feel, much concern for the young boy who grew up with them. His description should make us sit up and take notice. Why should he feel sorrow for his unavailable parents and nothing for himself as their child? On the face of it, it makes no sense. And yet, in flagrant or subtle form, such a description is shared by most traumatized children.

Billy feels his parents' pain precisely because they do not. And, burdened with their pain, he has little room left for empathy toward his own. Many names have been given to this odd inversion of empathy: multigenerational projection, scapegoating, altruistic surrender. The convolution of Billy's emotions is central to the nature of psychological trauma, providing the link between trauma and depression. Where did Billy's feelings go? Billy Jodein's lost connection to self suggests that in those nights out with friends or upstairs alone in his room he learned more than simply to cut off from his deepest emotions. He actively learned to despise them.

In depression, the childhood violence that had been leveled against the boy—whether physical or psychological, active or passive—takes up permanent habitation within him. The depressed man adopts a relationship to himself that mirrors and replicates the dynamics of his own early abuse. This phenomenon, which I call *empathic reversal*, is the link connecting trauma to depression. To understand the mechanism of empathic reversal, we must accept a disturbing truth—that trauma intrinsically involves fusion between the offender and his victim. In the very moment of damage, some form of unholy intimacy occurs, in part because trauma always involves a failure of boundaries. In *active trauma*, a child's boundaries are violated. The parent is uncontained, out of control. In *passive trauma*, the parent neglects the child's needs; the boundary between parent and child is too rigid, impenetrable. Both are instances of boundary dysfunction. Most often, childhood trauma results from a layering of both kinds of boundary failure, as in the case of a father who is so stimulated by his adolescent daughter's sexuality that he will no longer touch her, or the case of a mother who neglects to set appropriate limits on her son's temper and then blows up at him herself.

When a child is traumatized—by a parent who is either negligent or out of control—his first and most profound response will be to take responsibility for the failing parent. When a child comes face to face with a caregiver's pathology, that child will do whatever he must to reinstate the caregiver's psychological equilibrium. A child's need to preserve his attachment, his willingness to contort himself into whatever shape the parent needs him to be in during such moments represents one of the least recognized, most pervasive, and most powerful psychological forces in human development. Trauma expert Judith Herman notes that: "Even more than adults, children who develop in [a] climate of domination develop pathological attachments to those who abuse and neglect them, attachments that they will strive to maintain even at the sacrifice of their own welfare, their own reality, or their lives." The child's need to regulate his parent is as fundamental as his own instinct for survival. In fact, it is a direct manifestation of that instinct, for the simple reason that each child relies on his parents' capacity to function in order to survive. As Herman suggests, in extreme cases, the need to preserve the attachment to an abusing parent may even supersede self-preservation.

Increased imprinting to abusing objects has been documented in birds, dogs, and monkeys. But of all the species on the earth, human children have the most protracted period of dependency. Children remain at the mercy of adult providers for an extraordinarily long time. One of the distinguishing characteristics of persistent, "mild" childhood trauma is that, unlike a terrorist bomb or a devastating hurricane, damage is delivered to the child by the hands of those on whom he relies. Safety fluctuates, often capriciously, with danger. Love alternates with contempt. The child remains in an excruciatingly confusing and precarious position. In such instances, both as a result of the boundary failure and as an unconscious coping strategy, the child will take the feelings that the parent is not handling responsibly into his being. Along with whatever other feeling-states may be involved—anger, pain, lust, fear—it is inevitable that one of the feeling-states transmitted to children in such traumatic moments will be the feeling of shame. Herman summarizes:

> All of the abused child's psychological adaptions serve the fundamental purpose of preserving her primary attachment to her parents in the face of daily evidence of their malice, helplessness, or indifference. By developing a contaminated, stigmatized identity, the child victim takes the evil of the abuser into herself and thereby preserves her attachment. Because the inner sense of badness (shame) preserves a relationship, it is not readily given up even after the abuse has stopped; rather, it becomes a stable part of the child's personality structure. Simarlarly, adult survivors who have escaped from abusive situations continue to view themselves with contempt and to take upon themselves the shame and guilt of their abusers. The profound sense of inner badness becomes the core around which the abused child's identity is formed, and it persists into adult life.

When a parent traumatizes a child, he is in a state of shamelessness. If the injurer felt appropriate shame, he would contain his harmful behavior. The shame a parent does not consciously feel will be absorbed, along with other unconscious feelings, by the child. Pia Mellody has called these transmitted states *carried shame* and *carried feeling.* They are the means by which the wound, the legacy of pain, is passed from father to son, mother to son, across generations. Carried feeling and carried shame are the psychological seeds of depression.

Projective identification is the term modern psychiatry has given to the phenomenon of carried feeling. Psychoanalytic theory emphasizes the projecting person's repudiation of his own feelings. The process is described as one wherein a person injects into another the disowned aspects of his own personality. When my father took a strap to me he beat into me his unacknowledged misery. My father hated and punished his own weak, dependent child in me, and I absorbed into my psyche both the hated and the hate-filled parts of him. I took on his sadness, depression, and rage. In the jargon of psychiatry, I "accepted" his projection. Like many of my patients, I can dimly remember the actual experience of that absorption. As my father raged, out of control, I can recall feeling, like Billy, terribly sad, almost nostalgic. In the midst of his brutality, I most strongly sensed, even as a young child, the urgency of his fragility, his pathos. I felt sorry for him. As a therapist, whenever I hear a depressed man tell me that he feels sorry for one or both of his parents, I know I am in the presence of carried feelings. A healthy parent, barring some true catastrophe, does not bid for his child's pity.

The paradox is that at the same time the child internalizes carried shame, he also takes in the offender's rage, his shamelessness. All traumatic acts are simultaneously *disempowering* and *falsely empowering*. No matter how badly a caregiver treats a child, he also models, through example, a shameless way of being in the world. His actions say to the boy: "You, too, can behave as I do when you become a man." In this tragic moment, the very forces that betray the boy, forces he most often finds abhorrent, come to live inside him.

In *The Prince of Tides*, Tom, the narrator, remembers the brutal eve of his father, Henry's, departure for Korea. Henry flies into a rage, knocks down little Tom, turns on his wife for trying to protect her son, and beats Tom's older brother bloody. Tom recalls his childhood reaction to the violence: "I looked up and saw my father shaking my mother, her eyes brimming with tears, with humiliation. I never loved anyone as much as I loved her in that moment. I looked at my father, at his back to me, and I felt the creation of hate in one of the soul's dark porches, felt it scream out its birth in a black, forbidden ecstasy."

The unpleasant fact that must be faced about trauma is that, in the very moment of victimization, a version of the same violence that hurts the child from without comes to "scream out its birth" from within. And that birth is permanent. From this night forward, Tom, if stressed enough, is capable of turning on someone in rage, just as his father did. With chilling irony, Henry's rage stealthily enters his son through the very door of Tom's repulsion. Whether called social learning, modeling, identification, or absorbed energy, the raging force surrounding Tom is pulled into his very being, becoming a part of him from this point forward for the rest of his life. There is no escaping this process.

Looking at the dynamics of depression in men, one is first drawn to the disowned boy—the relational, "feminine" aspects of self that men learn to repudiate. The imaginative personification of that lost boy is a useful technique for helping a depressed man recover those parts of himself our culture has "invited" him to suppress. But moments like the one described in *The Prince of Tides* suggest that if we are to personify internal aspects of the self, we should not think of one inner boy, but two. One part of Tom identifies with his frightened mother, while another, less conscious part, identifies with his angry father. One part of my patient Billy was traumatized by his father's rage, while another part of him took it in as a model. The psychiatric term for this internalization of the offender is *identification with the aggressor*. It is the dynamic behind the abused child's, the battered wife's, or the political prisoner's idealization of his own tormentors. In rare instances, as in the case of Patty Hearst, it is the motive behind a captive's attempt to transform herself into becoming like her own captors. When Elie Wiesel finds himself furious at his father for the stupidity of being beaten by an Auschwitz guard, Wiesel has absorbed the guard's perspective. When I found myself mistrustful of Eddie for his awkwardness, or when my brother grew furious with me for "causing trouble" in our family, we have adopted the offender's point of view. Billy, feeling sorry for his parents, takes on their attitude of contempt for his own pain.

Traditional ideas of children as either identified with mother or father are too simplistic. Children do not internalize wholesale, static qualities, like masculinity, femininity, or any other fixed characteristic. Children internalize interactions. They internalize what they see and what they themselves experience firsthand.

What Billy takes in, as would any child in his circumstances, is neither the identity of abuser nor abusee, but the interactive theme of abuse itself. As he matures, the theme of abuse may have a variety of permutations. Billy may become a demanding, angry manager to his staff and a frightened victim to his boss. He may find himself startlingly contemptuous of his wife and cruelly treated by his own son. The roles Billy may play in enacting the drama will shift, but the drama itself, the internalized dynamic of violence, will follow him throughout his life—unless he heals.

Violence—internalized, most probably, by Billy's parents in their own childhoods—spilled out, night after night, into their tortured marriage. Too preoccupied with their warfare to care for their child, Billy's parents' emotional neglect became a shaming force that convinced their son that he was unworthy of their attention. Young Billy's absorption of his parents' implicit contempt for him became a virulent force in his own life, years later and hundreds of miles from home. Billy's self-loathing, his feelings of powerlessness and shame, are the component parts of the disorder we call depression. Billy has learned to despise himself.

"Don't think it was all my father," Billy says angrily in a session a few months into our treatment. To my knowledge, I had never indicated that I had, but I keep quiet.

"My mother was in this up to her neck," he sneers. "It was both of them. All the way." He shifts in his chair, jittery. "I mean, my mother likes having her own way. Believe me."

"So, what would happen if she didn't get it?" I ask him.

"She'd pout," he answers quickly.

"Meaning?"

"Just that," he tells me. "She'd go off in a corner and sit there. Not talk to anybody. Literally."

"Not talk to anybody," I repeat. "Like you, for instance?"

"Like me, especially," he answers.

I lean forward, close to him, trying to understand. "She wouldn't talk to you?" I ask. "Answer you?"

Billy nods. He seems far off, and nervous.

"For how long?" I try bringing him back.

He shrugs, affecting carelessness.

"How long, Billy?" I ask, more sternly.

"Days," he says with a shrug. "A few weeks, maybe."

Billy's demeanor is muted, impatient, as if he had someplace better to be, as if I were bothering him with my questions. He hasn't been like this with me for a while.

"Wait a minute." I lean toward him again. "Your mother would refuse to talk to you, give you the silent treatment, for weeks at a time?"

Billy nods again, indifferent. But I can see that he is shaken. Talking about being shut out by his mother is upsetting him.

"How old were you?" I ask him.

He shrugs. "Four, five, I don't know. Forever." He turns from me.

"And what would your father do?" I persist.

"Get mad mostly," he says.

"At her?" I ask.

Billy smiles. "No," he says. "At me. Like, for setting her off."

We pause for a moment, thinking.

"So," I say at last, "she wouldn't talk to you—sometimes for weeks at a time—and then he would come in and blame *you* for it?"

Billy nods, staring away from me, looking over my office.

"What are you feeling, right now?" I ask him.

Billy fidgets. He swings his feet in the chair, like a ten-year-old. His eyes shoot around the room. "Is this really *necessary?*" he asks, eyes darting.

"What's going on?" I ask again.

With a physical *whoosh*, Billy sweeps out of his chair and crosses to the other side of the room.

"Billy?" I say.

"Hey!" he snarls. "Hey! I don't like what you're doing to me!"

"Describe it," I say quickly. "Describe what's going on in your body."

Billy shakes his head, as if he's trying to clear it.

"Bill?" I ask, wanting him to talk.

"Light-headed," he tells me. "Dizzy, like buzzing."

"What else?" I urge.

"My fingers are weird. Like an MSG rush."

"You're having some anxiety, Billy," I tell him.

"*You're having some anxiety,*" Billy mocks. "Cool! Great! Hey, we're *really* making some progress, now!"

"What were you remembering?" I ask him.

"When?" he says.

"Before the anxiety."

Billy paces. "I remember," he muses, still in motion, "I remember . . . Aw, *shit!*" he exclaims.

"Go on, Billy," I say quickly. "Keep talking."

He laughs, edgy, a little out of control. "I remember *this,*" he tells me. "I remember *this!*"

"What do you mean?" I ask.

"This *state,*" he tells me, almost laughing again. "Hyper, like this. She would be sitting there, or cooking, or whatever—talking to one of her girlfriends. Whatever. But not to me—just not to me. And I would get so fucking *agitated.*"

"Go on," I say.

"I remember"—Billy's tears start to come, even while he moves—"I used to twirl around her, just like this"—he stretches out his hands—a little boy. "I used to say, '*Mommy, I'm a top! Look at me! I'm a top!*'" Billy starts crying, his nose running, but he doesn't slow down. I want to tell him to wipe his nose, but I don't want to stop him. "I used to sing this little song to her," he says. "This stupid little song."

"Sing it," I tell him.

"You've got to be fucked," he says.

"Tell me, then," I say.

Billy stretches his arms out and sings, "I'm Popeye the Sailor Man. I live in a garbage can." Billy cries in earnest, big, messy. He looks like he wants to sit down again but isn't sure how to get back. I usher him into his chair.

"I used to . . ." he tries to continue.

I hand him some tissues, which he clutches.

"When we were alone and she wouldn't respond like that . . . I mean, what must I have been, four, five?"

"Breathe," I say softly.

"I used to *slam* my fingers in a drawer." He starts sobbing. "I used to slam my fingers in the *fucking* drawer, okay? And then I'd show her." He doubles over. "I'd show her my bloody fingers."

With my hand on his back, I press Billy forward as he sobs. "Let it go, Billy," I keep repeating—a mantra, a nursery rhyme. "Just release it. Let it go."

At four years old, Billy Jodein did not deserve to live in a garbage can, or feel that he belonged in one. And, while Billy might be the first to deny the full import of his little ditty, I found it chilling—an outward manifestation of his carried shame. When, as that little boy, Billy slammed his fingers in the drawer, he dramatized the relationship between perpetrator and victim, which he had internalized. Billy had grown to despise his own vulnerable flesh, just as his father had despised his mother and his mother had grown to despise her son. In that moment, Billy enacted several roles simultaneously. He punished the vulnerable part of himself—his shame. He acted out the vengeful, raging part of himself—the offender. He dramatized to his mother the hurt he felt as a result of her abandonment. And yet, at the same time, he joined with her in a kind of spiritual union by adopting her punishing stance toward himself. These are the essential dynamics of depression.

If *empathic reversal*—the process of taking on the offender's perspective and losing empathy for one's own—is the process by which trauma becomes depression, reversing that reversal—reestablishing empathy for the vulnerable child within and creating distance, a healthy judgment toward the offender—lies at the core of recovery. From the first moments a depressed man enters my office, most of the actions I take are aimed at reconnecting the dismembered, pained self and challenging the toxic, internalized offender. First, the harsh force of shamelessness and the grandiose defenses must be confronted and stilled. If the anger and pain are directed away from the self, as is usually the case in covert depression, the addictive defenses and the irresponsible behaviors must stop, allowing the underlying depression to surface. If the harsh, offending energy is directed inward, as it is in overt depression, it, too, must be stilled. The vulnerable part of the self must be protected, encouraged, and nurtured. Both internal children—the wounded boy and the harsh boy—must learn nuanced maturity and responsibility.

Contrary to some "inner child" work currently in vogue, the goal of therapy with depressed men rarely aims at granting further license to either of these immature aspects of self. Often without their conscious awareness, these regressed ego states may already be running—and ruining—men's lives. But denying their existence, refusing to deal with these already fragmented parts of the self, is also not a solution. By bringing the man into a conscious, healthy relationship with these unintegrated yet potent aspects of self, therapy attempts to enhance, or in some cases, to bring into being for the first time, a functioning internal adult.

My work with Billy was representative of many depressed men's recovery process. Both of the immature parts of him—the disavowed, vulnerable boy, and the aggressive, harsh boy—had to be faced. Billy's overt depression was an endless reiteration of the relationship between these two internal forces—one young and torturing, one young and tortured. In the same way that I have found it useful to personify the disowned, vulnerable boy, I now worked with Billy, through visualization, first to unearth and then modify the relationship between both of these aspects of self. Billy's first introduction to such imaginative role-play occurred in the presence of forty-three men.

Although I had some experience leading men's groups, I would never have had the courage, left to my own resources, to put together a "men's gathering" involving close to fifty people. This was the inspiration of my friend and colleague Dr. Jack Sternbach, who has been running men's groups of every imaginable size, shape, and format, for over twenty-five years—long before they became fashionable. Now in his sixties, Jack has taught me a great deal about men and how to help them. Sitting Buddha-like on the floor, he opens up the final evening in our series. For six consecutive Fridays, from 5:00 to 11:30 P.M., forty-three men have come together to support one another in deep psychological work.

"For the rest of our evening together," Jack says, looking into the faces of men we have come to know well in a brief time, "we invoke a spirit of acceptance. Our work tonight is sacred work. This place has become a sacred place, where differences will be honored, not run from. Where tensions between us and within us will be held without judgment in loving witness."

In groups small and large, these men—challenging, loving, sustaining one another—reopen old wounds and confront old defenses with a speed and a depth, almost a thirst, I have rarely seen. It was invigorating to collaborate at such velocity with an older colleague I trusted. And it was important for the group, so they told us, to witness our working relationship.

One of my quiet pleasures in this series has been watching Billy's jaw drop, sometimes metaphorically, sometimes literally, as the cadre of men around him—some three times his age—plunged to a depth of emotional exploration he could scarcely have imagined. In this final evening, Billy surprises both Jack and me by volunteering to "take the hot seat" himself. Because of my history with Billy, Jack and I agree that I will assist him.

While the men gather around us, sitting or reclining on the floor, Billy and I sit next to one another, facing out toward an empty chair four feet in front of us. That chair has been the repository, over these evenings, of envisioned mothers, fathers, bullies, and molesters, good and bad parts of the self, scoundrels and kings. It awaits our work.

"How are you doing?" I ask Billy, settling in next to him.

"Nervous." He smiles.

"Yeah, me too," I say, a little tense myself. "Quite a crowd."

Billy laughs softly. "I feel mixed about that."

"Go ahead," I invite him.

"Well, I'm nervous, believe me. But I also feel buoyed up. *Like, I feel their energy, man,*" he clowns. Some men laugh. "No, really, though," he continues, "like floating in the ocean."

"It's called support," I say.

"Well, I like it," he says.

"That's good," I say. "It's a good thing to like." I ask Billy if he would allow me to help him move into light trance, a state of relaxation, in which he could do some of the imaginative work he has seen others engage in. He gives his permission. I direct him to close his eyes and scan his body for areas of tension. Billy identifies tension in his eyes and in the back of his neck. After exploring the possible messages of these sensations, I make a suggestion:

"Why don't you bring that 'held up' feeling into your body," I advise, "and circulate it around to the tense places inside?"

Billy looks in my direction with his closed eyes. "I will if you will," he smiles.

"Now that's a good idea," I answer.

Slowly, Billy and I descend into the work. As Billy's trance deepens, he first retells and then gradually reexperiences some early, painful memories. Quietly following his lead, I urge Billy on as he winds his way back, carefully, inevitably, to the five-year-old boy with bloody fingers. Billy finds it difficult to sit still in the chair when the agitation comes over him again. Intense, physical restlessness courses through his body.

"I have to get up!" he wails at one point, as if he were caged.

"Go! Go!" I tell him. "Move around! We can still work." Permission to move seems to calm him enough to enable him to remain seated as the feelings of intense agitation wash over him. Together, we search for the abandoned young boy at their center.

"Billy," I say, "I want you to turn your mind's eye—which is located up around the center of your forehead—inside so that you're looking down into the cavity of your body. And in your imagination, I want you to go down into that agitated feeling in your gut, deep inside that, and see if you can locate that little five-year-old, that hurt boy."

Billy takes a long time, brows furrowed, searching. Then, he smiles softly and nods without speaking. The outward signs of his agitation subside.

"You've got him?" I ask. "You've made contact?"

"Well," he says, "sort of."

"Sort of," I reflect.

Billy smiles, not the self-conscious, mocking smile I have known, but a simple, happy, smile I have seen more frequently in these evenings together. "I've got his foot!" Billy tells us. Several men softly whoop their approval.

I pause for a minute. "You mean you've made contact," I ask "but . . ."

"I *know* he's there," Billy answers, "but he's only showing me the tip of his shoe."

"The tip of his shoe," I say, impressed. "Well, that's good. That's good!"

"He won't let me see him," Billy tells us. "But he will let me know that he's there."

"Kind of coy," I observe.

"Shy, I'd say," Billy corrects me.

"That's just fine," I tell him. And it is fine. Billy's ability to establish even this much contact with his hurt self is an impressive accomplishment. Many of the depressed men I treat are so disassociated from their own vulnerability that it takes several sessions, sometimes even months, before the wounded boy will show himself at all. Other men hold that part of themselves in so much contempt that, once contacted, the man wants us to banish the imagined boy to a place as far removed from him as possible. Generally, I have found that the vulnerable boy will show himself when and to the degree that it is safe for him to do so. As I work with the man to tame and soften his harsh energy—his internalized contempt—the vulnerable self will begin to peek out. For initial, light trance work, the tip of a shoe is not a bad start.

"Bill," I say. "Can you ask the boy what it means that he'll show you his shoe and nothing more? Can you ask him that?"

"Aloud?" Billy asks.

"Yeah," I answer. "Aloud."

Billy squares off, pushing through the natural embarrassment of such an odd public exercise. The men around us draw in a little closer. "Terry wants to know," he begins cautiously, "what it means that you'll show your shoe to me and nothing more." Billy furrows his brow, intensely concentrated.

"What's he say?" I ask. "How does he answer that?"

"He won't say," Billy frowns, angry. He starts tapping his feet. The expression on his face darkens.

"Billy?" I ask.

He remains silent for a few moments, brows squeezed together, as if he is peering hard at something. Then he leans back, frustrated and annoyed. "He's *gone*," Billy tells me, upset. "Took off somewhere."

"You sound angry," I tell him.

"I wanted to do some *work* here tonight." Billy's movements in the chair grow agitated. I wonder if he feels inadequate in front of the other men, or rejected by the little boy. I wonder if his feelings are hurt. "I'm not in the *mood* for bullshit games." For the first time in a while, Billy sneers. "*Little shit*," he mumbles.

That grabs my attention. "Excuse me?" I say. "What did you just mutter?"

"What?" Billy says.

"Just then," I say. "Just now. Under your breath. What did you say?"

Billy thinks for a minute. Some of the guys start to stir, but Jack shushes them.

"Little shit," Billy recalls.

"That's it," I tell him. "That's what we want. Who's that for?"

"Little shit?" he asks. "Him, I guess," he shrugs. "You know, the kid."

I drape my arm behind Billy's chair, inch up a bit closer to him.

"Say it again," I tell him softly.

"Little shit," he repeats, without much conviction.

"Louder," I say. "Like you did last time. Like you mean it."

"Little shit," he sneers, quietly.

"Again," I say. "*Louder!*"

"Little shit." His voice rises. "Little *shit!*" he begins to shout. "Little *fucker!*"

"That's it."

"Little *fucker!*" Louder.

We pause for a moment, sitting together. "You feel that?" I ask him.

Billy nods.

"That rage?" I say.

"Oh, yeah," he nods again. The rawness of Billy's anger hits me like a wave as I sit next to him. Billy slouches, his eyes intent on mine. Just as we had begun to personify and develop a relationship with the wounded part of Billy, we now had an opening to do the same imaginative work with his contempt, his harsh child—the internalized aggressor.

"Billy," I ask, "can you scan inside your body, just like you did before, for this energy, now? This 'little shit' energy?"

He nods.

"Where is it?" I ask him. "Can you say? Where is it inside your body?"

Billy answers immediately. "Up here," he says, indicating his furrowed brow. "In my head, like a headache."

"It hurts?" I ask.

"No, not pain, really," he answers. "Just pressure. All those thoughts."

"A lot of thoughts?" I reflect. Another pause. With his permission, I rest my hand on his shoulder. "What I'd like you to do now, Bill, is to go up into that pressure, up in your head, and see if there's some image or presence connected to that 'little shit' voice, that energy."

Billy has seen other men do this work and he knows what I'm after. For several minutes he remains utterly still, serious, focused. Then, suddenly, he breaks into a huge, warm smile.

"Something's come to you?" I ask him.

He nods, enthusiastic.

"Go ahead," I urge.

"Like, I guessed that we were about to put that little boy, you know, that little five-year-old, up into that empty chair?" he begins.

"The vulnerable boy," I say. "Uh-huh."

"And so," he goes on, "I have this image of—sort of—that boy. Like he's all tied up. Tied to the chair. Like an Indian war whoop kinda thing. And dancing around him is this—this is the thing up in my head, the 'little shit' thing. Well . . ." he pauses. "It's this gorilla."

Although Billy can't see me, it's my turn to smile. "A *gorilla!*" I say, delighted.

"Yeah," he answers, pleased with himself.

"Well, well, well!" I remark. "So, what's it doing?"

Billy answers easily, "It's, like, dancing around the boy. You know, beating its chest. Being threatening. You know. Its, like . . . a gorilla."

Over the years, all manner of metaphors for the internal harsh child have spilled into my office—sharks, bloody force fields, Hitlers, monsters. In comparison, Billy's dancing gorilla seemed almost whimsical, relatively benign.

"Is it saying anything?" I ask Billy.

"Well . . ." Billy shifts in his chair. "Actually, yes," he says. Suddenly, all the warmth of the preceding moment drains from his face. Billy sits up straight in his chair. He looks grim.

"Billy," I ask, "what are you feeling, now?"

"Nothing," he replies too quickly. "I'm steeling myself is all."

"For what?" I ask.

"For whom," he corrects. "I'm steeling myself from him, for the onslaught of the gorilla."

I lean my hand against his shoulder blades. "What is he saying, Bill," I ask, "as he dances around? What are his messages to that young boy?"

Billy is quiet a long few moments, his jaw set firm.

"Billy?" I ask.

"I'm not sure I want to get into all that," he answers.

"In front of these guys?" I ask, thinking that he is embarrassed.

He shakes his head. "In front of myself," he answers. He seems close to tears.

"Well," I say. "You can pass on the question. You look like some pain is coming up right now, Billy."

"No," he shakes his head. "I don't want to pass. Let's do it."

"Sure?" I ask.

He nods, hands folded in his lap.

"Okay, Billy," I tell him, softly. "Take a good look at the gorilla and when you feel ready, tell me what he's saying to that boy."

Billy sighs, a long, protracted exhalation, the sound of a burden beyond years. "He says all the things I say. All the things I say to myself."

"All the shame messages," I prompt.

"It's like sticks in a fire. It's like, he's burning that boy up. At the stake. And each thing he says, it's just one more stick in the fire."

"So, what's he say," I prompt softly, "specifically?"

Then I and forty-three other men watch Billy transform. His face grows black and his snarl turns into a kind of a hoarse growl.

"Little *shit*," he spits out. "*Fucking little whiner.*"

I put a hand on his shoulder. "Go on," I urge softly. "Let's hear it."

"You're *fat*." He needs little prompting. "A fat *pig*. A *big blobby pig. Pimply faced, ugly.* You little *asshole. Stupid. Unloving.* All you *care* about is *yourself* anyway—"

"Billy," I interrupt.

He stops on a dime, emotionless, as if I had pulled out a plug.

"I would like you to ask the gorilla inside your head if he'd be willing to come out and sit with us in that chair, tonight."

"Now?" Billy asks. "Out loud? I feel stupid."

"Whatever," I say.

"Can I say it's you who wants him to come out?" Billy asks.

"Sure."

Billy squares his shoulders, takes a minute to marshal his resources, and then he begins. "Terry says he wants to know if you'd be willing to come out and join us in that empty chair over there," he says, arms clamped over his chest.

"Well?" I inquire.

He smiles. "Well, it's interesting," he tells us. "At first he was all blustery, you know, '*Fuck you, I'm not doing anything for you.*' But then he just settled down."

"He's sort of a blustery character," I reflect.

He nods.

"A lotta bark," I add.

"A big chest beater," he tells me, some of the warmth back in his voice.

"So, okay, let's bring him up into the room. Now," I ask, "should we move the chair? Should he come closer to you? Or would you feel more comfortable with him at some distance?"

"That's funny, too," Billy tells me. "When I was thinking we would bring up that boy, that little boy, I actually wanted the chair placed way back. Like, I didn't want him that close to me. Like, he'd leak on me or something. But this guy, this gorilla, I don't actually mind him."

Billy is obviously more closely identified with the internal aggressor than he is with the vulnerable boy, but I don't bring this up at the moment. "So, the chair's okay where it is?" I ask. "A little closer? Keep your eyes closed, just visualize it."

"Closer," he says. "I don't know why I think this is funny. I should be afraid of this force in me, but it just makes me smile, somehow."

"That's good," I assure him. "That's a good sign." We fuss with the chair until it's at just the right distance. "Okay," I say. "Tell him to come out, now."

Billy does, and in a magic consensual moment, all forty-three of us feel the presence of Billy's gorilla inhabit the empty chair.

Eyes still closed, Billy grins.

"What's he doing?" I ask. "The gorilla?"

"He's just *sitting* there," Billy tells us. "Very casual. Like, one leg swung over the other. Happy as a clam. He's *really* happy to be here. Like, '*Hi, guys!*' " Billy waves. Some men wave back, despite Billy's closed eyes. The whole room feels warm. We're all having fun.

"I'll be damned," I say. "Well, what happened to all of those horrible messages?"

"Oh, I don't know," Billy tells me. "They're all still there, I guess. Just not now."

"Hmm," I muse, at a momentary loss. "Well, Billy, is there anything you want to say to this guy, now that he's here?"

"Not me, boss," Billy answers. "You wanted him. This is your show."

"It's on me?" I ask.

"Uh-huh."

"Well, all right, then. I'll help out," I say, thinking fast. "But there is one thing you have to tell him yourself."

"What's that?" Billy asks.

I lean closely into him, my hand on his back. "You have to tell him to stop torturing that little boy," I say.

Billy Jodein faces his imaginary adversary.

"Billy," I say. "I'd like you to tell him to sit up straight and to wipe the smirk off his face. Tell him this is a serious matter."

Billy does so, aloud.

"And now?" I ask him.

"Better," Billy tells me. "He's listening. He's taking it in."

"Tell him, now," I say. "Use your own words. I'll help if you need me. Tell him to lay off that boy."

Billy opens his mouth to speak but nothing comes out. He tries again and his shoulders start shaking. He begins to cry, bewildered, undone by the potency of his own reaction.

I lean in close beside him. "Do it, Billy," I say to him.

"Listen, *you*," he addresses the gorilla through his tears. "I'm not fooled by you. I know what you do to me. I know how much you hate me."

"Good, Billy," I say. "Keep going."

Eyes shut tight, Billy points to the empty chair. "I am not going to let you push me around any longer."

"Say that again," I urge, softly. "Like you mean it."

"I will *not* let you push me around any longer," he says.

"Again," I say. "Louder."

"I will *not* let you push me around any *longer*," he repeats, his voice rising.

Like a catechism, Billy and I move into a call and response.

"I will not let you invade my thoughts," I prompt.

"I will *not* let you invade my thoughts," he repeats.

"I will not let you torture my heart," I say.

"I will *not* let you torture my heart," he repeats.

"I will not let you drain all my energy and keep me from life," I tell him.

"I have a *right*," Billy answers. "I have a *right* to live!" He doubles over in pain. "Leave me alone, for Christ's sake," he says. "Let me live!"

"What's he doing now?" I ask after a time. "Our friend?"

"Nothing," Billy tells me, wiping off his face. "He's just listening. Like, contrite."

"Good," I say. "That's good." We sit for a few minutes together, silent. I ask Billy if he'd be willing to hear some of my theories concerning the nature of his relationship to the gorilla. He is happy to oblige me.

"Can I tell you, for starters, why I think you feel so warm toward him?" I ask Billy.

He nods.

"Because that gorilla," I say, "that harsh, judging part of you— It's the closest you got to having a parent."

"What do you mean?" Billy asks.

"What I mean," I tell him, "is that if you look hard enough at that gorilla, really look into him, I think you'll find he's just another kid—living inside you. Just another immature part of you. And, in many ways, this is the part of you that tried bringing you up."

"You mean, like, standards and all?" he asks.

"That's exactly what I mean. The standards, the rules, and also the contempt. It's all part of the same package. This is the perfectionist part of you that you have used to judge yourself by."

Billy laughs, weakly. "Well," he says. "It's hairy."

"I guess it is," I agree.

"I have a hairy superego," he tells me.

"It's not your superego, Billy," I tell him. "It's just a kid. Just another kid."

Billy blows his nose, taking it all in. He turns to face the empty chair.

"So, now what do I do with him?" he asks, after awhile.

"Well, that's a good question," I tell him. "I think you may have already started."

"Get to know him?" he tries.

"Uh-huh," I agree. "Get to know him. Defuse him. Demote him."

Billy sticks his thumbs in his belt. It is obvious from his posture, his tone, that he already feels better. He thinks for a while, in no hurry to leave or resolve things prematurely. Finally, he rocks back in his chair and says in his mocking deep baritone. "You're on notice, Ape. I'm takin' over this psyche. There's only room in this brain for one grown-up person." The men around us cheer.

"And who would that be?" I ask him.

"Hey, you're lookin at 'im," Billy answers. "Believe me."

Did Billy Jodein's depression remit after one session with an imaginary gorilla? Of course not. But, like the overture of a symphony, the work he did with the support of a room full of men announced the themes we would focus on for the rest of his treatment. Billy began, as he once cleverly put it, "to turn off the repeating apes in my head." He began to limit, with tenderness, the harsh, relentless part of him. He learned how to cherish, rather than to act out, his own needs and vulnerabilities. He found himself able to attend to the voice of the long-ignored boy. In these ways, he was becoming a good parent to himself. After practicing each day, over and over again, he has gotten better at it. Just like most of the men I work with. Just as I have.

*   *   *

In *Listening to Prozac*, psychiatrist Peter Kramer notes that Prozac and its relatives are equally effective in treating both depression and obsessive-compulsive disorders. He observes that this dual effect challenges traditional views, which saw depression and obsessive disorders as two discrete disease entities. I agree that depression is not a discrete entity. It cannot be treated as if it were bacteria or simply a genetic disorder. Anyone who has listened closely to the voices of depressed men themselves would not be surprised to learn that one medication can treat both depression and obsessive disorders. Depression is an obsessive disorder. A depressed person is endlessly caught in the chains of his rehearsed inadequacies. Billy Jodein learned to break free of the shaming-shamed dialogue. Many other approaches might have helped Billy gain relief from his acute symptoms. But I am not certain they would have taken on as their goal the transformation of Billy's relationship to himself. This focus on relationship does not intend to deny or minimize the role of biology in a case like Billy's, nor to disregard important advances in the use of medication. I often recommend medication to depressed men. And I am delighted, even tantalized, by new possibilities of ever more subtle treatments for covert depression. Research has already developed pharmacological help in some cases of traumatic disorders, addictions, and disorders of violence. But I consider medication and other symptom-focused remedies as platforms that allow the man to do the therapeutic work, not as panaceas obviating the need for it. An unhappy, immature, relationally unskilled man on medication becomes, at best, a happier immature, relationally unskilled man.

Understanding the relationship between depression in men and the terms of masculinity itself allows us to place Billy's torment in context. Neither of Billy's two internalized roles, vulnerable boy or harsh boy, victim or perpetrator, is gender-neutral. In this culture, the lost boy, the shame-ridden, wounded victim, is "feminine." The punishing judge, the better-than, perfectionist offender, is "masculine." When our culture teaches boys to repudiate the "feminine" in themselves, to hold that part of themselves in contempt, we teach them to split themselves in half. Each half takes on an assigned role—roles that look very much like traditional gender stereotypes. The boy learns to go "better than" himself, to bring the dynamic of contempt into his own psyche. The dialogue between those two internalized roles often becomes the inner discourse we call depression.

This perspective enables us to metaphorically draw a line down the center of a piece of paper creating two columns. On one side, we list the "feminine," the lost boy, overt depression, shame, and victimization. On the other, we list the "masculine," the harsh boy, covert depression, grandiosity, and offense. The relationship between these two columns at once describes relations between men and women in our changing, but still sexist, culture and also the internal dynamic of depression.

Boys do not internalize either masculinity or femininity. Instead, what many of our sons internalize is a pattern in which women and womanish things—including half of the boy's own being—are held as inferior. Recovery comes when a man learns to embrace, remember, and cherish his own full humanity. This is neither an easy nor a very popular task. Society rewards self-objectification in men. It gives men privilege. It reinforces their superiority. And it shows little mercy for men if they fail in the performance of their role. But the price of that performance is an inward sickness, a sickness that depressed men, like the symptom bearers of a disordered family, carry for us all.

Any substantive healing must address that inward sickness. Emotional recovery is not about medical procedures. Psychotherapy at its best has never been a science, nor even an art, but a morality, in the classic sense of the word. Therapy is fundamentally a process that helps people discover how they must live. Depression in men is not just a disease; it is the consequence of a wrong turn, a path poorly chosen. And recovery demands the discipline of reworking that wrong turn, over and over again.

In the poem "Healing," D. H. Lawrence writes:

I am not a mechanism, an assembly of various sections.
And it is not because the mechanism is working wrongly, that I am
    ill.
I am ill because of wounds to the soul, to the deep emotional self
and the wounds to the soul take a long, long time, only time can help
and patience, and a certain difficult repentance,
long, difficult repentance, realization of life's mistake, and the freeing
    oneself
from the endless repetition of the mistake
which mankind at large has chosen to sanctify.

Recovery from depression requires, in Lawrence's words, "a certain difficult repentance." The root of the term *repentance* is *to return*. Repentance, and its companion word, *sin*, were originally associated with archery. To "sin" meant to miss the mark, and "repentance" meant to return to it. "Recovery" seems a paltry word for the mark depressed men set their sights on, their point of return. A man who is willing to drop down as far and work as hard as young Billy did is after bigger game than relief from an illness. A man willing to permanently alter the terms of his internal dialogue—to transmute the dynamic of wounded boy and harsh boy, feminine and masculine, shame and grandiosity, inside himself— seeks nothing less than a transformation in the way that he lives, the values he lives by. Such a journey goes beyond recovery. It is alchemy. It is a quest.

CHAPTER NINE

Balance Prevails:
Healing the Legacy

Through the mechanism of *carried shame* and *carried feelings*, the unresolved pain of previous generations operates in families like an emotional debt. We either face it or we leverage our children with it. When a man stands up to depression, the site of his battle may be inside his own head, but the struggle he wages has repercussions far beyond him. A man who transforms the internalized voice of contempt resists violence lying close to the heart of patriarchy itself. Such a man serves as a breakwall. The waves of pain that may have wreaked havoc across generations spill over him and lose their virulent force—sparing his children. The "difficult repentance" such a man undertakes protects those who follow him. And his healing is a spiritual gift to those who came before. The reclaimed lost boy such a man discovers—the unearthed emotional, creative part of him—may not be merely the child of his own youth, but the lost child of his father's youth, or even of his father's father.

Each man is a bridge, spanning in his lifetime all of the images and traditions about masculinity inherited from past generations and bestowing—or inflicting—his own retelling of the tale on those who ensue. Unresolved depression often passes from father to son, despite the father's best intentions, like a toxic, unacknowledged patrimony. Conversely, when a man transforms the internalized discourse of violence, he does more than relieve his own depression. He breaks the chain, interrupting the path of depression's transmission to the next generation. Recovery transforms legacies.

When a depressed man has trouble remembering why he should follow "the dark path," take up the arduous work of recovery, I ask him about his relationship to his father. And then I ask about his own kids.

"Do the work," I will often say to such a man. "Face this pain, now, or pass it on to your children, just as it was passed on to you."

Virtually every depressed man I have worked with knows what I am speaking about. Many of the men I treat would never tough out the process of therapy for their own sake. But men have been trained to be good soldiers, and many are willing to experience the pain they have spent lives running from for the sake of their children. I call these men *relational heroes.* Like the great adventurers of old, they are willing to descend to the depths and encounter their monsters. They want to be better fathers than they had. They want the legacy of physical or psychological violence to stop.

Thirty-five-year-old Jonathan Ballinger, a mechanic and recovering alcoholic, did not remember the fear he had felt as a child raised by two severe love addicts and alcoholics. Jonathan's parents spent most of their days and nights drinking with each other, fighting with each other, and then making up. Their son and his three sisters were, by and large, left to fend for themselves. Jonathan did not remember his childhood terror until we began working together. Before entering therapy, what Jonathan mostly did with the dread he did not recall was instill it in those close to him. He referred himself a few days after he slapped his wife, Carlisle, in front of their four-year-old daughter, Elise.

"You know what?" Jonathan told me in our first meeting. "I maybe could have stood it, hitting Carli, sick as that is. But when I saw Elise standing there watching what I did to her mother . . . this little girl . . . shit."

Jonathan had been sober for almost eight years and his recovery from alcohol has been courageous. But he needed to go further—down into the unhealed trauma he carried inside like a reservoir of rage, fear, and loneliness. Along with alcoholism, Jonathan had to confront his own love addiction, and his rageaholism—if he was to render himself fit to maintain a family and break the chain of violence from one generation to the next.

When I first met Jonathan, I was struck by the desperation in his voice. He did not want to lose his wife and he did not want to hurt his child. There existed within him a space between his sense of himself and the offensive behaviors with which he had been raised. He was not wholly identified with that aggression—so long as he did not feel stressed. Jonathan reacted to fear and helplessness, however, by lashing out. Helplessness forced Jonathan into proximity with the vulnerable parts of himself. In such moments, he warded off the threatening emergence of childhood pain and depression with rage. The harsh part of him swelled with power as he sensed increased vulnerability in others. Like most batterers, Jonathan medicated the few seconds of shame that broke through to consciousness with the narcotic of dominance.

One of the characteristics of traditional masculinity that served us as a resource in our therapy was an appetite for hard work. Jonathan came from a blue-collar Canadian community where men worked diligently for the sake of their families. And Jonathan worked diligently in therapy for the sake of his. He kept a journal, secured a sponsor, went back into meetings, read everything I recommended, and came in with thoughtful reactions to it all. Having grown up unattended to and unlistened to, it was as if we had unleashed a dammed-up river. I told Jon to write, and he wrote. I told him to pay attention to his dreams, and he kept a dream log. I told him to stop lashing out and instead to strive toward remembering his childhood, and Jonathan started coming unglued. Memory did not return to Jon, it rolled over him, gathering him up in a torrential flood.

He stepped up his therapy to twice a week—chain-smoking, hyper, not sleeping, refusing medication. "Fuck medication, man— pardon, my French," he swirled around me, one session. Somehow, I felt as though he were nervously pacing even though we were both sitting down. "I have spent my whole life afraid. Afraid to open the drawers. Afraid of the bogey man. Looking down the end of a bottle. Hitting my own wife." He begins to tear. "I mean, Carli's the best thing that ever happened to me. I know that. Hey, I'm an asshole but I'm not an idiot."

"Go on, Jon," I tell him.

"I want to *feel it*, man. I don't care if it sucks. I'm like a woman in labor—'Hey, don't give me no drugs. I'm goin' natural! Just don't hurt the baby!' "

For a few weeks, I worried that Jon was headed toward mania, but as the memories, and, more important, as the feelings began flooding in, his wild intensity deepened into grief.

"I feel like what therapy is—is you hold your hand in fire," he says, settling into the pain. "And you will yourself to not pull it out. You just keep it there for as long as you can. And then when you can't stand it anymore, you take a break until the next time."

"What are you feeling now as you say that?" I ask, pulling my chair next to him.

He shakes his head, turning inward.

"Jon?" I ask.

"I'm not sure I can go through with all this," he says quietly.

"You can stop it, Jon," I tell him. "Slow it down. You're at the wheel."

He shakes his head vehemently. "I know that," he says. "But I won't. Not anymore. This isn't a big martyr thing, just . . . It's true, I'm not sure I want to open up all these feelings. But I can't just shut them all off again. I can't do that to them. It's like, these feelings—this pain and all the rest of it—it's like they're my children. They're my little babies that never had a chance to speak and I can't shut them back up again. I can't do that."

Later, I ask, "How's your marriage these days?" glancing at Carli.

"It's better," she answers, looking at Jon.

"You getting any sleep?" I ask him.

"That's better, too—a little," Carli answers for him again, not patronizingly, more like a manager, the trainer taking questions ringside while the athlete catches his breath.

"And how's Elise?" I ask Jon.

"Hey," he smiles. "Check this out." He pulls out a folded piece of paper and hands it to me. In a child's crayon, a blossom of mixed colors: *a,b,c,d.,e,f,g* . . . and a little note: *I lov dad.*

"You keep that with you?" I ask him.

"Like a rosary, brother," he says.

I pat his shoulder. "You're a good man, Jon," I answer softly.

By equating pain and vulnerability with the repudiated and devalued "feminine," traditional socialization places boys and men in double jeopardy. First it requires a wholesale psychological excision, then it teaches men not to admit their ache, like the pain of an amputee, for the lost parts of themselves. It teaches men not to deal with their damage. But, to get to the Grail, a man must pass through the Wasteland. The path to the repudiated, hurt boy is a dark path through pain.

Just as the forces that push boys toward "masculinity" and the forces that push boys toward depression are inextricably bound to one another, so, too, recovery impels a collision, not just with depression, but also with the terms of masculinity itself. When a man reconsiders performance-based esteem, when he reaches into his own heart to unearth and form a relationship with the emotional parts of himself, when he takes on responsibilities for psychological self-care as well as the psychological care of others, he breaks with the terms of traditional masculinity. Today, men are often being asked to add these new challenges to the old "job description." And, with varying degrees of success, a great many men are attempting to change. For most, the hard work of adjusting to new role expectations is gradual and voluntary. But for overtly and covertly depressed men, the challenge of reconstructing masculinity, the terms they have lived by, is often immediate and necessary. When depression is at its most extreme, characterized by suicidality, severe substance abuse, or violence, reconfiguring the terms of masculinity can become a matter of life and death. Unresolved depression may represent a threat not just to the well-being of the man himself, but to those around him. "Those who cannot remember the past are condemned to repeat it," George Santayana wrote. Men who do not turn to face their own pain are too often prone to inflict it on others.

Therapists working with combat veterans have reported that when a man is subjected to trauma he sustains a double injury. The trauma itself is often compounded by the soldier's sense of having been "emasculated." To be a victim, overwhelmed by pain, is synonymous with being unmanned. The therapist must deal with both the injury and then with the further complication of the man's "crisis in masculinity."

Researcher David Lisak empirically tested the relationship between the traditional terms of masculinity and men's reactions to trauma. He gathered a sample of about two hundred fifty young men who admitted to a history of physical or sexual abuse as children and compared this group to a sample of men, matched in age and socioeconomic background, without such histories. The information he compiled regarding the men's attitudes about masculinity led him to hypothesize that, if it was indeed true that trauma threw men into crisis concerning their own manliness, then the traumatized group would show signs of "compensating" for their secret doubts about themselves. Lisak guessed that the traumatized group would salve their hidden insecurities with heightened fidelity to the traditional male role. They would be more rigidly "male"—more conservative, more homophobic, less willing to admit weakness. To his surprise, Lisak found that the group with abuse histories proved to be significantly less rigidly masculine than the control group of nonabused men—slightly less "macho," less traditional, less denying of "feminine" traits.

In search of a clearer understanding of his unexpected findings, Lisak began dividing the group of abused men by a number of variables. He divided the group by factors like age, race, social status, type of abuse they had suffered, and age at which the abuse had occurred. None of these factors yielded any significant data. Then he divided the group based on the subjects' self-reports concerning abusive behavior toward others. When Lisak applied this variable, the cohort, as if by magic, parted into two. Those abused men who reported becoming, at some point in their lives, offenders themselves, tested out as "hypermasculine," just as Lisak had supposed that they would. These offending men were profoundly traditional in their self-concepts and views, and highly intolerant of deviation in themselves or others.

Lisak's results were initially confusing because the other half of the cohort, the group of abused but nonabusing men, tested out as so far removed from conventional masculinity that they skewed the rest of the sample. These nonabusing men proved to be radically untraditional in both the ways that they envisioned themselves and in their concepts about the male role—far more unconventional than the cohort of "normal" controls. Lisak concluded from his data that trauma in men, even if experienced in childhood, does, as clinicians had suspected, pose a "crisis in masculinity." Lisak went on to suggest two distinct possible outcomes of that crisis. In one, the victim responds to feelings of unmanliness by "overcompensating," by clinging ever more strongly to traditional terms. Such men, the research suggests, may be dangerous. The coupling of an abused boy's unresolved hurt mixed with a grown man's power produces a volatile compound. In the other outcome of the crisis in masculinity, the men, rather than moving into shamed feelings of inadequacy, question the traditional terms of masculinity itself. Instead of raising the bridge, they divert the river. Having found themselves "unmanned," these men rewrite the criteria for manhood.

My reading of Lisak's research is that the group of abused and abusing men responded to their trauma with a preponderance of "identification with the aggressor." If I were to work with them clinically, I would look for covert depression, issues of false empowerment, and a pronounced, relatively violent, internal harsh child. By contrast, the group of abused but nonabusing men somehow managed—either by their own extraordinary efforts, with help from therapy, or by sheer force of grace—to rework the terms of masculinity. If I were to work clinically with these men, I would expect to see in them, along with whatever damage remained, some platform for a functioning internal adult. These men have resolved, at least to some degree, the issue of *empathic reversal* that lies at the heart of both trauma and depression. Somehow they were able to distance themselves from their abusers and to embrace parts of themselves that even the "normal" group of controls still held in some degree of contempt. I consider these men to be heroes. Lisak's conclusion resonates closely with my own. Since the interplay between shame and grandiosity is the dynamic linking trauma, depression, and gender, a man attempting to resolve either trauma or depression must confront and transform the legacy of masculinity itself. Conversely, a man who refuses to rework that legacy is prone to enact it.

The violence that abused boys absorb into their being acts like a storage battery, charged with the contempt and shamelessness of the boy's abuser. The harsh child also takes in the general force of contempt for the "feminine" that is rampant in our culture at large. The discharge of that stored contempt may be a danger to both the boy and to others. In study after study, traumatized boys are shown to "act out," becoming disruptive, rebellious, and physically assaultive. Boys on the receiving end of violence quickly learn to dish it out. Abused sons must come to grips with their trauma, either on their own or with help, if they are not to become abusive fathers. Contrary to the overwrought concerns about "family values," research clearly indicates that boys raised in healthy, loving families without fathers do not reveal appreciable signs of psychological ill health. Boys with abusive or neglectful fathers, on the other hand, are another matter. Too often, what fathers bequeath to their children is their own unacknowledged pain, and, in instances of violence, an entitlement to inflict it on others. The frightening reality that must be faced is that when a boy is emotionally or physically abused by his father, one avenue for obtaining closeness with him, for absolving the father and uniting with him, is to become him.

*   *   *

Tracy Deagen was one of the most violent men I have met outside the walls of a prison or an insane asylum. And, like all violent men, he was raised in violence. His father was that relatively rare breed of man known in psychiatry as "functionally psychotic." He went off to work each day, had friends of a sort, went to church. No one knew that he punished his children's petty infractions with strategically placed applications of scalding water, or by inflicting pain on their pets. No one suspected that the father insisted all of the children assist him in such "family discipline," forcing them to take turns holding one another down. People around the Deagens were unaware of all these things—until the children grew old enough to explode all over their little town.

I met Tracy in family therapy after his younger sister, Dori, was hospitalized. Dori had reacted to her mother's scheduled abdominal surgery by slicing open her own belly. After weeks in a medical unit, she was physically healed enough to be transferred to the psychiatric floor to which I consulted. Tracy's older brother, Will—upset, evidently, about his sister's hospitalization—broke into another local hospital, where he raped a nurse and stole narcotics.

Tracy, a beefy, baby-faced man in his early thirties, told me that, throughout his high school years, his favorite pastime was engaging in near homicidal roadside brawls. He would cruise the highway for a victim, the way a covertly depressed sex addict might cruise pickup joints—compulsively, on an almost daily basis. He frequently changed locales so as not to excite too much interest in any one police precinct. His routine was simple. He would deliberately drive like a madman until he managed to incite another driver. He would roll down his window, and begin trading insults. At the right moment, he would dare the other driver to the side of the road to "settle things like a man." Sometimes he had to cruise the streets for a whole day before he attracted a "taker." But he almost always found what he was looking for. The instant Tracy's "mark" stepped out onto the asphalt, Tracy beat him to a bloody pulp. Always. Then, he would drive home and wash up, sometimes wondering if he had killed the man. He told me in one session that he still wondered.

At first, I thought it abundantly clear that Tracy was symbolically killing, over and over again, the abusive father he was too frightened to oppose directly. But Tracy, a very bright man who could be chillingly lucid about actions he had little interest in stopping, told me that I was dead wrong. "When I was out there stompin' those guys," he corrects me, "I never felt so close to my father. It was the only time I felt at peace with him in my life."

"So, then," I ask, "who was it you were stomping out there on the highway?"

Tracy leans forward menacingly. "They were *pussies*, man. Every last one of them," he says. "Fuckin' fags. Limp motherfuckers. You see what I'm saying? I *liked* it. They *deserved* to bleed. Am I making you uncomfortable?" he asks me with glittering eyes.

"Do you mean to?" I answer, not budging.

"No." He smiles. "Not at all."

Tracy felt at peace with his father because, as he mercilessly beat up strangers, he could enjoy, for a brief moment, a kind of spiritual union with him. On the highway, Tracy became the omnipotent father, and his victims became the abused child he had learned to despise. Tracy had agreed to see me alone, after his sister was discharged, because of a recent incident that had disturbed even him. A few months before meeting me he had, in a fit of rage one afternoon, picked his four-year-old son up over his head. He had found himself about to hurl the boy across the room into a glass wall unit.

"The thing about it that scared me, man, was that the only reason I stopped was because I'd bust up the wall system. I mean, I spent a whole week putting up that system," Tracy told me.

I referred Tracy Deagen to a psychiatrist I worked with for medication and further treatment. At that point in my career, my issues of abuse and my feelings toward my own father were too unhealed for me to treat men as violent as Tracy. I was too revolted to be of use to him. Tracy went on medication, but he soon dropped out of treatment. My colleague and I reported him for suspected child abuse, as we were mandated to do. Tracy fled with his family to Canada, and we haven't heard of him since. I have no idea what happened to his son.

*　　　*　　　*

I do not know if I could be of any more help to Tracy Deagen today than I was almost twenty years ago. But at least I know what I would try. I now look to the one simple formula that runs through virtually all of my work with depressed men: to heal the dynamic of violence, one must repair one's relationship to the self, learn to reparent the self. One must bolster—or, in some cases, create—a platform of maturity, an internal adult. One must limit the aggression of the harsh child, and nurture, without indulgence, the emergence of the vulnerable boy. If a man will not accept the demanding challenge of "reengineering himself," as one patient put it, for his own sake, I ask if he would be willing to do it for the sake of his children. I never had the opportunity to offer Tracy Deagen that invitation, because I didn't know enough then even to formulate it. A few decades later, however, I was able to help another depressed man step out of the path of his father's footsteps.

Though neither as sick, nor as violent as Tracy's dad, Damian Ash's father flew into rages at him and his mother every time his business took a downturn. Jim Ash would find something wrong with his son and go after him. Margaret would insert herself between them, and the adults would fight viciously among themselves. After trying in vain to get them to stop, little Damian would eventually flee in search of someone else to be with.

Thirty years later, Damian's marriage looked frighteningly like his own parents'. In Wednesday night group, Damian succinctly described the emergency couples therapy session his wife had asked for the previous week. "Terry thinks that since I've been on the hot seat trying to sell my business, I've regressed to acting like an asshole again. Wouldn't you say that about sums it up?" he asks.

"Well . . ." I equivocate.

"Oh, c'mon," he says. "Who's kidding who? I'm acting just like my father. I know it. And the worst of it is, I've started to lose it in front of the kids. I don't give a shit anymore, really. I just get so caught up in it."

I suggest to Damian that he carry a picture of his children for one week in his breast pocket. When the anger starts sweeping over him, he is to go somewhere private, take out the picture, and stare at his kids' faces. He is to think about his father and the hurt and fear his father's rage caused in him. Then, staring directly into his children's eyes, he is to say, aloud: "I am giving myself license to act abusively just like my dad. I know this is going to really hurt you kids, but I really don't care. Indulging my anger is more important to me, right now, than you are." After saying that, he was to picture his father at his most repulsive and violent and say, again, out loud: "Dad, this one's for you!"

The following week, Damian reports to us that, though he is "still not exactly Mr. Pleasant," he has managed to contain his rage.

"Give me a percentage," I ask him.

"About not being angry?" he asks.

"About not acting like a jerk," I reply.

"Report on improvement," Damian answers in mock solemnity. "Feeling angry—ten percent better. Acting like an asshole—ninety percent better."

The other men clap their approval.

"Don't let that ten percent grab ya," tweaks Steven.

"Thanks, Dad," answers Doug.

"Welcome back from the brink," says Tom.

In containing his harsh child, Damian broke with the entitlement his father had demonstrated and pulled back from the edge of enacting harm. He learned to hold still long enough to identify his vulnerabilities, the feelings of fear, inadequacy, and shame that emerged as he faced the sale of his business. He even went so far as to learn how to ask his wife for comfort and support. In so doing, Damian began to manage both the aggressive and the insecure parts of himself.

Just as confronting the harsh child involves several generations, so, too, unearthing the lost relational, the vulnerable boy, is both a personal quest and also a drama that may span across generations. Henry Duvall cured his depression and released his four sons from its legacy when he uncovered the creative, lost boy that had been driven underground—not by Henry, or even by Henry's father, but by Henry's grandfather.

White-haired, diminutive, dressed in an expensive blue suit with a magenta shirt and a daring burgundy bow tie, Henry Duvall looks every inch like the well-known designer that he is. He leans forward, hands folded in his lap, eyebrows arched, and confides to me in his slow, thick Louisiana drawl.

"In a word," he breathes, "I believe I may be sufferin' from an unresolved Edifice Complex."

At sixty-three, after decades of staving off pain with a dazzling career and liberal amounts of alcohol, Henry's chronic, unacknowledged depression has reached up to immobilize him. He can barely function. Feeling tortured in his native Baton Rouge, Henry availed himself of what is known in psychiatry as "the geographic cure." But after an initial "high," changing cities had only made Henry feel worse.

"*To Carthage then I came, burning, burning, burning, burning,*" Henry quotes T. S. Eliot. He looks up at me, attentive. "I needed to plunge into this northern town," he says. "My body *thirsted* for it. I longed to hear the ring of cobblestones under my feet." The same cobblestones that Henry's father had traversed years before, until his father was, "like Macbeth from the womb, 'untimely ripped.' " Although he couldn't articulate it, the lost boy Henry Duvall burned for, the one he had come to Boston in search of, was not so much his own as the one that had been stolen from his father.

Per Duvall, Henry's grandfather, was a stern, pious figure—a shrewd businessman, a respected churchgoer, and, like Duvalls before him, a force in local politics. Those in Per's immediate circle were somewhat taken aback when Per, at the age of fifty-two, fell in love with and married a beauty from North Carolina. "Which," Henry explained, "back in those days, might as well have been Paris, France." Deirdre had, in fact, lived abroad and part of Per's adoration for her derived, despite himself, from the charm of her "cultivated" ways.

Per's family and friends warned him against his frivolous attachment, urging him instead to "marry plain," settle down with one of the "local girls." Nothing good would come of such "airs." And they proved to be right. Deirdre was a faithful wife and a model companion, a kind friend, a dedicated mother. She filled their one child, Nolen—"Noley," as everyone called him—with all of the art, music, and literature his little head could hold. Noley adored his beautiful, talented mother even more than his father did. Per, from a long line of bankers, was not the most expressive of men. It was not surprising that a woman of such a "high constitution," would divert some of her needs for affection into the close relationship with her child. No matter how sad or lonely Deirdre might be, Noley could always cheer her.

The first sign of disaster occurred when young Noley announced his intention to apply to Harvard University, declining to matriculate at the local college, which had served Duvall men of previous generations. Many difficult nights ensued before Noley, with quiet support from his mother, received his father's reluctant blessing. Early in the following year, Noley imprudently informed his parents in a letter that, "Stimulated by the intoxicating Atmosphere of Cambridge Society," he had "discovered himself as an Artist"—to be precise, a painter. Noley had no intentions of following in his father's business, nor any other business for that matter. He had felt compelled to let them know as soon as he could.

Without a moment's thought Per gathered a group of five other men, three of Noley's uncles and two friends. Wasting no time, this "posse," as Henry called them, swept into Boston and literally strongarmed young Noley back to Baton Rouge—where he had belonged all along, as far as they were concerned. Deirdre looked on helplessly as her son railed, despaired, and finally caved in.

Nolen Duvall never did graduate from college. He attempted a few desultory passes at the local school, but he did not do very well in them. He was the only Duvall man on record to fail in obtaining a degree of some kind. If that was an act of protest, it was Noley's last. He entered his father's bank and showed an unexpected aptitude for finance. Unlike his father, he married a local girl, "a thoroughly conventional, nice Southern woman." And, at the age of twenty-three, Noley lapsed into a chronic, rather mean state of grim depression.

"I can not recall my father once smiling," Henry tells me. "Or reading a book, or asking a question of me. He showed no interest in my upbringing whatsoever and precious little interest in anything or anyone else."

Noley died at fifty-eight, "for no particular reason anyone could ascertain." And, despite a few words to the contrary, it seemed fairly clear to Henry that his father's death came as no great loss to anyone other than, perhaps, Henry's grandmother, Deirdre. Noley's mother had stood with her grandson at Noley's funeral, squeezing Henry's hand, repeating over and over again: "Your father was simply too good for this world."

That had not been Henry's experience of him.

As Henry deluged me with fragments of poems and literary allusions, I was reminded of a poem myself, by Rilke, which I brought in one day to share with him. The poem is about a quest.

> Sometimes a man stands up during supper
> and walks outdoors, and keeps on walking,
> because of a church that stands somewhere in the East.
>
> And his children say blessings on him as if he were dead.
>
> And another man, who remains inside his own house,
> dies there, inside the dishes and the glasses,
> so that his children have to go far out into the world
> toward that same church, which he forgot.

Noley had psychologically died "inside the dishes and the glasses" of Baton Rouge and I suspected that Henry had come to Boston in an effort to revive him.

"How did you first become involved with art and design?" I ask Henry one session.

"Oh, I don't know," he replies. "The apocryphal tale in the family is that, as a young lad, I was playing out in the schoolyard one day and someone handed me a fat piece of chalk. Supposedly, instead of drawing a hopscotch board or some similar thing, I sketched the rough outlines of a cathedral." Henry shrugs, at once proud of the tale and at the same time disowning it.

"A cathedral," I wondered out loud, "or the towers of a university?"

At fifty-two, about the age Per had been when he fell in love with the exotic Deirdre, Henry Duvall "squandered the whole of my family's resources on what I thought at the time was a brilliant adventure."

Henry bought a building. "Well, it is rather more than a building," he allows. In fact, the old Victorian office building Henry purchased inhabited an entire city block. It is one of the few structures of its kind left standing anywhere in the world.

"I had always adored it," Henry told me. "It is far and away Baton Rouge's saving grace as far as I am concerned."

As a child, Henry spent hours, sketchpad in hand, drawing that building. These were some of the happiest moments in Henry's lonely childhood. "In many ways," Henry tells me, "that stupid building became my best friend. I mean, think of it. It was always there, utterly reliable. A neglected thing of beauty. I remember feeling about it that it relied upon my sensibility." Henry smiles, an utterly charming, self-deprecating man. "In a whirl of pathetic delusion, no doubt, I came to believe in my young heart that this damned building depended upon me."

When the inevitable developers threatened to tear the thing down, decades later, Henry, in a wild moment of spontaneity, dumped his entire family fortune into saving it. He bought it and spent six years lovingly restoring it with the help of his four teenage sons.

For six years, he and his family spent every spare moment in the building, which had become, in their affectionate vernacular, "Henry's Folly." They picnicked and partied in the building. Not uncommonly, in the midst of some tough assignment, Henry and the boys camped out in the building.

By the time Henry was approaching sixty, the boys were all grown and had gone off on their own. The real estate market plummeted to dizzying depths, and Henry's Folly had lost so much money that foreclosure seemed a near certainty. Henry Duvall sank into a despair that no amount of drinking or quarreling with his wife could distract him from. In his own eyes he was a failure, wasting a fortune it had taken generations to amass with one colossally stupid fiasco, robbing his children—whom he adored more than life itself—of the comfort and security that were rightfully theirs.

Antidepressant medication helped Henry a little, but a fresh perspective helped even more. Over the course of several months, Henry and I began to construct a different version of the story he had been telling himself these past few years. In the new version that gradually evolved, Henry was not a loser; he was a quester. And, in this new version he had not robbed his four sons. He had saved them.

"Tell me," I ask Henry one session. "What is the one thing in your life about which you are decidedly the most proud?"

"Oh," Henry answers without hesitation, "my boys. My four boys are far and away my greatest creation."

"Tell me about them," I ask.

"Well," Henry warms. "They are marvelous young men, all four of them. Each in his own way, mind you. All of them quite sensitive fellows . . ."

"Like their grandfather," I interject.

"Well . . ." Henry pauses. "As he might have been at one time, I suppose."

"Go on," I urge. "Tell me more about them."

Henry paints, in his usual elegant prose, vivid portraits of each of them. What all four sons have in common, I quickly learn, is art. Their years camped out together in the belly of Henry's Folly was not idle time. Each of Henry's sons, now all in their twenties, has become quite well recognized in his particular medium. Three of the boys have been awarded grants and the fourth is already showing in galleries.

"You don't get it, do you?" I marvel at Henry. "Even though I'm sure they've tried to tell you."

"I don't get what?" Henry asks, ever polite.

"That you gave this to them," I say. "Your passion; your daring. Your love of art."

"Well, I . . . " Henry begins.

"Where did they get it from?" I press. "Per?"

Henry Duvall and I begin a lengthy conversation concerning the uses of disaster. "There is a place," I inform him, "a dark wasteland a man has to cross if he is ever to get to the Grail."

"And you're saying I am in the Wasteland?" Henry asks.

"Oh, Henry." I smile. "You're more than in it. You purchased it."

Henry reciprocates by introducing me to the work of the brilliant photographer Diane Arbus, who succumbed to depression early in her career and took her own life.

"Arbus was drawn to 'freaks,' " Henry explains, showing me her work one session. Excited, energized, we stare down into the pages of the book like two detectives tracking a lead. "Siamese twins," Henry points out to me, "circus people—the 'deformed.' I once read an interview in which she was asked about her fascination with these faces. I will always remember what she said. She said that most of us live out our whole lives with a secret conviction that catastrophe lurks just round the corner. Do you know that feeling?" he asks.

I nod.

"The people she photographed," he continues, "have already had theirs. The disaster has come. It's all over. Arbus found these people liberated in some spiritual sense. Wise."

"You are wise, Henry," I tell him.

"Well, I . . ." he begins.

"No," I say. "It's true. Take it in. There's something attractive about sitting with you here, at ground zero. You know, you are like Oedipus," I tell him. "I know, you always joke about it, but you really are in that same postcatastrophic state as the subjects of these photographs. You are like Oedipus at the very end."

In a later session, we pursue the same theme. I remind Henry that Oedipus's story doesn't end with the play *Oedipus Rex*. "That's just where Freud finished the story, but it's not the real end. *Rex* is the middle play of a trilogy," I say. "In the final play, Oedipus is a saint. Blind, led by a young boy, he travels from place to place wherever there is famine or drought. And, wherever he goes, the land becomes fertile again. He is a hero, Henry. He went all the way down, like you. Spent it all. Like every great hero. He undoes himself, just as you did. But then he emerges again even more whole."

I sent Henry and his wife back to Baton Rouge to celebrate Henry's Folly. I suggested that he apologize to his sons for acting like a big failure these past years. He was to tell them that he had discovered he had done something in his life that Noley had not been capable of. He had thrown their family money into the winds and taught his sons, instead, to treasure their hearts.

Henry and his wife decided not to return from Baton Rouge. Henry took back the reins of the design firm he had left behind and, later that summer, Henry and his sons threw a huge tenth-year celebration for the building—their "last hurrah." In discussing the circumstances of the building's expected demise, one of Henry's cousins, a banker, hit on a novel scheme combining elements of funding for the building as an historical site with financing through floated bonds. So far, the plan seems to have worked. Like all great hero tales, Henry's has ended in victory.

Before he parted, I suggested that Henry visit his father's grave with his four sons. I asked him to introduce the boys to the grandfather none could remember, and paint their portraits to Noley as precisely and as lovingly as he had painted them to me. Then he was to introduce Noley to his grandchildren, one by one. Henry was to stress whatever positive legacy he could from his father and pass it on to his sons. If he could find it in his heart, he was to let go of his anger at his father, forgive him his limitations, and ask for Noley's blessing for himself, for his sons, and for their art. Henry promised to do this.

With typical panache, Henry Duvall sent me a two-sentence follow-up about six months after his departure for Baton Rouge. Henry's report to me consisted of one artfully mounted prescription for Zoloft—unfilled—along with the following note: *"Oedipus has returned, in triumph, to Thebes. Blessings to you and your family."*

Henry Duvall's depression dissolved when he began to see himself not as inadequate to the legacy of his father, but as transforming that legacy—when he rewrote the story of his descent from a tale of failure to a hero's journey. Many sons burdened with carried depression need to plunge into the heart of their own pain in order to find and confront not just their own, but their father's unacknowledged depression. Because male depression is so often a carried feeling, recovery frequently involves, or at least invokes, several generations of men. This pattern is suggested again and again in myth and in art. The hero descends, has a revivifying encounter with his haunted father, and transforms. Aeneas drops down into the underworld in search of his dead father, who tells him, in their fateful encounter, that Aeneas himself will father kings.

In the film *Field of Dreams*, a modern version of this common myth, Kevin Costner moves heaven and earth to encounter his father's lost vitality. Costner plows down a cornfield to make room for a baseball diamond, puts his home up for foreclosure, and follows the advice of a voice rising up out of the earth intoning, "If you build it, he will come." The "he" who comes to Costner in the film's closing scene is his own dead father, but not the old, caustic man he remembers. It is Costner's father as a young man, a new baseball player full of wild dreams. With the vulnerability of a child, Costner asks the apparition—"Hey, do you wanna play catch?" The ball tossed lightly between them passes like a symbol of redemption. The connection Costner establishes with his father's lost child heals an absence that had plagued him throughout the film. I call this unearthing and healing of the father's pain, in actuality or in imagination, *spiritually healing our fathers*. It is the work—done in the presence of the father if he is available, or, if not, on one's own—of rediscovering the vitality and relationality, the vulnerability, that the father has lost.

In the prototypical quest story, *The Quest for the Holy Grail*, Joseph of Arimathea, the Fisher King, lies bleeding. He has been injured by a lance in his groin—the place of generativity—and his lesions fester and rot. Half dead, half alive, he suffers while the kingdom around him decays. So, Thebes lies in ruin before young Oedipus. So, Denmark lies in ruin before young Hamlet. The young knight's quest begins with the wounds of the sick king, the father, the burden of toxic patrimony. It is up to the son to restore the lost life of his father. This is his task; what the quest is about.

As for most sons of depressed fathers, my profound, mad wish to heal my dad was fundamentally selfish. I wanted to restore him so that I might feel some relief from the burden of his pain inside me. I wanted to remove the lance from his groin to prevent it from festering in mine. This is true for many children, whether they know it or not. Most children of depressed parents wish to heal their parents in order to divest themselves of the carried feelings and shame which they have absorbed. And like Henry Duvall, the lost boy I yearned for had not been vanquished by my father, but by his.

I was not consciously aware of my longings to rescue my father. I was most aware of despising him—for his violence, certainly, but, more than that, for his ineffectiveness. I knew my father was a loser, and for that I held him in utter contempt. I imagined that when I despised my father for his incompetence in the world, I distinguished myself from him. I did not suspect that, in my very disdain, I was never more thoroughly like him. I judged my father in much the same way he judged his father before him. The raw emotions I thought were unique to me were, in fact, absorbed, unsettled energies from lives before mine. For my father the pettiest transaction with an uncooperative world could become a test of wills—an occasion to stage the drama of his angry victimization. I remember when I was in college, watching my father try to wrestle a pair of chairs into the trunk of my old beat-up car on a sweltering afternoon in late August.

"We'll just tie the trunk closed, Dad," I offered.

"Nonsense," he said, showing off, perhaps, for my school friends who'd gathered for a ride back to college with me. In the glare of the sun, Dad made us all stand around and watch for well over an hour while he struggled with his impossible task, cursing, bumping his head, pinching his fingers.

"Now, Edgar," my mom sighed when she finally came outside and put a stop to it.

"What's with the damned chairs?" one of my friends said pulling me aside.

"It's not the chairs," said another knowingly. "It's his manhood."

"Well, someone should tell him his manhood won't fit in the trunk," replied the first. "It's too big." We all laughed.

I glanced over at my father, sweating, his huge potbelly thrust forward. He seemed so wretched to me. That's how it always was between us. The more ridiculous and abusive he became, the more pathetic he seemed. While on the surface we met in direct antagonism, underneath, like an undertow, I felt the pull of his covert depression.

We are at my brother's house in Raleigh, North Carolina. I am in the first years of my new marriage to Belinda, a gutsy, soulful woman who came from a background as difficult as my own, and who dragged me from psychoanalytic work into family therapy and, later, into training with Pia Mellody. Belinda and I are both "retreads" together, psychological bootstrappers, up from the depths.

Cold blackness has been my companion for decades. Through my teens and twenties, my unwillingness to sit still inside that darkness drove me into drug abuse, wildly inappropriate relationships, risk taking, and petty crime. I have been married and divorced once, almost completed a doctoral program, driven cabs, written bad novels, and, finally, been washed up on the shore of psychotherapy—as both patient and trainee—just in time for my thirties. I did not have a job in which my earnings were higher than the official poverty line until I was thirty-one. Many of my old friends "in the scene" are either dead or in mental institutions. And yet, here I am, at thirty-seven, a long way from a time in which it wasn't clear whether I would survive. I have a career, a wife, and a child on the way—the first of our generation.

"Well, Dad," I say, showing him the ultrasound shot of his soon-to-be grandson, "are you excited about becoming a grandfather?"

"No." Dad cocks a supercilious eyebrow.

Stunned, although I should have known better, I pursue. "You mean you don't care about my having a child?"

"Not particularly," he dismisses me.

I can feel the blood rush up into my face. "That's a hell of a response, Dad," I begin.

He shrugs.

I turn on him. "Why not?" I say.

"Why not, what?" he asks, blandly.

I am shaking. "*Why* don't you care?"

He looks at me full in the face. "Why should I?"

"Because it's my son, you asshole," I tell him.

He looks beyond me, pauses. "What's one more bastard in the world?" he asks.

It takes all my restraint not to hit him. "Listen, you fool," I breathe, speaking quietly, my face pushed up against his. "You may think that you are a bastard. You may even think if you want that I'm a bastard. But my son *has* a father, do you understand? He has a father. And you will *never* use that language toward him again. Never. If he means that little to you, you don't have to see him. You or Mom. You think on it. You want to mess with me, you want to mess with Mom, so be it. But you will cherish this child or I won't let you within twenty feet of him, do you understand me?"

He returns my grimace, furious to be talked to this way. "Listen, you little snot," he begins.

"This conversation is over," I tell him.

He changes tacks, laughs. "Jesus, Terry, you're always so *sensitive.*"

"Yeah, Dad. I'm sensitive. Call my son a bastard and I get sensitive."

"Its just an expression, 'poor bastard.' You're always reading into things, making a problem—"

"Fuck you, Dad. You just think it over." And I slam out of the house.

It's cold outside. Late December. Not bitter, like Boston, but cold enough. I take a turn around the little pond in the park behind my brother's house and come back a half hour later, a little calmer. As I step through the door the tension in the house is palpable. My brother fusses with setting the table, angry, I imagine, that I have caused yet another family scene. Belinda shoots me a concerned look. My father and mother glance at each other. Something unspoken passes between them.

"Don't take off your coat," my father tells me, reaching into the closet. "Let's go for a walk."

I nod in agreement, wary, not sure what to do. This is the first time my father has ever asked to walk with me, the first time in recent memory he has asked me to do anything. We walk together around the pond, huddled against the damp chill.

"Here," he says, pointing to a stone bench overlooking the water. "Sit down."

I burrow deep into my jacket, hands in my pockets.

My father looks out at the water. Suddenly, I want a cigarette, to sit and smoke together like we used to do before we both gave it up. I hadn't wanted one in years. "Sometimes I say things I don't mean," he begins. "They don't come out the way that I intend them to."

I can't look at him. "Maybe you should think before you open your—"

"Listen," he says softly. "It would be better if you just listened."

I bite back the words, look out over the water, gray and condensed looking under December clouds, like slag.

"You kids have no idea what it was like back then. The Depression," he begins.

I want to tell him I have heard all this before, but the therapist in me knows to shut up and wait.

"When I say things I don't mean, rough things, I guess . . . it isn't that . . . I'm just . . ." He sighs. "I'm not like other people," he says. "I know that."

"What do you mean, Dad?" I ask.

"I know that people feel things I don't. They have needs I just don't seem to have. I'm just not much of a people person, I guess."

Hearing his words I smile to myself. *Not much of a people person.* I can hear my mother's influence in the phrase. "Do you really think you're so different?" I ask.

He nods. "Yes," he says. "Yes, I do." We look out at the water together for a while. "I know it makes me seem rough sometimes. Because I don't get it. I don't get people's feelings, sometimes. But, well, your mother's working on it."

"Like, what don't you get, Dad? I mean—"

He cuts me off abruptly. "When my mother died," he begins, awkwardly. I can tell he has rehearsed this, practiced saying it in his head. "When my mother died I was seven years old." He pauses. "A door shut inside me. I remember it. I can almost remember closing it. Anyway, from that time onward I never opened it again. Can you understand that, Terry? I would read things in books, novels and such, about falling in love, friendships. I know people feel that, but—"

"What about Mom?" I cut in.

"Oh, she feels a lot," he says.

"No, I mean. Did you not fall in love with her?"

He thinks for a while, weighing his loyalties. "I love your mother and you two boys more than I have ever loved anyone," he equivocates.

I look for a while out at the dead water. Its feels strange to be having this conversation with him at thirty-seven, to hear him finally admit things I have been trying my whole life to address. Imagining such a scene, I had always envisioned happiness. A bird calls out and I look up. A flock of geese fly overhead. Watching them, a torpid emptiness steals over me, a fatigue. "What was she like?" I ask my father.

"Who?" he asks.

"Your mother."

"Oh," he pauses, "I don't know." He answers slowly. "I barely remember."

"Do you remember anything?" I ask.

He concentrates. "I think she was nice," he tells me. "I mean, I've heard she was. Of course, one would hear that. But, I think she really was. Warm, they tell me." He looks at me, alarmed.

"Terry," he says, "why are you crying?"

"Just keep talking, Dad." I stare up at the geese.

He reaches in his pockets for tissues, but comes up short.

"Dad," I ask suddenly, realizing that after all these years of silence, I can ask him anything. "Dad, what was her name?"

"Her name?" he asks, startled. "I never told you?"

"No, Dad. You haven't talked about any of this," I say.

"Well, that's an exaggeration, Terry. I remember—"

"Dad," I interrupt.

He stops. Sighs. "Mathilde," he tells me. "I really think I must have told you. *Tobias* in Hebrew."

I stare at him. "Tobias," I say, startled. "She has my name."

He smiles at me, indulgently. "No, Terry," he says. "You have hers."

I am both pleased and taken aback at the thought of being the namesake of his dead mother. I burrow deeper into my jacket, resisting an impulse to tuck myself into his side for a hug like I used to when I was little. I am taller than he is now. I feel suddenly aware of the two of us, in public, sitting together. I am embarrassed by my tears.

"There's something else I want to tell you," my father says, rather grimly. "Your mother thinks I need to talk with you about this."

I wait. He clears his throat.

"You know, your grandfather and I, we never really got along very well."

I hadn't known that, particularly. I knew we never saw much of him, or my father's brother, Phil. But I never knew why.

My father looks out over the still water and squints, as if into the sun. "Something happened," he tells me.

I wait, afraid to speak, afraid to break the spell and send him back behind his wall of silence for another thirty years.

"Something bad," he says.

"Go on, Dad," I say softly.

"My father, Abe, was a weak man," he tells me. "A passive man. I hated that in him. I still do."

"What happened, Dad?" I urge him on.

"Well, you know we were all broken up," he answers, "the family. After my mother died, my father just went to pieces. He lost the store. He couldn't hold down a job. It was the Depression, Terry. I mean, people were starving around us. People were hungry. Do you know what it's like to be really hungry?" He sounds angry, as if I were at fault, but he catches himself. "We all went to Sylvie's, Aunt Sylvie, and then I got thrown out."

"Yes," I say. "I remember."

My father bends down to scoop up a twig in his meaty hands. He breaks it, absently, and breaks it again. "He never once tried to stand up for me," he says.

"Go on, Dad," I urge as he falters.

"I didn't want to tell you this before because we thought it important that you had a positive relationship with your grandparents, you understand?"

I nod.

"But, I guess you're old enough now." He pauses. We wait in silence for a minute or two. "One day when I was about nine or ten, Philip must have been six or seven . . . I don't know where Sylvie was, I honestly can't remember all of the details. Anyway, she must have been off somewhere or maybe he even arranged it that way, I don't know." He stops.

"Go on," I say, again.

"We were alone, the three of us," he continues. "And, he told me to get into Sylvie's car, that he would drive me back to Grandpa's, his father's, where I lived. I was surprised, because I always walked or rode the bus. But I got in. And he made Phil get in too, in the backseat. He told Phil to lie down and go to sleep. And he told me to close my eyes and rest, too. But I didn't. Something was wrong. I knew it right away. I could feel it."

I look into my father's face, but he is far from me.

"My father turned on the engine," he tells me, "the ignition of the car. And then, he put his arm around me and told me to rest. And that was that. That was all there was to it. Just that." He sums up a moment that altered his life. "I remember," Dad tells me, "he stared out the window, the windshield, and when I tried talking to him, he wouldn't answer. I think that was the most frightening part. The way he wouldn't answer. 'Shh,' he kept saying to me, like, 'Go to bed, shh.' When he wouldn't respond, I tried to get out, but he held me. He had his arm around my shoulders, like a hug. But he was strong, holding me down, not even looking at me." My father bends down to stare at the ground. I think he has begun to cry, but he hasn't. "When I felt him hold me down like that, I knew," he tells me. "Young as I was, I knew. He was going to kill me. He was going to kill us all. I could smell the gas by now. He must have plugged up the door in the garage, somehow. The whole place started to stink."

"What did you do?" I ask.

"I started screaming, to, like, wake him up," he answers. "Then, I started hitting him, beating him, really, kicking and biting—anything." He falls silent. "I don't remember much else, to be honest. I think I broke a window, broke it with my foot. I don't remember actually doing it, but I remember its being broken. And I got him to unlock the doors. I think the window roused him for a moment, and I got him to let us go."

"What did you do?" I asked.

"I grabbed Phil. That I remember. I knew I had to get us both out of there. Phil was scared. He was so little. I dragged him back with me to my grandfather's, carried him mostly. Phil was struggling with me and crying the whole time. He wanted to go back to Sylvie's. He wanted his father. Dad came and got him the next day. I wanted Phil to stay with me, but he wanted Dad, and they went back together." My father falls silent for a long time. Neither of us moves.

"I never spoke to my father again," he says quietly. "After that. I mean, 'Hi, How are ya? How's the weather?' That sort of thing, but never, really. Not like a father. Not like anyone. He was a stranger. Up to the day that he died."

"Did he ever try talking to you about it?" I ask.

My dad shakes his head. "Never," he says.

I want to put my arm around his shoulders, but something in him stops me. "What about Phil?" I ask.

"Phil doesn't remember. He doesn't want to hear it, either. I think he was mad at me because I wanted him to stay with me."

"You just wanted to protect him, Dad," I say.

"Yeah, well." He smiles. "I don't think he was old enough to understand that."

"And who knows what they said about you, back at Sylvie's." I say.

"I never went back to Sylvie's," he tells me. "After that day, I didn't want to. Phil and I . . . we kind of drifted. We never spoke much again either, to tell you the truth."

"You must have missed him, Dad," I say softly. "You must have missed your little brother."

My father bends his head and does not speak. Sitting beside one another on the stone bench, we share a moment of incredible softness, such as I had rarely known. I want to reach up and hug him. I want to kiss his cheek, but I am afraid he will flinch at my touch and, somehow, at that moment, I couldn't bear it if he did.

"I'm sorry, Dad," I say lamely.

"Your mother and Les and you," he says, hoarse, fighting back tears. "You're the most precious things to me. The most precious things. Don't let the way I talk fool you."

"Okay, Dad," I say.

We sit for a while, both of us equally at a loss. Then, without a word, we stand up. He pauses—maybe to embrace me or shake my hand. I can't tell what he wants.

"Let's go back," he says at last. "They'll be worried about us."

I follow him back into the house.

Sometimes it takes generations to heal.

When my father was about nine years old, just before the family split up, he got himself a paper route, a job grown men were fighting over. He woke up each morning at 4:45 and worked for two hours, always looking to expand his territory, always eager. After six or seven months, he had saved enough money to buy a used bicycle. He tried to persuade his father that this was not a frivolous purchase. On the bike, he could cover three times the territory he canvassed on foot. He could bring in more money for all of them. Abe forbade it and my strong-headed father went out one day and bought a bike anyway. In front of my father's eyes, Abe took a sledgehammer and smashed the bike into unrecognizability.

"Deliver papers on that!" my father remembers him saying when he was done.

By the time I reached high school, my means of self-medication—drugs and jazz and minor skirmishes with the law—took up so much of my attention that there was nothing left over for school. I was truant as often as not, skimming artfully, like a stealth bomber avoiding radar, as low to the ground of expulsion as possible without actually hitting it. My grades were far too poor for a real college, and so I did time for a year at Atlantic Community College. I pulled up my grades, and got accepted that spring to Rutgers, New Jersey's state university.

My father marched me down to the bank and loaded me up with as many school loans as they would give me.

"Can't start too early building a good credit rating," he told me.

Even though I was leveraged up to the hilt and had been offered a work-study scholarship at Rutgers, Dad got scared at the last minute that my going to college might cost him something, and he forbade it. A two-year school was good enough, he said. If I wanted more I could do it myself. I pointed out that I was doing Rutgers myself and then he pointed out that, judging from my academic performance over the years, it wasn't clear that I would be bright enough to handle a "real" college, anyway.

Shouting escalated to screaming and then to blows. I was already nineteen years old. It was the last time my father was physical with me. We punched each other a few times and then locked hands, wrestling on the floor, while my mother shrieked hysterically. I was crying. Fighting him, I felt like I was drowning in water, clawing for air. Drugs were getting the upper hand in my life and I vaguely knew it. A few of my friends had already died. I feared that if I didn't get out of Atlantic City, I might be joining them.

My father and I cursed and sweated through our violent embrace, gripping each other's hands like locked wrestlers, taking turns holding one another back from doing damage. At times, a wave of rage would pass through me and I would truly want to kill him, desperate to hurt him, while he bent back my fingers. Then the wave would pass through him and it was all I could do to protect myself. We rolled around like that, on the floor, Prometheus and his eagle, for a good half hour, and then, for no apparent reason, we just stopped. We picked ourselves up and stared at each other, our chests heaving, our faces red—pugnacious and bewildered. I stormed out of the house, out to the beach I always fled to. Out to my friends and their drugs. My wrists ached where they had been bent back. My breath felt coarse and raspy. But I knew I had won.

My parents dropped me off at my dorm at Rutgers the following September. I had cajoled my way into a single room, the height of luxury. A twenty- by eighteen-foot cinder block cell, spare enough for a monk, would be my new home. And from there, the world. I never went home again. I remember the thrill of my own bed, my own walls. I had made it out of Atlantic City. More than alive, I had escaped intact.

My mother kissed me and went out to the car. My father hung back to hand me an unexpected six hundred dollars.

"That's emergency money," he told me. "Don't spend it and call home in a jam. There's nothing left for you."

"Thanks, Dad." I hugged him.

My father stuck his hands in his trousers and looked around with satisfaction at my cinder block walls, his great potbelly protruding before him, as if swelling with pride. "A college man," he said, as though the whole thing had been his idea. "You're a real college man now."

I nodded happily, eager for him to leave.

"Remember this one piece of advice from the old man." He chucked me under the chin. "Keep your hands in your pockets and your pecker dry."

"Yes, Dad," I said, sunnily. To this day, I have no idea what he meant.

I watched my parents drive off in the rusted Chevy I had spent much of my high school years begging them to get rid of. My obese mother turned around to peer at me through the back window with her famous "million-dollar smile." I could see the sheen of sweat on her face through the glass and a salmon-colored kerchief trailing from her hand, bobbing up and down in farewell.

"I hate passivity, dependency!" my father had said that day on the bench near my brother's house. My father must have found some way to wall himself off from the fact that, abrasive and ineffectual, he had been fired from most of his jobs. It was my mother—obese, an utter baby at home, despised by us all—who kept the family going, first through her modest earnings as a nurse; then by becoming an administrator; finally, by running a 250-bed nursing home. My father hated dependency the way Brer Rabbit hated the brier patch. But he never knew it. He had about as much consciousness about these matters as a hit-and-run driver. My father overtly adopted a better-than position while he covertly played out a drama of increasing reliance on his wife. Ever arrogant, ever superior, he condescendingly projected the unacknowledged, hurt child in him onto others—most notably his wife and his kids. But he simultaneously acted out that unacknowledged thirst to be cared for in ways that grew more and more desperate. He switched from design to fine art, sold real estate, traded stock, gambled on the futures market with cash drawn from thirty different credit cards. In his later years, my father had no career, no money, no friends, no causes he believed in. His art had failed him, his financial schemes had failed him. And, in his late fifties, Lou Gehrig's disease, ALS, began its assault on the rest of him.

I don't know what force of violence my grandfather internalized to bring such oppression to bear on himself and his family. Abe was dead by the time I was old enough to have talked to him about it. But I know that the eagle of depression that gnawed at my soul went back at least two generations. The carried shame my father took in was so vast, so profound, that it compromised his capacity to succeed, to feel, to live at all. Although decades passed before he finally succumbed, one might say that my father never fully made it out of Abe's car that afternoon, that, from that day forward, he never quite granted himself permission to survive.

For reasons that are a matter of grace, I was filled, early on, with an impulse to turn and face the dark forces that took both these men down. For years, I walked alongside the edge of their abyss, but I never quite fell. Balance prevailed. I had an instinct not to follow in their footsteps.

As was true for my father and me, for Henry Duvall and his children, and for all of the men that I treat, recovery from overt and covert depression acts like a circuit breaker. Healing interrupts the legacy of depression's transmission from parent to child. Like the young knight who must find himself by bringing rest to an anguished king, depressed men, by healing themselves, bring peace to their ancestors and protection to their offspring. Sometimes, when tracking the history of a family that has suffered severe loss, political oppression, migration, or devastation, I can actually see in which generation the force of violence entered the family and began its rampage. More often, as in the case of my father and grandfather, violence gripped the family earlier than I can trace. In the sagas of grandfathers, grandmothers, uncles and aunts, depression's toll—alcoholism, failed relationships, violence—sweeps through the family like a fire in the woods.

The hero's journey is not for the benefit of the hero alone. It is for the benefit of his community. The monsters he slays, the trials he endures, are for the relief of the ills of his people. It is not a search for personal glory. It is a search for restoration. The path of recovery is a demanding one. Left to oneself, one might well shrink from it. But few of the depressed men I see are left to themselves. They have wives, partners, friends. And they have children. The challenge recovery from depression poses to them can seem frighteningly vast at times, but the stakes are very high.

My father never completed his quest. In the end, Abe's depression exacted its toll on them both. My father left it for me to bridge the violence he absorbed and the care—the assumption of basic trust—my own children now live by. Dad never made it over his prison wall. But he wanted me and my brother to. Even as I watched brutal passions pull him down, I understood that the best part of him wanted more than for his sons to survive. He wanted us to surpass him.

CHAPTER TEN

Crossing the Wasteland:
Healing Ourselves

With remarkable delicacy, Jeffrey Robinson propels his great bulk through my doorway, balanced on small dancer's feet. Decades ago, Jeffrey—now in his fifties and looking like a linebacker gone to fat—came close to winning a state championship in ballroom dancing. All that remains of his former passion is an indelible grace in his movements and a penchant for glove-leather shoes. Despite huge quantities of medication and several attempts at therapy, overt depression has drained away all the energy that once fueled Jeffrey's rumbas and tangos, pulling him into deep social isolation. It has been years since he dated anyone. He has very few friends, seen irregularly. No particular interests or hobbies. Jeffrey describes himself simply as "a machine." He works as an insurance broker in a large, well-respected firm where, for twenty-some years, he has been considered steadfast and reliable if not inspired. On evenings and weekends, he returns home and "unplugs"—a word he uses to describe his almost total paralysis.

"So, what do you do all day long?" I ask him. "Walk me through a typical Saturday."

Jeffrey looks up at me through thick glasses that make his blue eyes seem to float.

"But it's just like I've told you," he answers. "I don't do anything. I putter around the house. I nap sometimes. The day goes."

"And if I were to install myself in your house with a video camera?" I persist. "If I were to film you passing the day, what would the camera record?"

Jeffrey sighs, strained by the effort of having to think this hard. After staring at his folded hands for a moment, his head snaps up, and he stares at me decisively.

"I eat," he says, his jaw set. "That's what you'd see me doing all day. I sit in front of my TV set and I eat." He sounds furious.

"What are you feeling, right now?" I ask him.

"I hate it," he says.

"Go on," I prompt.

"You call this a life?" He turns from me. "It's embarrassing just to describe it."

"You're feeling some shame about it?" I ask.

"Oh, *please*," he snaps back.

"Well," I pursue. "Are you? Or anger?"

"I don't have any feelings," he almost shouts. "Don't you get it? Shame? Anger? That'd be a step up. I go to work. I go home. I'm like a battery on *charge*, like a recorder on *standby*. I'm in sleep mode. Then I go to work again and pretend to be alive for a while."

"You don't sound like someone with no feelings right now," I challenge. "You sound angry. Angry about what's happened to you."

"I'm just . . ." he looks at me. "I'm just . . ." And then he collapses. I watch it happen, watch the energy drain from him. He caves in like a rag doll.

"Jeffrey," I call to him. "Jeffrey, what just happened? It's like the wind just spilled out of your sail."

Jeffrey stares down at his lap, his folded hands, unable, or unwilling, to reply.

Jeffrey had a history of psychological injury, although, as is often the case, his trauma was passive and far from abject. Jeffrey's father died in a car accident when he was quite young and Jeffrey did not really remember him. Sally, his mother, managed to support them both on a combination of her husband's insurance and her earnings as a legal secretary. They were able to keep their big old Victorian house in Dorchester—the house Jeffrey still lives in.

Jeffrey remembers his mother with warmth and affection. She was funny, good-hearted, well liked by just about everyone—most of the time.

"What does that mean?" I ask. " 'Most of the time.' "

Hesitantly, Jeffrey recalls his mother at other times, odd, confusing instances.

"I wouldn't recall these at all," he tells me, "if it weren't for my previous therapies."

"Good," I answer. "What have you figured out?"

He shifts in his chair. "Well, I haven't figured anything out, exactly," he hedges. "But I have managed to recall a lot."

"A lot of what?" I pursue.

He looks up at me through his thick glasses. "A lot of her being strange," he says. "Mostly, she was great," he quickly adds. "Don't get me wrong."

"Okay," I assure him.

"But then there were these other things." He drifts off for a moment. "I used to wonder—with these other therapists—if she was, you know . . . mad."

"Oh," I breathe.

"If she had some sort of disorder, like, maybe, manic-depressive disease," he continues. "But, I think there may be a simpler explanation. I mean, whether that's true or not about being bipolar."

"Can you give me—" I begin.

"I think she was drinking," he continues, undaunted. "That's what I've started to think about it, in retrospect. I think that those times, those odd times when she acted so weird, she was drunk."

Jeffrey remembers the details. "I can tell you the first time I 'got it' that there was something wrong," he begins. "I must have been six, maybe seven."

"Go on," I say.

"We were in Woolworth's," Jeffrey recalls, shifting his large frame in his chair, absently patting the thinning, white hair that tops his square, ruddy face. "We used to go there every Thursday afternoon. 'Our little outing,' she would call it. It was sort of a big deal. She'd put me in this little blazer, you know. And we'd go sit at the luncheon counter at Woolworth's. I'd have a hot dog and an ice cream soda."

"It sounds nice," I venture.

Jeffrey nods. "Generally speaking," he agrees. "But then there was this one afternoon when, I remember, she got into this huge fight with the guy at the counter about my hot dog." Jeffrey smiles. "Like, my hot dog was burnt or something. It wasn't fit for me to eat. And she and this guy start going at it. She really starts yelling at this guy. I mean, looking back, I'm sure he was being stubborn, too. But, the point is, everyone was staring at us. The whole store. And I remember trying to pull her away, you know, like, '*Ma, shut up, already.*' Not that I actually said that, of course. But the thing of it is, the hot dog was fine. Honestly, it was no different from any other hot dog I've ever eaten."

"Do, you remember how you felt, Jeffrey?" I ask.

He creases his pant leg between thumb and forefinger. "Well, mostly embarrassed," he answers. "You know—someone come dig a hole and roll it up after me."

"Like, you wanted to disappear?" I ask.

"Umm," he nods.

"That sounds like more than embarrassment," I tell him. "Sounds like shame. Like you picked up her shame. We call that *carried feelings.*"

"Well, Jesus. I mean, it was a little *weird,*" he answers.

"It does sound confusing," I agree. "Do you remember being scared?"

He shakes his head. "Not scared, exactly," he answers. "More like, I don't know, just confused. Like, *Invasion of the Body Snatchers* kinda thing."

"Like: 'Where did she go?' " I say.

"Yeah," he agrees. "We'd be standing at a street corner and the light would turn green and she wouldn't move. Just stand there . . ."

"She was unplugged," I offer.

"I'd have to give her a poke or something. Get her started up again." As Jeffrey speaks, he becomes more animated than I've yet seen him.

"Did you ever try to talk to her about it?" I ask him.

"About the change in her?" he asks, and then leans back, smiling. "Yeah," he says. "Once."

Looking back to that one afternoon he dared confront his mother, Jeffrey now realizes that his mother was hosting a drinking party.

"Her girlfriends would come over for cards and stuff—this was early in the day, mind you. And, in hindsight, I guess, they must all have been passing the cup pretty good. They would get loud, lots of laughter. It was kind of nice, in a way. But my mother would get weird, the way she did. I remember . . ." he falters.

"Go on," I tell him.

"Well, there was this one time, I must have been eight or so. Not much older than the Woolworth's thing. I said, 'Ma, how come you're acting so funny?' " Jeffrey falls silent.

"And how did she respond?" I prompt.

"She didn't say anything," he recalls. "I think that's what got to me. She just whisked me right out of the house. Onto the front steps. And then she locked the door behind me."

"So much for confronting your mom," I say.

"I didn't know what hit me," he remembers, his voice sounding small. "I was out there all day, listening to them, Mom and her girlfriends. I was hysterical at first, but she just ignored me. After a while, I gave up."

"What did you do for food?" I was curious. "The bathroom?"

"I don't remember," he answers. "Peed in the bushes, I guess."

"Jeffrey," I ask. "Would you be willing to try a different kind of therapy format than what we've been using?"

"What do you mean?" he answers. "What do I have to do?"

After a brief explanation, Jeffrey agrees to close his eyes. "I want you to picture that little boy," I tell him. "Playing by himself on the front lawn."

"Why?" Jeffrey asks, without opening his eyes.

"I'm going to ask you to make contact with him," I answer.

Jeffrey sits bolt upright, looking straight at me. "No way!" he says.

"You have a strong reaction," I note.

"Forget it!"

"Okay, fine," I say, quickly, meaning it. "You're in control, Jeffrey. Can I just ask you—"

"I don't want to make contact with that child," he says, in a rush. "I put that kid behind me a *long* time ago."

"What are you feeling, now, Jeffrey?"

"I'm not feeling anything, and I'm not going to feel anything."

"Okay," I soothe. "It's good that you can—"

"I don't want to get within ten feet of that boy, is that clear enough?" he says.

"Couldn't be clearer," I answer.

"I *hate* that boy," Jeffrey mutters.

"Say what?" I ask.

"Nothing. Forget it," he answers.

"Say it, Jeffrey," I insist.

"I hate that boy," he repeats dutifully, like a ten-year-old.

I lean close to him. "Why?" I ask him.

"I just don't want it, that's all."

"Don't want what?" I ask. "What would you feel if you were to let it in?"

"I think I've had enough loneliness for one lifetime," he snaps at me, angry.

"Is that what it is?" I ask. "Is it loneliness that you would have to let in?"

Jeffrey folds his arms over his chest with a grunt and leans back in his chair, refusing to answer. We sit for a long time together, side by side. We stare, in silence, at the bland, soothing landscapes that hang on my wall. Clouds have come up during the session and my little office has grown dark. I should get up and turn on a lamp. But inertia locks me into my chair and I just sit there. Jeffrey feels pushed by me, I know, and he's angry about it. As our silence unfolds, I find myself softening toward him, becoming apologetic.

"It's just that your life," I say gently, "the way it is now. It already is so lonely."

"That's just the thing," he tells me. "Maybe it is lonely. I won't argue the point. But I don't feel it, understand? I don't have to feel the pain of it."

Softly, I ask, "Is that okay with you, Jeffrey? Is the life you're leading now really okay?"

He lets out one of his huge, burdened sighs.

"Jeffrey?" I ask again.

"That's it, isn't it?" he answers, defeated.

"That's what?" I ask.

"You either feel it or live it, right? The pain. Either feel it or live it. Isn't that what you're going to say to me?"

"I wish there were easier options," I tell him. "I really do."

Another sigh. "The thing of it is," Jeffrey tells me, "if I were to agree to do this, I would have to think there was an end to it. That I could get to the other side."

"I don't think your feelings will hurt you," I answer.

"Its not just that," he corrects me. "It's that, as a therapist, you think there's something worth having on the other end of all this. That there's another side to begin with. But I'm not convinced of that. You may have had your ups and downs, Terry. But you don't know what it's like to be without hope. That's the big difference between you and me."

I get up to turn on the little lamp perched on top of my filing cabinet. "We may not be as different as you think," I reply.

Like Dante and Virgil standing together on the broad plain of Hell, looking down into the concentric circles of the Inferno, Jeffrey Robinson and I perch on the rim of his personal wasteland. We speak, almost abstractly, like two merchants weighing an object for purchase, of the pros and cons of his possible descent, the hardest work of his life. Jeffrey and I are at one of the critical junctures in healing the depressed man's relationship to himself—the moment he decides to stop his flight and face his own condition. Once a man resolves to take up his hero's journey, real therapy can begin. Our descent occurs in three phases. First, the addictive defenses must stop. Then, the dysfunctional patterns in the man's relationship to himself must be attended to. Finally, buried early trauma must reemerge and, as much as possible, be released.

When a man relies on the defenses employed in covert depression, he places himself in the hazardous position of trying to ameliorate the pain of alienation in ways that leave him more alienated than he was at the start. For some, the covert defenses take on a life of their own, intensifying in a downward spiral. Other covertly depressed men, like Jeffrey, appear to stabilize in their misery.

Traditionally, emphasis is placed on the distinction between an abusive use of a substance and a true addiction. In my work with covertly depressed men, the distinction between abusive and addictive dependency means relatively little. Whenever a man turns to an external prop for self-esteem regulation, he is involved in the defensive structures of covert depression. Narcissus at his well is an addict. For simplicity's sake, I label dependency on any self-esteem "dialysis machine," addictive dependency. What I call addiction and what psychoanalytically oriented therapists would call a "self disorder" or a "narcissistic dependency" are synonymous.

There are some advantages to expanding the definition of addiction to include not only classically defined addictions per se, but also any form of external self-esteem regulation, and self-medication. This broad perspective on covert defenses allows me to scan for a host of "mild" compulsions that are generally seen as so trivial, or even as so laudable, that their role in disguising and stabilizing hidden depression is overlooked. Just about anything can be used as an addictive defense—spending, food, work, achievement, exercise, computer games. When a man with covert depression uses something we normally think of as benign, or even as positive, like work or exercise, it seems almost laughable to insist on questioning the function of that activity in his life. But ordinary activities used as a defense against depression can have wide-ranging consequences.

It took almost six months of seeing no improvement in Jeffrey's condition before it occurred to me to ask him what he imagined would happen if he agreed to eat sensibly and unplug his TV. Jeffrey experienced a mild anxiety attack within a few seconds of my simply posing the question. It took another four weeks before Jeffrey gathered the strength to consult a nutritionist, agree to an eating plan, and—armed with increased dosages of anti-anxiety medications—turn off his television. The initial depression and fear that rose up in him were so overwhelming, that, by the second day of the weekend, Jeffrey brought himself down to the local emergency room. His reaction was proof positive, as far as I was concerned, that we should hold off trying to treat his depression until we treated his addictive use of television and food.

Jeffrey's psychological and physiological "cold sweat withdrawal" was as real and frightening to him as any drug detox. But, with support from me and from a men's group he joined, Jeffrey persevered. The cure for the addictive defenses of covert depression is simple in theory, miserable to experience. All one need do to stop such defenses is decide to stop them—then, with ample support, withstand the withdrawal. Almost a year passed before Jeffrey stabilized in his newfound "sobriety." But within a few months of his commitment, movement appeared in areas of his life that had been frozen for decades. Jeffrey began working out. At his health club, he made a few friends. Through his friends, he signed up for an outdoor activity or two, then a class at the local adult education program. By the end of the year, Jeffrey had rediscovered cooking and hiking, and had begun again, despite embarrassment at his weight gain, to dance. For almost twenty years, Jeffrey's depression had defeated both him and the clinicians who tried to help him. It would have defeated us as well, had he not had the daring, one day, to unplug his defense rather than himself.

Jeffrey's disfunctionality was obvious. No one in his right mind would try to argue that Jeffrey's life, as it was, was successful. For many other men, however, the means of addictive defense are so close to our culture's "normal" expectations of masculinity, that, while I may see them as suffering, they see themselves as some of life's winners. These men have not had the good fortune to pass through catastrophe, as had Jeffrey, or Henry Duvall. These outwardly accomplished men, running from inward emptiness, often reap ever greater rewards from the culture the more out of touch they become. The more they acquire, the bigger their deals, the more society reinforces their performance-based esteem. The message that professionally successful, powerful, or wealthy men truly are better than others is ubiquitous. The false empowerment that often contributed to setting up these men's lonely drivenness becomes ratified by everyone around them, except, perhaps, those who must try to live with them. These modern Narcissuses mirror society's antirelational values. They frequently have little motivation to change, and the subtle cost to them is often outweighed by disastrous consequences to those around them.

At fifty-six, Russell Whiteston is at the top of his game. He has won national kudos as a pediatric orthopedist, having spearheaded new preventative measures that could improve the lives of thousands of children. He is a much sought after national lecturer, with a booming medical practice at home. He has more money than he knows what to do with, a lovely wife, five beautiful children, and a twenty-eight-year-old mistress. The delicate balance of Russell's demanding life was disrupted when his mistress, Georgina, left her husband in order to be available to marry Russ. Unfortunately, marrying Georgina would first require of Russ that he leave Diane, his current wife, and the three kids who still live at home with them. Russell has moved out of his house to think things over—although, judging by the hours he tells me he's keeping with Georgina, one wonders how much thinking he has time for.

In a private session, Russ implores me not to mistake him for one of those "middle-aged guys who make life decisions led by their genitals." His relationship with Georgina, he insists, is "a matter of the heart."

"What happened to the heart in your thirty-year marriage?" I ask him.

Russell confesses to having been unhappy in his marriage for years. Diane was not nearly as affectionate as he wished, their sex life not nearly as exciting. Over the years, their interests have diverged. Diane tells a slightly different story.

"When I first met Russell thirty-three years ago," she tells me, "I knew that he would always have another mistress—orthopedic surgery. And that was all right with me. I went into this with open eyes. But over the years it has completely consumed him."

For the past five years, Russ has worked every evening until eight or nine o'clock. And he has traveled almost every weekend. "If he is home for dinner one night in twelve," Diane tells me, "that's a lot."

If work has always been Russ's drug, the intoxication of his new-found celebrity has became his obsession. In meetings and conventions, on boards and programs, flying to important conferences all over the world, fighting (as he is the first to point out) the "good fight" for improved health in our children, Russ seems utterly unwilling to modulate the flood of performance-based esteem. He basks in his glory like a junkie with an unlimited supply. Meanwhile, his family life has completely corroded. Frustrated, helpless, and angry, Diane has transformed into a nagging, bitter woman. And Russell, almost sixty, surveying the wreckage his workaholism created, contemplates a course of action a number of well-off, middle-aged men seem to take—disposing of his wife. For the moment, Russ seems bent on trading Diane in for a young, adoring, willing new partner, a woman who works for him, travels with him, and who would be delighted to become the doctor's new wife.

Russ spreads his hands in a pleading gesture. "I'm tired of people trying to lay their guilt trips on me," he warns. "I have been a good boy all my life. Worked like a dog, raised five children. I never once cheated on my wife. And, believe me, the opportunity was there. But, here I am, fifty-six years old. Sure, I could go back into the marriage and put up with it, deal with her lack of affection, give up the companionship I feel with Georgina, the things we share, the excitement. But what have I got left? Fifteen years, eighteen years maybe? Don't I *deserve*, too? Do I have no *right* to be happy?"

I ask Russ if, over the course of thirty-one years, he ever voiced his dissatisfactions to Diane, ever talked about their sex life, ever told her he needed more affection. Did he address any issue or work in any way to better their marriage?

"Well . . ." he grows sheepish. "You know, I had other priorities."

Russell Whiteston doesn't know the first thing about cultivating and sustaining an intimate relationship. He let his marriage to Diane go to rot and now he drinks in the glow of his new infatuation. He is not disturbed by a thirty-year age difference between him and Georgina, nor does he worry that Georgina might not stand by him later when she is in her thirties and he faces his seventies. And the kicker is that, given the differences in his and Georgina's financial situations, their status, and resources, Russell may be right.

At this point, Russell has virtually no interest in improving his marriage. Between national praise at work and an exciting, compliant mistress, at home, he is thoroughly self-medicated. The fact that even now he suffers from high blood pressure, high cholesterol, gout, "a small ulcer," and monthly fits of black despair—none of which he will go into treatment for—is something he'd rather not "dwell upon." None of the men in Russell's family lived to be older than sixty-five. I do not expect he will be an exception.

There is so much societal tolerance for the defensive maneuvers that fragment Russell's family and wear down his own body and mind that the odds of turning him around seem virtually nonexistent. It has all gone on far too long in this family. I will do my best to see them through the transition, find support for Diane, counsel their children, and help them remain civilized. But unless Russ wakes up, my hands are tied. Treatment will be relegated to damage control. And I strongly suspect that his kids will face problems of their own when they hit young adulthood.

Those who do not turn to face their pain are prone to impose it. Russell Whiteston is not a bad man. In many ways he is a kind, decent man. He is just no one I would recommend getting close to.

The degree to which a man relies upon addictive defenses to ward off depression determines the degree of his abusiveness or irresponsibility toward others. A covertly depressed man cannot afford to be fully responsive to those around him because his primary need lies in maintaining his defense, his emotional "prosthesis." It is not uncommon for a man's need for performance-based esteem to become so compulsive that it not only gets in the way of his relationships, it even gets in the way of his performance.

Kyle Jarmine was a free-lance computer software engineer with all of the right qualifications to become a successful entrepreneur. He had gone to high-powered schools in both engineering and in business and was generally considered something just shy of a genius. Yet, by the time I first met him, Kyle's perfectionism had pulled him to the brink of bankruptcy. Repeatedly, he slaved on small projects, polishing them far beyond what was necessary to satisfy his customers, adopting, whether he knew it or not, a sly, supercilious attitude implying that he cared more about quality than did those who had hired him. Between his poor time allocation and implicit arrogance, Kyle was quickly running a promising business into the ground. Never quite realizing that he was upsetting his customers rather than impressing them, Kyle's primary relationship was not to their needs, but to his own prowess. Until he learned healthier forms of self-esteem, Kyle was on a collision course with his own insensitivity.

Like Narcissus's paralysis at the well, the defenses of covert depression dry up a man's capacity to respond to his environment. But, though the damage done in covert depression is most evident in a man's external relationships, the origin of his distress lies within. While Narcissus was incapable of loving another, the source of his incapacity lay in his lack of self-knowledge. What the defenses in covert depression medicate is the pain of the man's poor relationship to himself.

Edward Khantzian, the father of the *self-medication hypothesis*, speaks of addictions as attempts to "correct" for flaws in the user's ego capacities. In contrast to earlier psychiatric formulations of substance abuse as "sensation seeking," unconscious self-destruction, or obsession with pleasure, Khantzian and others currently writing on the psychology of addiction speak of substance abuse as a desperate strategy for dealing with self "dysregulation." Khantzian's research on both alcoholics and drug abusers led him to focus on four cardinal areas of dysregulation: difficulty in maintaining healthy self-esteem; difficulty in regulating one's feelings; difficulty in exercising self-care; and difficulty in sustaining connection to others. What Khantzian does not attempt to address is the connection between these impairments and the kinds of traumas, renunciations, and atrophied skills that lie at the heart of masculine socialization. Traditional socialization of boys diminishes the capacity to esteem the self without going up into grandiosity or down into shame. Traditional masculinization teaches boys to replace inherent self-worth with performance-based esteem. It insists that boys disown vulnerable feelings (which could help them connect), while reinforcing their entitlement to express anger. It teaches boys to renounce their true needs in the service of achievement, and at the same time blunts their sensitivity to reading the needs of others. The damage to self that Khantzian describes can be summed up as *damage in relatedness.* And if disconnection from self and others creates suffering, then learning and practicing the art of reconnection can relieve it.

The addictive defenses in covert depression must be quieted in order to gain access to a man's heart. Once he agrees to give up his armor, as Jeffrey was able to do, the next step lies in assessing and treating the man's connection to himself, his "self disorder." Since I see maturity ("ego functions," in psychiatric language) as a relationship between the man and himself, that relationship can be worked on directly just like any other relationship. Education and a few basic techniques help increase the man's capacity to esteem himself, set appropriate boundaries, identify and share his feelings. In imaginative work, the client forms a relationship with the immature parts of his personality—the two inner children. He learns to bring the strengthened "functional adult" part of him out to nurture and contain those younger aspects of self. In so doing, the dynamic of internalized violence is ameliorated. But the dramatic personifications of these multiple parts of the depressed man's psyche is only one aspect of bringing his relationship to self into recovery. Learning to bring the "functional adult" to bear on moments of immaturity is not a one-time ritual performed in my office. It is a practice the man must repeat each day of his life.

Jeffrey tells me in one session that every time he is turned down by a potential dance partner, he is flooded with shame. He feels old, fat, clumsy, and unappealing. Within seconds he regresses to the state of that eight-year-old boy standing on the other side of his mother's locked door. In times past, that hurt, vulnerable part of Jeffrey he could scarcely acknowledge would have driven him to flee from the dance floor, toward the comfort of food or television. Now Jeffrey has learned to access another part of his psyche, a more mature aspect of self, to both nurture and contain his immature impulses. I call such a healing instance a moment of *relational heroism*. Relational heroism occurs when every muscle and nerve in one's body pulls one toward reenacting one's usual dysfunctional pattern, but through sheer force of discipline or grace, one lifts oneself off the well-worn track toward behaviors that are more vulnerable, more cherishing, more mature. Just as the boyhood trauma that sets up depression occurs not in one dramatic incident, but in transactions repeated hundreds upon hundreds of times, so, too, recovery is comprised of countless small victories.

Each time Jonathan, instead of slapping his wife, Carli, in the presence of their four-year-old, Elise, pulls out the note his daughter wrote to him and uses it as a circuit breaker, quelling his rage, he engages in a moment of relational heroism. Each time Damian Ash looks at his kids' photographs and reminds himself not to lash out at his wife in the way he saw his father lash out at his mother, he is a relational hero. Each time Jeffrey Robinson feels the physical flood of agitation, depression, and shame sweep over his body but does not run from his dance class, he has learned to give to himself the functional parenting he never received. Such moments lie at the heart of the recovery process.

Jeffrey once teased me that our therapy felt like couples counseling between himself and himself. He threw out the line to tweak me, but, in truth, I felt flattered by it. How does a man like Jeffrey learn to do for himself what his parents could not? He learns from therapy and he learns from other men and women in recovery.

*   *   *

Thinking of maturity as a daily *practice* is a radical departure from traditional psychotherapy in which the man's difficulties in relating to himself is envisioned as *character pathology, ego dysfunction,* or *structural deficits.* His "developmental arrest" is seen as deeply embedded. Therapy is viewed as providing a "corrective emotional experience" via an intense relationship to the therapist. The therapist essentially reparents the patient, and the patient, over years of therapy, gradually internalizes new, benevolent "interjects" that modify his structural damage. Such a process is extremely labor intensive, often requiring several visits a week for many years.

Rather than attempt to reparent the depressed men I work with, I teach them how to reparent themselves. I do not see relational skills as static entities toward which one has a passive, helpless relationship. They are activities. Self-esteem, for example, is not something one *has;* it is something one *does.* And it is something one can learn to do better. I call this part of recovery work the *practice of relational maturity.* Treatment involves assessment, instruction, and exercise. First the man and I evaluate his strengths and weaknesses. Then I give him a few simple tools to use in work on himself. Finally, he goes off to practice and reports his progress for fine-tuning and for my support. My role is more that of a coach than that of a traditional, transference-based therapist. I tell the families I work with, only half facetiously, to think of me as their maturity and intimacy personal trainer.

Pia Mellody has devised a five-point grid that I find practical and comprehensive. It consists of five self functions: self-esteem, self-protection, self-knowledge, self-care, and self-moderation. Since I view these functions as operations rather than entities, the men I work with can be taught how to boost their level of skill in these areas. They can become relationally *fit.* Jeffrey has now learned a few simple techniques of self management to deal with those uncomfortable moments when he feels rejected and shame filled. Jeffrey can now close his eyes for a moment, breathe deeply, remind himself that, in his fifties, he is too old to be abandoned. He might imagine himself encircling that internal eight-year-old with his adult wisdom, nourishment, and love. "I am enough and I matter," he might repeat to himself, quieting his rising panic. "Whether I am accepted or rejected, right now, the person whose job it is to cherish me is me."

Men like Jeffrey learn the internal technology of first recognizing and then bringing themselves up from shame states; of recognizing and then bringing themselves down from grandiose states. The depressed man's relationship to self-esteem becomes proactive, as does his relationship to boundaries, getting in touch with his feelings, dependency, and moderation. In moments like the one Jeffrey describes, the depressed men I work with learn to do therapy on themselves, over and over again, seven days a week. Our work together doesn't transform them so much as give them concrete tools with which to transform themselves.

Treating covert depression is like peeling back the layers of an onion. Underneath the covertly depressed man's addictive defenses lies the pain of a faulty relationship to himself. And at the core of this self-disorder lies the unresolved pain of childhood trauma. Healing from depression unpeels these three layers in three phases: sobriety, the practice of relational maturity, and trauma release. Trauma release work generally occurs after the client has unplugged his addictive defenses and has enhanced his ego capacities to the point where he can manage the pain such release work inevitably unleashes. In trauma release work, the depressed man forms a relationship with both of the wounded, immature parts of him—the vulnerable child and the harsh child. He redresses the empathic reversal that rests at the core of his depression, identifying with the injured child and disidentifying with the aggressor. In a safe, supportive environment, he reexperiences the pain and the often extraordinary shame of traumatic interactions. Finally, he "gives back"—releases—the carried shame and carried feelings he internalized in such moments, extruding them, unburdening himself of them, often permanently.

*　　　*　　　*

"When you locked me out of the house"—eyes closed, Jeffrey Robinson addresses his imagined mother—"you shamed me. When you ignored my cries and my shouts, you implicitly *shamed* me. You told me by your actions that I was not worth attending to. You behaved shamelessly in your drunkenness, and I took in that shame. And I have felt depressed and unworthy for the rest of my life."

"Go on," I urge, my hand on his back.

"When you did that to me, Mother, I felt like I was disgusting. I felt like I *deserved* to be abandoned because I was so unlovable. And I have felt disgusting and unlovable ever since . . . every day of my life." Jeffrey begins to cry.

"Don't fight it, Jeffrey," I tell him.

"I am *tired* of feeling disgusting for you," he goes on. "I am *tired* of feeling unlovable, unworthy. It was *you* who were incapable of love at that moment, not *me!*"

"And about that I am angry," I coach.

"It's true," he says, back straight, deep in the reliving of the pain. "About that I am angry, Mother."

"Again," I say, "*louder.*"

"Mother, I am *angry,*" he says, with feeling. "I am *angry* for the sake of that little boy. I feel bad about your drinking. I wish you had done something about it. But I am still *angry* that you behaved like that to me. I don't *care* how drunk you were."

"I was a little boy," I coach.

"I was a little boy," Jeffrey tells his imagined mother.

"I was a precious, vulnerable little boy," I say.

"I was a precious, vulnerable . . . Ah, *Jesus!*" Jeffrey doubles over in pain and sobs. "*Jesus! Ah, Jesus!*" he cries.

"Let it go, Jeffrey," I soothe. "Just let it go."

Jeffrey Robinson remains on heavy dosages of medication. As our work progresses, as memory, and, later, feelings have returned to him, I have learned that the few "odd incidents" Jeffrey first recalled were hardly a few. They were the unacknowledged bulk of his childhood experience. Finally, Jeffrey has been able to talk to close family members about his mother's alcoholism.

Jeffrey may need to stay on medication for some time to come. The physiological consequences of his early, pervasive neglect may require chemical intervention for a few years, before his body will retrain itself, as it most often does. Even though Jeffrey must rely on medication, in terms of his capacity to function and enjoy life, and his connection to others and himself, his thirty-year depression is in full remission. First, he stopped the addictive defenses that stabilized his depression and held it in place. Second, he learned how to parent himself, nurture, guide, and contain himself, on a daily basis. Finally, he delved deep into his early darkness and released the introjected imagery, feelings, and shame he had taken in. Jeffrey Robinson is a hero. No less than Dante, Aeneas, Oedipus, he has descended. And he has emerged.

It is difficult to imagine how one could guide a path one has never taken. When I recall my own descent, I am flooded with gratitude for my Virgil, the one who went down beside me and kept me from harm as I now do for others. His name is Frank Paolito.

"I got stoned again, last night," I confess to my therapist. "I just couldn't help it."

"Pot?" Paolito asks.

I nod. "I know, in the way of things, it could be a lot worse. But, it keeps me up, now. Funny, it used to help me sleep, but now it just makes me agitated. And then the next day I'm so tired, so exhausted. It's already hard for me, doing this internship at the VA. It's already depressing. All those blasted men. What are you thinking?" I ask, suddenly, sharply.

Paolito shakes his head gently. "Nothing," he says. "Just listening."

"In another few days I'll—"

"Why?" Paolito interrupts. "Why did you ask, just then? Were you imagining something? Concerned about something?"

"About what you thought?" I ask.

"Hmm," he nods.

"Yeah. I guess. That you would be judging me," I say after a pause. "Junkie Terry, therapist-addict."

"Why would I think that?" he asks.

"Why wouldn't you?" I retort. "It's true."

Paolito smiles, the disheveled, crinkly smile I have grown so desirous and yet so afraid of. "Junkie Terry," he repeats. "That's *junk* as in *trash? Garbage?*"

I can feel the hot blush of pain rise to my face, but I staunchly hold back my tears.

"What are you feeling, now?" he asks, softly.

"Oh, you're too smart for me, Frank," I parry.

He leans almost imperceptibly forward. "Why would I judge you," he says, "for needing relief from the pain you carry inside?"

I find it harder to hold back my tears.

"Why would I feel anything, Terry? Except, perhaps, sad that you must do this to yourself?"

So it is with Paolito. Unlike the other therapists I had previously tried, and dropped in short order, Paolito—despite my numerous, clever invitations—refuses to engage with me in intellectual pirouettes. Like an immovable plumb line, he simply beams his affection for me, over and over again. And no matter how convoluted or complex I present myself as being to him, he simply smiles, a little wistfully, and loves me. I find the touch of his love excruciating.

"On the broad plain of Hell," I tell him one session, "where the unbaptized philosophers are, where Virgil himself resides, there is no torture. Who could torture Plato, Aristotle? But it is still Hell. While Dante speaks to the souls of the great thinkers, rain falls, and they flee in terror. Virgil explains to Dante that it is rain falling from Heaven and it burns the skin of the damned—even these great men—for the simple reason that they are not in Heaven and never will be. I feel your kindness toward me like that rain from Heaven, Paolito. It burns my skin."

"It's painful to let yourself trust," he answers with characteristic simplicity.

"It's painful to let myself feel anything at all," I reply.

*   *   *

A few months after my parents deposited me at Rutgers, when the thrill of my cinder block room and college sheets wore off, I had what would have been called in any decade other than the wild 1960s a nervous breakdown. Not unlike pudgy, disheveled Billy Jodein, the depression I had managed to hold at bay while I lived at home thoroughly overwhelmed me almost as soon as I escaped. I spent whole days in bed, paralyzed by depression, memorizing each crack in those cinder block walls. Every single day I contemplated suicide. At the end of each evening, I put myself to bed noting, almost ruefully, that I was still alive. Newfound friends and dorm mates are the ones I credit for my survival. They wanted to call my parents, but I wouldn't let them. They wanted to take me to the university hospital, but I wouldn't go. It's a wonder no one reported me to the school. Only in the anti-authoritarian sixties would they have tolerated my behavior as they did. My fellow students brought me food from the dining hall. They brought me notes from my reputed classes. They brought me—bless them— drugs to get me high.

That year was like being frozen in cold, except that I was frozen in pain. As in those nightmares when you can experience everything but you've lost control of your body, I remained lucid. In some ways, I have never felt as lucid before or since. My mind, like the world itself, felt crystalline, sharp, hard, and utterly devoid of warmth. It wasn't so much that I was paralyzed as that there was no longer any particular reason to move, to feed myself, to live at all. If I had been in the path of an oncoming car I probably would not have found the motivation to step out of the way.

And I loathed myself. I loathed myself for the state I was in. I loathed myself as an unlovable person. I felt there was something intrinsically monstrous about me, some rancid stink inside my soul that I had barely managed to cover over with the cheap perfume of my charm. I felt mostly dead and deserving of it. I had become an inanimate object to myself. I had somehow misplaced the knowledge that I was human.

A long, bleak winter finally became spring, and the empty, black frozenness that had encased me began, for no apparent reason, to break up like bits of ice. I did not know what had happened to me, and I did not know why it had stopped. It came one day, like thick cloud cover. And then, months later, it lifted. I only knew this: that nothing on God's earth would bring me voluntarily back to that place again.

And yet, here I was, years later, at thirty-one, letting this therapist coax me back into the pain. Frank Paolito was old enough, smart enough, and secure enough within himself to resist my seductive sparring. He cherished me. And he had one goal in mind—to help me learn how to cherish myself. I drank in his fondness for me, despite myself. And, like buried metal rising toward some huge, magnetic force, the pain I had spent my life running from broke the surface to greet his implacably benevolent gaze.

In college, my pain overwhelmed me, unbidden. This time, I let myself drop into it. I remember the morning I touched bottom. It was in about our third year of twice-a-week therapy. The depression I had run from most of my life, I was willing myself to allow, although the discomfort and fear I felt were almost unendurable. For a few weeks, we had been talking about medication, even, perhaps, a brief hospitalization. That day, I called in sick to my internship at the VA. I just couldn't handle being there. After hours in bed, I managed to drag myself into the shower. I could not stop crying. I knew, in this controlled implosion called therapy, that I was reliving the bleak aloneness I'd felt throughout most of my childhood. Imagining Paolito by my side, I resolved to allow my feelings to surface and wash over me. I have never felt so achingly alone and afraid. I remember staying in the shower as waves and waves of emotional pain rolled over me. "You can do this," I kept repeating to myself. "You can do this. Don't run."

I remember being angry. Angry at my own depression, angry at the pain itself. I think I was pumping myself up with anger in order to withstand the horrible, yawning emptiness. I don't know how long I stayed bent over in the shower, not feeling the freezing cold water running over me. But for the first time in my life, I was not afraid. And after a while, a long while, the pain began to subside of its own accord. I became aware of the cold water splashing over me. I felt a little restless, almost bored, crouched over for however long it was. I was aware, slowly, that my legs ached and that I must have been shivering. I turned off the water and dried myself off, just as anyone else would. I looked at the mirror and shaved. The natural process had, for the moment, run its course.

Depression freezes, but sadness flows. It has an end. The thing I had spent so much time avoiding had just swept through me—and I was fine. In the healing safety of Paolito's company, my covert depression had became overt. My overt depression had transmuted into grief. And grief, I would come to understand, is depression's cure. By empathizing with the wounded part of me, bolstering the adult part of me, and adroitly sidestepping even the slightest alliance with my internalized hatred, Paolito modeled for me the healing of the empathic reversal that lay at the heart of my covert depression. He taught me, through his example, to cherish my own vulnerability, and to quietly disregard internalized messages of self-contempt. I know that I owe him my life, just as many of the men I work with let me know that they owe me theirs. The chain of toxic injury can be matched by a chain of grace and restoration.

Depression is not really a feeling; it is a condition of numbness, of nonfeeling. In my work with depressed men, I differentiate between states and feelings. States are global, diffuse, impersonal. One's relationship to a state is passive, disembodied. A state of depression just drops over someone, like bad weather as it did with me when I was in college. And, most often, in six to eight months, with or without treatment, for reasons no one really understands, acute depression usually dissipates. The bad weather blows away.

Feelings, in contrast to states, are specific, anchored in the body of one's experience. Depression is a state. Sadness and anger are feelings. Anxiety is a state. Fear is a feeling. Intoxication is a state. Happiness is a feeling. One feels *about* something. Feelings are embedded in relationships; thus, when one feels something about a relationship, one can take relieving action. Emotions are signals that emerge from the context of our interactions.

The cure for states is feelings. As I discovered that day in the shower, unlike states, which tend to congeal, feelings will run their own course in due time. Despite the often expressed male fear that, if one were to let oneself cry, one would never stop, tears, in fact, eventually taper off if one lets them. Feelings are not endless, but our numbing attempts to avoid them can last a lifetime.

The essence of recovery lies in the art of bringing a learned and practiced maturity (the functional adult) into relationship with immature, injured aspects of the self (both the vulnerable child and the harsh child). By acknowledging trauma and by repudiating identification with the aggressor, the internalized dynamic of violence is mended; the frozen state of depression breaks up, and simple, healing grief thaws the heart. Researchers have begin to track the footprints of these processes of restoration in the neurophysiology of our brains. New research on the biology of trauma suggests that what I have been calling the inner children and the functional adult are, most likely, discrete circuits in our neurochemistries. Neurological research also seems to support, and to help explain, the curative action of recovery.

Appreciating the nature of trauma memory is key to understanding a depressed man's recovery process. In a way, trauma memory is not memory at all; it is a form of reliving. Jeffrey is flooded by a physiological surge when he is rebuffed on the dance floor. In that instant, he is not a fifty-year-old man remembering the feelings he experienced as an eight-year-old boy. For a brief moment, Jeffrey *becomes* that boy. He looks out at the world, at the person who rejects him, through the lens of that abandoned child. He is "in his wound," in his child ego state. The technical term for this phenomenon is *state dependent recall.* When the combat veteran who hears a firecracker spins around as if he had a gun in his hands, he is not remembering combat; he is back in it.

Bessel van der Kolk summarizes the current literature on trauma memories:

> Research has shown that under ordinary conditions many trau-
> matized people, including rape victims, battered women, and
> abused children have fairly good psychosocial adjustment. How-
> ever, they do not respond to stress in the way that other people do.
> Under pressure they may feel or act as if they were being trauma-
> tized all over again. Thus, high states of arousal seem selectively to
> promote retrieval of traumatic memories, sensory information, or
> behaviors associated with previous traumatic experiences. The ten-
> dency of traumatized organisms to revert to irrelevant emergency
> behaviors in response to minor stress has been well documented in
> animals as well.

In laboratory experiments involving thermal brain scanning, researchers were able to trace heightened limbic system activation when Vietnam veterans were shown pictures of combat twenty years after their tours of duty. Limbic system activity quieted again, and higher cortical functions reactivated, soon after the stimulus was removed and the subjects were asked to put their experience into words.

Current research indicates that traumatic experience may be stored in a different part of the brain from the higher cortical systems, which make sense of them. Several researchers have distinguished the two different circuits of memory, calling one the *explicit*, the other the *implicit* memory system. The implicit memory system stores habitual responses, physiological responses, and emotional associations. The explicit memory system is responsible for the recall of facts, verbalizations, and the construction of explanatory frames. To put it simply, the implicit memory system experiences, the explicit memory system knows and explains. A host of studies now indicate that they function as distinct neurophysiological pathways. Explicit memory involves the prefrontal cortex, whereas implicit memory involves the limbic system, particularly the amygdala and the hippocampus. What neurobiological researchers have learned from physiology is consistent with what I, and others, have learned from clinical experience. Recovery means bringing these two systems together. Van der Kolk writes:

> The goal of treating post traumatic stress disorder is to help people live in the present, without feeling or behaving according to irrelevant demands belonging to the past. Psychologically, this means that traumatic experiences need to be located in time and place and differentiated from current reality.

Van der Kolk goes on to say that, in traumatized people, the body's hyperaroused state may be too great to allow talking therapy alone to be effective. He recommends, and I agree, that clinicians should feel free to rely upon medication when needed to give patients a stable platform from which they can undertake the hard work of psychotherapy. The drugs of choice for treating post traumatic stress disorder should come as no surprise. They are Prozac and its family, the "serotonin reuptake inhibitors." Serotonin has been identified as a critical agent in helping the septohippocampal system delay the "fight or flight" state of emergency hyperarousal. Serotonin is the same chemical whose imbalance is implicated in overt depression, impulsive aggression, "antisocial personalities," obsessive-compulsive disorder, and possibly some addictions. Our knowledge about serotonin is relatively crude, but the one thing that seems tantalizingly clear is that the track of serotonin imbalance correlates, in some manner, to self-esteem, to trauma, and to depression—both overt and covert. Researchers like Bessel van der Kolk, Robert Golden, and H. M. Van Praag have called for a questioning of psychiatry's fundamental idea of discrete disease entities. New research on psychobiology points toward a cluster of possible disorders and symptoms, ranging from depression to anxiety to aggression, which share a physiological signature—serotonin imbalance. As for recovery, the Prozac family seems to approximate chemically some of what healing work accomplishes emotionally and cognitively. It helps quiet the implicit memory system and strengthen the explicit memory system, or, said differently, it helps decrease the intensity of the wounded internal children and bolster the skills of the functional adult.

*   *   *

The relationship between psychological trauma and depression has been central to developmental theory since Freud. And yet—since Freud's own portentous decision to disbelieve his patients' reports of abuse—psychoanalytic theory has rigidly minimized the actuality of interpersonal violence. Trauma, while central, remained an abstract phenomenon. Only recently have the actual process of trauma, its repercussions, and its healing left the drawing room of unsupported theory to be brought into the laboratory for systematic study. Several influences have combined to focus our attention on the actual, rather than the imagined, process of trauma and recovery. The feminist movement exposed the reality of domestic violence toward women, and, then, by extension, toward children, correcting—close to one hundred years later—Freud's fateful mistake. In a grassroots movement, thousands of Vietnam veterans demanded that the post traumatic stress disorder from which they and their comrades suffered be legitimized, understood, and treated. Then the addictions recovery movement broadened its focus from an exclusive concern for the addict and the alcoholic to a concern for his spouse and his children. After including issues of "codependency" as well as the consequences of having been raised in an alcoholic home, the recovery movement took on the issue of childhood trauma. Finally, the growing medicalization of the field of psychiatry generated systematic exploration of trauma's biological consequences.

While each of these four different groups—feminists, veterans, Alcoholics Anonymous, and psychobiologists—has widely divergent orientations and languages, and while there is no shortage of political tensions between them, many of their actual observations about and techniques for dealing with trauma are remarkably consistent. There is a noteworthy resonance, for example, between Khantzian's description of the underlying disorder of self that fuels addiction, Pia Melody's five-point grid for looking at maturity, and Bessel van der Kolk and Judith Herman's description of *complex post traumatic stress disorder,* which they see as involving "chronic affect dysregulation, destructive behavior against self and others, learning disabilities, dissociative problems, somatization, and distortions in concepts about self and others." At the center of all of these descriptions is pain. And at the heart of pain is the legacy of childhood trauma.

Recovery from covert depression must involve three layers—the addictive defense; the underlying relational immaturity or disorder of self; and the childhood trauma that set the whole process in motion. The pain—the depression that the covertly depressed man seeks to escape—results from all three of these phenonomena. Childhood trauma leads to disorders of self-regulation, which can either be felt as overt depression or warded off, acted out, as covert depression. The final factor to be considered in this equation is gender. Both the types of abuse and neglect from which children suffer and their characteristic ways of dealing with it are gender dependent. Girls are pushed inward, boys are pushed outward. Some of this directionality may be inherently biological, but most agree that the process is a complex web of nature and nurture. Healing the spectrum of disorders plaguing girls and women currently has, at its core, the renewed assertion of self. Healing for boys and men has, at its core, the skills of reconnection. Until a man has halted the acting out of his distress, dealt with his relationship to himself, and brought his mature self to acknowledge and deal with early wounds that remain very much alive within him, he will be inescapably impaired in his capacity to sustain a fully satisfying relationship. As Jeffrey Robinson did, as Henry Duvall did, as I did, a depressed man must first learn to cherish and take care of himself. Only then will he be equipped to value and care for others.

CHAPTER ELEVEN

Learning Intimacy:
Healing Our Relationships

Narcissus leans over his well. Longingly, he reaches out for the creature who, he imagines, inhabits the water. He learns quickly that any attempt to grasp hold of the "sprite" he desires only causes it to disappear. And so, Ovid tells us, he "contents himself with sighs." But it turns out that Narcissus is not alone. In the gentle spring air, his lamentations are repeated by another—over and over again. Narcissus's mythological double is the figure Echo. Just as Narcissus is punished for the hubris, the pride of withholding his love, Echo is punished for the hubris of her deceptions. Ovid tells us that Juno deprives her of speech and places her beside the very well over which her love, the disconsolate Narcissus, pines. Ovid writes:

> Each time he cries, "Ah, me!" the nymph repeats
> "Ah me!"; and when he flails his arms and beats
> his shoulders, she repeats that hammering.
> His final words at the familiar pool
> when once he gazed into the waves,
> were these: "Dear boy, the one I loved in vain!"
> And what he said resounded in that place.
> And when he cried "Farewell! Farewell!" was just
> what Echo mimed.

Narcissus is so far removed from innate feeling, from authentic internal sensation, that he does not even recognize his own face.

Instead of the capacity to experience himself from the inside out, he seeks a desperate union with an external source of abundance, which he thinks will complete him. The price of his delusion is death. Unable to eat or sleep, like a severe addict in the final stages of obsession he wastes. With no capacity to speak her own words, Echo records and reiterates Narcissus's every sigh. If he is a reflection, she is the reflection of his reflection, the shadow of his shadow. Narcissus loses sensation, and the result is fatal paralysis. Echo loses her voice, and the result is also paralysis. Neither is capable of authentic relationship.

Like Narcissus and Echo, many of the relationships between depressed men and their spouses represent not an aberration but an exaggeration of the cultural norms for men and women. The same gender bifurcation that deprives men of their hearts deprives women of their voices, setting up a culturally sanctioned pas de deux in which the man's covert depression, his dependency on self-esteem props, is matched by his spouse's protectiveness, her often resentful dependency on him. Whenever this traditional quid pro quo unravels, the relationship, and sometimes the man himself, is thrown into crisis. It is often at such a juncture that I first meet him. Joe Hannigan's wife, for example, chose to confront her husband's depression, rather than try to protect him from it. And Barbara Hannigan's boldness triggered a crisis in Joe that was nearly fatal. I first met Joe the day after his six-year-old daughter nudged him back from the brink of suicide.

With his six-three frame and broad, ruddy face, Joseph Hannigan was as South Boston Irish as boiled dinner and just about that tough. A construction manager for a few of the larger commercial banks in New England, Joe was known as someone who could bring a job in on time and under budget despite union upsets and material shortfalls. He was a stocky, plain man, someone you would want by your side in an emergency. A few days before I first met him, Joe had spent his afternoon conducting a site inspection somewhere in the western part of the state. Afterward, he checked into the fanciest hotel in the area, chatted on the phone with his wife, typed a few last-minute notes on his laptop, and then lined up the 183 pills he had stockpiled for the last seven months. Arranging the pills in long, neat rows, Joe poured himself a tumbler full of Scotch to wash them down. At that point, the phone rang. It was six-year-old Allie, miffed that her father had said good night to Mom but not to her. And, by the way, she added, now that she had him on the phone, he *did* remember her school assembly on Friday, didn't he? The one in which she was slated to sing? He *was* planning on being there, wasn't he?

It had taken Joe months to work up his nerve for this date, and now here he was, outflanked by a first grader. Obviously, he could not tell her the truth. And he was far too decent a guy to tolerate the idea that the last thing he would say to his daughter would be a promise he never intended to keep.

"Dad?" Allie insisted.

Joe sighed. Of course he would be there, he reassured her. Joe later told me that in speaking that one sentence, he felt as if he were letting back into his being the whole of his life. He did not welcome the experience. He did not feel relieved. He felt obstructed.

Joe Hannigan sat on the edge of his hotel bed and sipped his tall Scotch for a long time, looking out over the lights of Springfield. After hours of drinking and staring, he finally decided that if he wasn't going to lie down and let depression roll over him—which was still his first choice—then he would just have to stand up and find some way to beat it back. He'd be damned if he was going to live as he had been living any longer. Joe picked up the phone and called a friend who called a friend who knew me.

Joe Hannigan's overt depression was a harvest reaped from a lifetime's reliance on performance-based esteem. Psychologically, Joe had been "the man of the house" since about the age of six or seven. Joe's father, William Hannigan, a first-generation Irish-American, had clawed his way up from the confines of his South Boston neighborhood, where he had begun as a laborer. Bill had started his own small construction company and he had done well enough to support himself and his family. He had done, as Joe put it, "an honest day's job." What made Bill's modest success seem remarkable was the depth of overt depression he waded through most of his days: Bill's "Black Irish," Joe's mother had called it. "Ah," she would sigh, "your Dad's Black Irish is bad today."

Joe remembered that there had been times, like after the death of Bill's father, when the "Black Irish" completely got the better of him. Times when his father would retire to bed, unable to sleep, and yet unable to eat or to rouse himself. But these periods were relatively short-lived. Mostly, Bill managed to drag himself out of bed in the morning, make it through his workday, and pull himself home, where he would collapse into the indulgent arms of the women—Joe's mother and aunts—who enfolded him in fluffed pillows, strong tea, and euphemisms.

"The only thing no one did for my father," Joe told me in one session, "was to ask him what he was so goddamned sad about to begin with."

Although she rarely let it show, it was a lonely life for Laureen, Joe's mother, and Joe, the oldest and still the most sensitive of the three boys, stepped into the breach as his mother's confidant, comfort, and friend. He told me that, as early as six or seven, he remembered "feeling sorry" for both of his parents. Like many falsely empowered children, Joe was more tuned in to his caretaker's feelings than to his own. And, as he grew up, Joe took on more and more paternal functions within the family. He cheered his dad, comforted his mom, and cared for, even disciplined, his younger brothers and sisters. Precocious Joe listened sympathetically to his mother's worries. He absorbed, as if through a permeable membrane, both of his parents' sadness. By the time Joe had reached his early teens, he was already working in his father's company. And, showing a keen sense of business acumen, he soon took over much of its day-to-day operations—to his father's great relief.

While William Hannigan had not made millions, his son did—at least for a time. Joe tells me he is happy that his father died of cancer while Hannigan Construction was still booming, in the early eighties. When the New England recession hit, years later, the construction business froze, and Joe was forced to sell off the company in chunks to pay the government, banks, and creditors. In his mid-forties, Joe had watched his life's work, and the work of his father, be carted off piece by piece.

Now, in his early fifties, Joe has tried to accommodate to the overt depression that has become his companion since the loss of his business. He has not adjusted well. The little pink tablets Joe had lined up into neat rows were Paxil, a Prozac-type antidepressant. They have not helped much. Neither have Joe's desultory attempts at therapy. Like his father before him, Joe manages to drag himself through his workday, only to collapse at home. It is as if, in penance for losing the company and "betraying" his dad, Joe has sentenced himself to become him.

"Even now, I'm not sure why I didn't go through with it," Joe confesses to me in our first telephone conversation.

"Why didn't you?" I take him up on the question.

"For Allie, I guess. My kid," he answers.

"And your wife?"

He pauses. "When can I see you?" he answers.

I tell Joe I can make room for him later that afternoon, but only on the condition that he come in with his wife.

He pauses again, annoyed. "Why?" he challenges.

"Have you told her about last night?" I guess.

Another pause. "I don't want to upset her." Joe sighs. Holding the phone away from my mouth, so do I. "Now, here is a guy," I think to myself, "who not eighteen hours ago was ready to desert his wife and child forever. But today he is afraid to upset her."

"I'll need to see you both," I reiterate.

Reluctantly, Joe agrees. We set up the appointment.

In an expensive plum wool suit, with long legs and cascading black hair, Barbara strides into my office looking burnished, handsome, and enraged. Between her good looks, obvious intelligence, and radiant contempt, I can see why a man might have trouble facing her.

"Let's get to the point." She quickly seizes control of the meeting. "I am absolutely furious with this man. Doctor—"

"Call me Terry," I begin, warmly.

"Whatever." She brushes it aside. "Listen. I am no stranger to depression myself. Like Joe, I have been on medication for years, right?" She casts a baleful eye at her husband, who nods almost imperceptibly, squeezing out the tiniest possible gesture of assent.

I squint at him. "Was that a 'yes'?" I ask him.

"Oh, *definitely.*" He smiles broadly at me, needling her.

I hold Joe's beaming gaze for a moment. In her chair, Barbara fumes. Joe smiles up at her provocatively. The hatred between them is palpable. Their rageful struggle—his seemingly passive, hers active—had such a grip on them both that Joe's near suicide—though real enough, I had no doubt—might be as much a move in their game as it was the result of his depression.

"Well, Joe?" she tries again. "Medication? Hello? Joe? Am I right?" Barbara's voice notches up a level.

Joe just smiles, staring intently at a chaotic pile of paper on my desk. "Say whatever you need to, Barbara." He thoroughly dismisses her.

Barbara exhales, crosses her arms, and leans back in her chair. We wait.

"Do you want to go on?" I finally ask her.

She shakes her head, her eyes filling up.

I hand her a box of tissues. "Can you say why you're crying?" I ask. Again, the head shake.

"She's pissed," Joe finally speaks. "I think she's so mad that I almost did it, at this point she's probably disappointed that I didn't."

That gets to her. She turns so swiftly that I think she's about to hit him—or bolt out of the room. Instead she says, "Right, Joe! I want you dead. That's the kind of *bitch* I am! I'm so *mean!* That's why I got pregnant again. Just because I hate you so much."

"Pregnant?" I venture.

"Every woman lets her husband knock her up before she offs him," Barbara continues.

"*Offs* him?" I ask.

"No, Joe"—Barbara ignores me—"I want you *alive.* I want to see you *suffer.* I want you to know just how it feels when I walk out on you. And the kids, too, Joe, both of them."

"You just try and take those kids, Barbara, and I—"

"Excuse me," I cut in, vying for their attention. "How long has this been going on?"

They both look at me, blankly. "What?" Joe asks.

"Mutual, escalating hatred," I pronounce each word slowly.

For a brief moment, they uncoil, sheepish like chastened kids, but it doesn't last long.

"I didn't really *do* it," Joe tells her out of the corner of his mouth, squinting up at me, like a kid with a homeroom monitor.

"Oh, Joe. *Joe.*" Barbara finally lets go. She begins to sob. All of the tension that she must have held in since she first heard the news releases. "You stupid, *stupid* man," she says, crying. "You *almost* did, didn't you? Don't you think *almost* should count? You didn't stop because of *me,*" she chokes out between tears. "It wasn't for *me!*"

"It wasn't about you, darling, one way or the other," Joe tries to comfort her.

Barbara doubles over in pain, deep, wracking sobs. When she can talk, she sits up. Her face is a mess. "Jesus, Joe!" she says at last. "Leave me alone with two kids—with your *child* growing inside me—but it's not about me. It's not about me?" She stares at him, suddenly bitter. "Why don't you take some *fucking* responsibility?" she growls.

I watch Joe harden, his jaw clamped down tight as he stares off into some middle distance. No doubt he has heard these words before.

"And don't you tell me that I hate him." Barbara turns on me.

"I'm *tired* of hearing how hateful I am. *You* live with him. See how much you love him." I clear my throat, about to say something, but she just continues. "I wish I *could* hate him, goddamn it," she says. "It would make my life easier if I could. *That's* the damn problem!" She blows her nose, wipes her eyes. Mascara drips down both her cheeks in dark, ragged splotches. Joe hands her more tissues. As she fusses, he softens. His gaze toward her warms. In her tailored clothes and perfect red nails, with wads of soggy Kleenex in her hand, Barbara looks endearingly undone. "Son of a bitch," she glances at her husband, who dares a slight, kind smile. "Son of a bitch," she mutters again, but it is clear that her rage is losing steam. Trying to stay angry, she stares at Joe, who gazes at her tenderly. She blows her nose again—a real honker. Despite themselves, they both laugh.

If they had never had kids, they probably would have survived. If the business hadn't fallen apart, they might even have been happy. In her twenties and early thirties, Barbara's depression had been severe at times, only recently abating with the help of a new generation of drugs and years of hard work in therapy. Her first pregnancy, however, had temporarily forced her off drugs. To her surprise, Barbara had made it through that period fairly well, but she had been frightened to death, needing desperately to lean on Joe. He had reacted to her increased dependency and to the responsibility of his first child by becoming more vehemently depressed than ever. Barbara could not help feeling that it was as if, consciously or not, when faced with inescapable family demands, Joe had almost willfully "out-depressed" her.

"Can you *imagine* what it was like?" she asks me in a later session. "Here I am, faced with my first baby. Scared out of my mind. Off medication. Sleep deprived. Trying to breast-feed. And having to meet Joe at his doctor's to discuss *his* possible hospitalization?"

"It wasn't a game," Joe meekly protests.

"It wasn't serious enough for you to get into real therapy *either*, Joe," she snaps back.

"Talking therapy doesn't help me," Joe tries.

"It would have helped *me*," Barbara answers. "If you'd gone into therapy it would have helped *me*. C'mon, Joe! If I'd been in your position, I would have gone to fucking faith healers. I *did* go to faith healers, well, naturopaths. You could have done *more*."

Joe shrugs, as if to say, *I did what I could.*

Having barely succeeded in righting themselves after the near disaster of Barbara's first pregnancy, they had courageously decided to have another child. Despite his best efforts Joe found himself sucked down once again into depression. Only now, it was compounded by his fear of Barbara. While Joe may have come to inhabit his father's role, a generation had passed between Joe's mother and his wife. Barbara had no interest in suffering in martyred silence as Laureen had. She'd made it clear that, as hardhearted as it might seem, if Joe slipped away again, as he had during the pregnancy with Allie, she would leave him.

Joe believed Barbara. Feeling powerless in the face of increasing despair, he was petrified of the inevitable showdown between them. In a convulsion of hurt, shame, and anger, he had come close to abandoning Barbara that night in his hotel room before she had a chance to abandon him. It was a sad, high-stakes game they were playing, and their children were due to pay the price if nothing intervened to stop them.

Over the years, Joe had tried cognitive, behavioral, and group therapies but without much success. None of the previous therapies had included Barbara or had placed Joe's depression in the context of his current relationships. I believed Joe when he told me that prior treatments for depression had all failed. And so we agreed not to treat Joe's depression. Much to Barbara's amusement, we contracted, instead, to treat Joe's false empowerment—the consequences of his grandiosity, his performance-based esteem, and his male privilege. Our contract began with the dishes.

*　　　*　　　*

As Barbara described it, Joe hadn't concerned himself with a dish in the house for years except to ask what she had in mind to put on it. Joe feebly protested. But even he could not recall the last time he had actually washed one. He was working upward of fifty hours a week, he explained, while Barbara was at home—

"Eating bonbons and doing my nails," she cut in.

"Here's the deal." I turn to Joe. "You have a couple of possibilities. One, you could finish the job you began a few days ago and kill yourself. Two, you could hang out as you are and let Barbara leave you. Three, you can stand up to this thing and start to push back. Which do you want?"

"I've been trying to fight this thing all along," Joe complains. "I thought that's what I already was doing."

"Well, let's see," I answer. "Let's start with the influence depression has come to exert on your life. Let's take a look at some of the things depression has taken from you. And let's see how it manages to do that."

Together, Joe and I begin to map out depression's influence, the tactics it uses to maintain its assault on his life. As our conversation unfolds, depression begins to take on character; it becomes a personified force, a cruel denominator intent on sucking the life out of him, as it had his father before him. This is a technique called "externalizing." Instead of locating the problem inside the man, making him a bad or defective person, I help the man relocate the problem as an attack from without. He can then chose to join with me, if he wants, to stand up and beat the enemy back.

Like a lot of experienced therapy veterans, Joe believed that once he "understood" his depression, his behaviors would transform for the better of their own accord. A common belief is that once the therapist and the client "resolve" the issue, then, the client is "freed up" to change his life. The problem was that, try though he might, Joe's feelings weren't budging. And medication wasn't making a huge difference. Joe might have been listening with all of his might to his Paxil, but it wasn't speaking up all that audibly.

The central principle guiding my work with depressed men like Joe is a simple one. If disconnection lies at the root of the ailment, reconnection relieves it. There are myriads of ways men in this culture commonly disconnect—from themselves and from those around them. Like his father before him, Joe had managed to maintain his breadwinner role but was thoroughly disconnected from emotional or even physical caretaking within his own family. At home, with both his wife and his daughter, Joe used depression like a wall of indifference. I could not predict whether we would have better luck than Joe's previous therapies in treating his overt depression. But there was little reason not to go after his wall.

Like a surgical reattachment of a torn limb, our therapy served to reconnect Joe to his family. Nerve by nerve, and vein by vein, we set up the alignments and let the tissue knit itself together again. We did not wait for Joe's feelings to change. Alcoholics Anonymous has a saying: "Fake it until you make it." If an alcoholic were to wait until he really felt like not having a drink, he could wait a long time. I believe that one first changes the behaviors, then, if one is lucky, the feelings follow. The same thing is true for couples therapy. If a man were to wait until he really felt like learning to be more communicative, the couple and I might sit and grow old together. Sometimes a man has to get up off the psychological couch and get going, whether he feels like it or not. This is called discipline.

A great many men have been falsely empowered by this culture's belief that discipline is not required in their domestic lives—relationships need not be actively worked on. "A man is the king of his castle," the old saying goes. And, while few modern men would have the temerity to state such a belief openly, a great many act on it.

I told Joe that I thought he was a victim of changing male roles, a near casualty in a time of transition. Like many depressed men—indeed, like many men generally—Joe was caught in what I call "the new job description." For his whole life, he had been raised with one set of skills and expectations and now, in his early fifties, he found himself on the brink of disaster unless he was willing to "reengineer."

*   *   *

The rigid gender roles we take for granted, the arrangement that contributed to the antagonism between Joe and Barbara, are actually a relatively recent development. Joe and Barbara were on the verge of divorce because of the unviability of roles we may think of as standing since time immemorial, but which, in fact, only came into being early in the twentieth century.

At about the turn of the century, the structural changes brought about by the industrial revolution reached into the heart of American families and changed their shape forever. In the previous age of family farms and cottage industries, households were organized equally around the tasks that served the group's well-being—cooking, education, tending the ill—and also the tasks that produced goods—gardening, raising livestock, making clothes. There was no great distinction between *family caretaking* and *family production*. While philosophical role distinctions did exist—women, for example, were the tender souls most suited to care for the sick—in practical terms, the activities of men and women, adults and children, even family members and servants routinely overlapped. The daily life of the household was marked by enormous fluidity in roles.

With the industrial revolution, production moved out of the home, and men moved with it into the growing urban areas. As men took on the role of wage earner, women and children became ever more dependent on the man's salary. It is at this moment that many of the divisions that we now take for granted first sprung into being: the division between work and leisure; between the domestic and the occupational; between public and private life; and the rigid polarity of sex roles. All of these divisions had previously existed to varying degrees in society's rhetoric. But now, for the first time, they dictated actual behaviors affecting the daily functioning of family life. Men and women's "separate spheres" moved out of the realm of salon philosophy to shape our most routine and intimate transactions.

From that time of rigidification to the present day—despite women's entry into the work force—the socioeconomic status of most families has been determined by the status of the male. To the degree to which the man succeeds, the family prospers. To the degree to which the man fails, the family suffers.

I believe that from the point of this great division, women and men began to engage in a deal, unconscious and nearly ubiquitous, a deal whose tracks had already been laid down by centuries of philosophy, but whose actual daily operation had never before been a palpable fact. Men agreed—for their and their family's well-being—to abdicate many of their deepest emotional needs in order to devote themselves to competition at work. Women agreed to abdicate many of their deepest achievement needs in order to devote themselves to the care of everything else, including their working husbands. I call this deal the *core collusion*. It is at this juncture that the roles of *man-the-breadwinner* and *woman-the-caretaker* were born. A women accomplished her new, critical role as the husband's ministering angel by seeing not just to his physical needs, but to his psychological needs as well. As psychiatrist Matt Dumont has written: "It does not matter much whether the returning male is a miner or a professor; his wife, knowingly or not, has the culturally defined task of reading his face for signs of dispair and doing her level best to get him back out there again the next day. Women are the cheerleaders of industrial society."

If the relationship of most traditional wives to their breadwinning men is one of caretaking, of "building up the male ego," then the wife's relationship to a depressed spouse represents a kind of caretaking doubled. Wives of depressed men tend to blame themselves; they try to cajole their husbands into getting help. They may nag; they may complain. But until things get truly dismal, they seldom put their foot down, as Barbara Hannigan finally did. Unfortunately, a woman's socially ingrained proclivity to avoid confrontation often provides a rich medium in which her husband's dysfunctionality may flourish and grow.

Joe turned his back on many family responsibilities and, for years, Barbara tried to work around it. It is not hard to understand Joe's wish for a moratorium on obligation. As a small boy, he had stepped into the vacuum left by his depressed father. Little Joe became, in many ways, his mother's emotional husband, his father's business partner, his siblings' father. The only person's needs Joe learned to ignore were his own. In trade for his own emotional betrayal, Joe received the payoff of grandiosity. Like many narcissistically wounded, successful men in our culture, Joe took a profound conviction of his own superiority out into the world, and the world rewarded him for it. But then Joe's luck faltered. He had made a grand showing until the day the whole thing came tumbling down around him. Since his sense of worth was synonymous with the success of the business, when it crashed, Joe's self-esteem bankrupted right along with it. He had based his whole life on conditional grandiosity, on the assumed success of performance-based esteem, and when his contract with the world collapsed, he had little recourse for self-sustenance. A severe, overt depression gripped him, held him for twenty years, and almost succeeded in killing him.

As is the case for a number of overtly depressed men, however, along with its misery, Joe's depression provided a means for stepping off the conveyor belt of the traditional male role. Joe no longer worked sixty to seventy hours a week. He no longer based his sense of value on the bottom line of his business. The problem was that he had not learned to base his sense of value on anything else, either. Joe had always played by the rules, been a good son, brother, employer. Life was supposed to reward him for this *valor*. Joe was caught between a vision of masculine competence he no longer fully believed in and shame at his own disbelief. Joe's depression was like a call of "uncle," a signal that said, "I've had enough." His disaster was crisis enough to knock him off the blind path he had followed. But it hadn't presented him with a new model, a different path. Joe's refusal to be the overfunctioning "sturdy oak" was a step in the right direction. But instead of negotiating or articulating his own needs, he simply refused to be responsible.

I told Joe that the six-year-old boy he had turned his back on was now staging a sit-down strike with a vengeance. That boy in him refused to function until he was acknowledged. The problem was that Joe's depression-as-protest was no more relationally skilled than his overfunctioning had been. Since Joe's needs were "acted out" rather than spoken, Barbara had no way of meeting them. And since Joe refused to talk about his problems, he forced Barbara, rather than asked her, to care for him. The wounded, neglected part of him refused to budge until it was finally acknowledged, while the falsely-empowered, grandiose part of him felt entitled simply to resign. Dragging Joe back into relationship meant developing, for the first time, a much-needed middle ground in which Joe could be responsible to others and in touch with himself at the same time, in which he could meet reasonable responsibilities and also ask for care.

Once the victorious knight slays the dragon, he rides off with the beautiful young princess. The man, through his accomplishments, finally wins back the relational riches he himself had been taught to abandon. These relational riches are most often embodied in the smiling, pristine face of an ideal woman who often remains elusive, slightly above, slightly out of reach. Novelist Tim O'Brien begins *The Things They Carried*, his acclaimed memoir of Vietnam, with this opening passage:

> First Lieutenant Jimmy Cross carried letters from a girl named Martha, a junior at Mount Sabastian College in New Jersey. They were not love letters, but Lieutenant Cross was hoping, so he kept them folded in plastic at the bottom of his rucksack. In the late afternoon, after a day's march, he would dig a foxhole, wash his hands under a canteen, unwrap the letters, hold them with the tips of his fingers, and spend the last hour of light pretending. He would imagine romantic camping trips into the White Mountains in New Hampshire. He would sometimes taste the envelope flaps, knowing her tongue had been there. More than anything, he wanted Martha to love him as he loved her. . . . She was a virgin, he was almost sure. She was an English major at Mount Sabastian, and she wrote beau-

tifully about her professors and roommates and midterm exams, about her respect for Chaucer and her great affection for Virginia Woolf. She often quoted lines of poetry; she never mentioned the war, except to say, Jimmy, take care of yourself. The letters weighed 10 ounces. They were signed Love, Martha.

Martha is the one Lieutenant Cross dreams of in his foxhole, the virgin he has sworn to serve and protect, the princess he fights for. She is normalcy, abundance, domesticity, the life amid "the dishes and the glass" from which he set out, only to yearn for it from far away on the front lines.

For generations, traditional men have been willing to slog their way through combat trenches, dirty, mean jobs, dangerous occupations, to sacrifice their health, even lie down and die, for the sake of their breadwinner roles. Men have enjoyed the "privilege," as more and more angry voices are rising to say, of killing themselves. In return, what men have been promised is an appreciative, saintly wife—a whore in the bedroom, a kitten on the living room couch, a scintillating cocktail companion, and a damn fine cook and homemaker. This is not a mature relationship. It is what I have taken to speak of with couples as *traditional emotional pornography*.

While some pornography is deliberately demeaning, all explicitly erotic material is not intrinsically violent toward women. But most pornography does play out in the arena of sexuality a broader male fantasy—a fantasy of women's boundless, joyful compliance.

The one thing never depicted in a pornographic film is a woman criticizing her lover or demanding something different from him. The essence of the pornographic vision of women is that they are so thoroughly "in sync" with the male, that the things that give him pleasure just happen to drive her wild as well. The clearest example of this male sexual fantasy is the movie *Deep Throat*, in which a woman's clitoris is located in the back of her mouth. Films and novels are full of vamps who expertly contort themselves into masculine wet dreams. I call these women *sexual mothers*, abundant goddesses like Mae West, Ava Gardner, and Marilyn Monroe.

The archetype of the sexual mother embodies a dream of being limitlessly given to; being perfectly nurtured, as a child is nurtured by a mother; being regarded as a perfect lover, perfect husband, someone's Prince Charming. This vision precludes a few nasty realities, like the negotiation of another's needs, doing things wrong and having to learn how to do them differently, struggling with moments of profound loneliness. Society teaches neither member of the couple how to deal with the raw pain that is a part of any real relationship, because it does not even acknowledge the existence of that pain. Stuffed with such romanticism, neither men nor women learn to vigorously negotiate their differences, because true harmony is seen as obviating difference.

Men like Joe Hannigan have been raised with the delusion that "their women" take active pleasure in demanding nothing from them. This is emotional pornography—the idea that a good woman is one who is happy to take care of—and leave alone—her breadwinning man.

Early in their development men learn to turn their backs on the voice of their own emotional needs as well as the vulnerabilities of others. In return, they expect—after the war has been fought, the deal effected, the trophy won—a vision of gratification that is often immature.

Women, traditionally barred from direct confrontation, have learned the "feminine wiles" of management. Women's protectiveness is inherently condescending, a sisterly solidarity that says, "We know better. We must look after these children we have married." For all their vaunted superiority, a great many men intuit that their wives are managing them. Women, in this culture, have been taught to be indirect, manipulative, and silent, while men have been taught to ignore their women, punish them, or feel wounded by them if they dare speak out. Neither Narcissus nor Echo is well equipped by traditional socialization to take his or her place at the negotiation table. Barbara Hannigan vacillates between being silent about her needs and screaming them out in a rage when she finally blows up. Her work is to learn assertion without aggression. Joe needs to wake up to the responsibility of listening, of bringing himself to the negotiation table to begin with.

*   *   *

Joe began helping Barbara around the house, whether he felt depressed or not. He began listening to her at the end of a day rather than dozing off in front of the evening news. Taking a renewed interest in his daughter, he planned activities for the three of them. Joe reported that none of these efforts was terribly difficult, once he committed to making them. His capacity to be disciplined and to learn quickly were positive resources drawn from the traditional male role. I have found that often, once men understand that the old roles are no longer working, once they submit to the necessity of having to change, they are most often excellent students. Men are raised to be good workers. Once they realize that they must work on themselves and on their relationships, they can usually carry it off. My faith in men's capacity to relearn and reemphasize relational qualities is rooted in the understanding that we human beings are far more similar than dissimilar. And the range of skills and behaviors available to each sex is much broader and more flexible than we once believed.

While our polarized vision of men and women carries some undeniable truth, this easy dichotomy obscures how nuanced and how plastic real human attributes are. A generation of parents who have tried to raise "nonsexist" children have been overwhelmed by the apparent psychological differences in little boys and little girls. "Anyone having both daughters and sons *knows* that boys and girls have a completely different feel to them!" is a sentiment I hear over and over again. Meanwhile, magazine and newspaper headlines scream out new research findings on an almost weekly basis "proving" that boys and girls are structurally, inescapably different— with different hormones, different math capabilities, different brains. But the idea that the dichotomy that causes so much suffering in both genders represents an inevitable unfolding of biological destiny does a disservice to our understanding of both nature and nurture, and lends little hope for real change beyond learning to live with our differences. The idea that men can never be as emotional or as related as women lets Joe off a hook both he and his family would be better off leaving him on. Yes, there are structural differences between men and women, but the real picture is by no means as simple as one might think.

There is some indication, for example, that human males are, if anything, *more* emotional than human females. Male babies have been shown consistently to exhibit greater separation distress when they are left by their mothers, to be more excitable, more easily disturbed, and harder to comfort. And the male's comparative sensitivity to emotion may carry through, in some ways, into adulthood. In a fascinating project attempting to map out the physiological correlates to marital interactions, John Gottman "wired" a sample of couples and measured their physiological responses while they communicated. Gottman found that his male sample showed on the whole a greater physiological response to emotional arousal than his female sample, and the men took longer to return to their physiological baseline once aroused. The aversion of many men to strong emotion, Gottman speculates, may not be the result of a diminished capacity to feel, as has been commonly believed, but just the reverse. Because men may bring a heightened biological sensitivity to the experience of feeling, strong emotion might be experienced as aversive, as physiologically overwhelming. Whether or not one agrees with Gottman's conclusion, such research represents just one example of the ways in which scrutiny reveals our biological differences to be infinitely more complex than headline-grabbing stereotypes about them.

Focus on wholesale differences between the sexes blunts the extraordinary variation between members of each. It also fails to acknowledge that when circumstances change, each gender seems able to access qualities generally linked to the other. And, finally, it does not take into account that biological tendencies may be amended. Just because some human trait is "biological" does not mean, necessarily, that it is acceptable. One could make a case that racism is an extension of xenophobia, the contempt for strangers, and thus may have strong biological roots. But, one rarely hears a passive, fatalistic acceptance of racism. An often cited example of evidence for the biological basis of complex human behaviors is the phenomenon of assault by stepfathers on stepchildren. Ape, wolf, and human males all show remarkably consistent rates of attack toward the proximate offspring of others. There are well-docu-mented evolutionary reasons why males might prefer rearing those who carry their own genes. But I have yet to hear anyone claim that we should accept the inevitability of attack and molesta-tion in blended families because men are just biologically wired for that behavior. There is, in humans, a force whose job it is to ame-liorate raw biological tendencies. We call it civilization.

In twenty years of work with men and their families, I have come to see men's struggles with redeveloping neglected emotional and relational skills as about on a par with women's struggles to redevelop assertive, instrumental skills. Generally, it seems about as difficult for the sons of Narcissus to open up and listen as it is for the daughters of Echo to speak.

Barbara Hannigan began warming up as the sincerity of Joe's efforts became apparent. The bickering that had marked their marriage for years started to subside. More than the renewed rela-tionship with Barbara, however, it was falling in love with his daughter, Allie, that melted Joe's heart.

"I had no idea she was this great," he enthused in one of our final sessions. "I mean, while I was off in my fog, she has just become such a *charmer*!"

As Barbara entered her last trimester, she found herself relying on Joe more and more. And he had managed to shake off the lethargy of his depression enough to be counted on. Joe actually found himself getting excited at the prospect of his next child.

"It will be an interesting experience to really be there for this one," he told me. "I feel like I missed out on it last time. It was a walk through."

Patricia Hannigan was born about seven months after I had first met Joe and Barbara. Chubby and ruddy complexioned, she was the spitting image of her proud father. "I feel like I just about deliv-ered this one myself," Joe boasted a few weeks after her arrival.

"It sounds," I told him, "as if you and Tricia have both had something of a birth experience."

Three months after Tricia's delivery, sleep deprived from sharing night duties with wife, Joe has never felt better. He has tapered his medication to about half of his accustomed dose, and he plans to keep it there.

In the men I treat there is often an initial resistance, a kind of shudder, at having to give up the traditional notion that a man need not work much, either emotionally or physically, in his own home, but most of the depressed men I work with are grateful to find new courses of action that actually improve their family's lives. They are pleased to be with a happier partner in a more loving household. I have also found that a great many men want more for themselves as well. They want to experience themselves more fully, even if it means encountering pain. Just as many depressed women are tired of their oppression and willing to risk security to begin asserting their needs, many depressed men are tired of their disconnection and ready to tolerate the humility, the fall from hubris, implicit in listening to the needs of others.

"What does it mean," Joe and Barbara ask me one visit, Tricia drooling between them, "when the pain-in-the-butt factor around getting ourselves to these sessions begins to outweigh our urge to come?"

"Generally, I'd say that it means we're finished," I answer.

"That's what we figured," Joe says. He swoops down to wipe off Tricia's milky face with an old cloth diaper. "Slime child." He smiles at her, poking a finger at her tummy. Tricia vaguely reaches out for her father's huge finger and gurgles.

"Hard to imagine." Barbara looks at her husband and child.

"Yeah." Joe peeks up at his tired wife, flashing his kind, apologetic smile. "Tell me about it," he says.

*   *   *

Both forms of depression in men, overt and covert, frequently evoke in mates an urge to protect their husbands. If overtly depressed men often implicitly demand care, covertly depressed men often implicitly demand dysfunctionality. The spouse of a covertly depressed man may offer herself up as a scapegoat, expressing his projected vulnerabilities for him. This is a phenomenon called *adult-to-adult carried feelings*.

In decades of research, British psychiatrist Julian Hafner has detailed the sometimes devastating effects on male partners when women patients recover from phobias and anxiety disorders. A huge number of phobic women's husbands begin to show signs of addiction, pathological jealousy, violence, and, most commonly, overt depression, when their wives' level of functioning rises. Hafner's research supplies empirical evidence for one of the axioms of family therapy: a force exists that allows one person to stabilize the psychological equilibrium of another—if she is willing to contort herself into the shape required to accomplish the task.

Any woman knows that few strategies serve to "build up" a male more effectively than her own appearance of helplessness. Some women seem willing to keep their covertly depressed men strong by becoming less functional than their partners. Such self-sacrifice does not belong simply to a lunatic fringe. Married women are consistently reported on a number of sociological measures as less happy, less well adjusted, more anxious, more overtly depressed, and generally more neurotic than either married men or single women, while single men are the most at-risk population in the nation for both physical and psychological health problems. The huge discrepancy concerning the effects of married life on men and women has led pioneer sociologist Jessie Bernard to speak of "his" and "hers" marriages. Bernard reviews dozens of studies and government statistics on health and concludes that contemporary marriage appears to be beneficial to the well-being of men and detrimental to that of women.

*   *   *

Judy first came into treatment because of an anxiety disorder that seized her right after her mother died. As her condition grew more difficult to manage, her husband, Tom, was enlisted as her driver, food shopper, payer of bills. Judy became Tom's full-time occupation, which worked out, in a way, because Tom had been laid off from work about four months prior to Judy's first attack. Tom refused to join in our sessions. I met him in the waiting room, where he sat patiently reading old magazines. He was polite and aloof. I facilitated a referral for Judy to a behavioral treatment program specializing in panic disorders. That program, coupled with a brief run on some new medication, cleared her anxiety within a few months. I was not surprised, however, to hear from Judy again a little later. The panic attacks had returned. I questioned Judy closely about her and Tom's well-being in the months that she had been in remission. It wasn't until our third session that Judy told me that Tom was drinking heavily since she had gone back to work.

"It's just so hard for him to sit alone all day, while I go off," she cried.

"So, you've found a way to keep him company and give him a job all at one go," I told her. I asked if she would invite him to join us and let me talk to Tom myself, a suggestion she had refused before.

Judy thanked me profusely for my help and insight. She promised to "think on it" and let me know in our next session. I never heard from her again. Living with panic attacks and agoraphobia, evidently, frightened her less than the prospect of encountering the full brunt of whatever Tom carried inside.

If Jessie Bernard and dozens of sociologists who have followed her are correct, than a wife like Judy is an extreme version of the many women who are willing to become symptomatic themselves while their husband's symptoms decrease. These women carry the "dysfunction" of vulnerability itself—any kind of emotional vulnerability. What streams up to the surface in many of the husbands in Hafner's study is the needy, depressed, little boy those men, like Joe Hannigan, tried to disown in early childhood. No one benefits when women protect depressed men's disconnection in this way.

*　　　*　　　*

If ever a deal was cut between a man and a women, my parents had such an arrangement. Dad was the brilliant, abrasive artist, the 6 foot 2, 280-pound *enfant terrible*. Living his frustrated life out first in grim Camden, New Jersey, and then in honky-tonk Atlantic City; he was a pearl before swine, a Prometheus among cretins. My mother was lucky to have him—such a talented, intelligent man. My mother—obese, disfigured by blindness in one eye, afraid to drive, afraid to take classes, afraid of public speaking— leaned on "my Edgar" like an oversized doll. And yet, when not at home, Mom was capable of supervising a 250-bed nursing home.

"It's all because of your father," she would demur. "I'd be com- pletely *lost* without him."

Mom was "his baby," and Dad was her "star." And the more he raged, abused her, put her down, the more she dug in, went off to her work, and kept us alive.

Looking back, I suppose I should have been grateful to her, but I wasn't. Like everyone else in the family, I despised my mother. Not in any particularly flagrant way. She just didn't count. As with her girth, my mother buried herself so deeply within her role, in the performance of mothering, that there was no way to "get at" her, to touch her or to be touched by her. In all of our years together, I can- not recall many moments of authentic conversation between us. She was so preoccupied with keeping Dad stable, that anything from the children that threatened to pierce the surface, to demand real contact, any demonstration of pain, or mess, or need, left her literally blank. She would turn and walk away from us as though she had not heard.

In large part, Mother carried the family shame, as I learned to do when I grew up. But she was not just a scapegoat. Mother partici- pated, in her own, disowned way, in the violence of our family. My father was a brute, a force of nature, as mindless and, in a way, as predictable as some large beast one had the misfortune of disturb- ing. But the injury I felt from my mother went deeper. It was more a puncture than a gash. It felt more personal and more cruel. Like many children from chaotic homes, even though my father was the flagrant abuser, my most unresolved feelings are reserved for the parent who refused to protect me. While I know intellectually that my feelings toward her might be unfair, they nevertheless remain less forgiving than those toward my dad. My father lashed out at us on impulse, thoughtlessly, but I could watch my mother *decide* to abandon us. I could feel her waver for an instant between husband and child and then retreat from all of us. I could see it in her eyes.

In preparation for the ritual beatings, Mother would be brought into the room to watch. They had learned somewhere that it was important to present a united front to the children. As I was strapped, I would plead with my mother, at first with words and later, as I grew older, with just my eyes. I would beg her to help me, to get him off me. And I would watch as the light of consciousness left her. Staring straight at me, brazenly, as if in a dare, I could see my mother vacate. It was an oddly intimate moment, almost obscene, as if she were showing me some wanton part of herself I had no business glimpsing.

Where did she go? That question plagued me. When she decided to abandon me to him, when the light in her eyes went out like that, where did she go? To some chill territory, I sensed, to which it would not be in my best interests to follow.

Looking back, I now realize that my poor mother, caught between my father and me, probably was as dissociated in her own way as I was. But I was too young to realize that at the time. I think my mother spent a good amount of her time dissociated—each time my father savaged her, in private or public, barked at her, called her stupid. And all the while she must have been thinking— to the degree to which she allowed herself thought at all—that she was protecting him, crating him against the harsh knocks life had given him, keeping him present and sane for all of us. And perhaps she was.

As the years went by, mixed in with their love was a rancor that poisoned them both. Bickering, snarling, loving, enmeshed, like two armless people trying to rise by leaning against one another's backs, they fought their way through their life. Toward the end, they were so chaotic that, as a joke in our teenage years, my brother and I would time how long it took them to make their way from our living room out to the car. Their average was forty-three minutes.

"Leah!" Dad would yell for her to hurry.

"Now, don't be a horse's ass, Edgar!"

"Jesus!" he'd shout.

"Edgar, where are you going with that magazine? I'm ready!"

"I just have to stop off at the bathroom."

"Now?"

"When you have to go, you have to go."

"I don't know if I will live long without him," my mother told me the day we buried this needed, hated man. And she was right. She did not long survive him.

When I am faced with a family in which there is a depressed woman, my first move is to empower the woman. When I am faced with a family in which there is a depressed man, before beginning work with the man, my first move is to empower the woman. To help a depressed woman means facilitating her rise against the forces of oppression that surround her. To help a depressed man, one needs to invite him to step up to increased relational responsibility, a move he may not be inclined to make if his partner allows him to avoid it.

My father was blasted out of the relational as a young boy— frozen out of connection by the death of his mother, fragmented out by the breakup of his family, traumatized out by the horror of the Depression, and then almost physically annihilated by his own father's hand. It would have taken an extraordinary woman to insist that my father relearn the skills of connection again. My mother was not up to it. Struggling with her own depression, with virtually no economic or cultural support for standing up to him, my mother did what women of her generation learned to do. She managed him as best she could, and she endured.

*　　　*　　　*

Joe Hannigan almost killed himself rather than submit to the pain and indignity of fully entering into the relational. He was overwhelmed with a sense of hopeless inadequacy; he was angry and entitled. He did not know how to satisfy Barbara, and he just did not want to "give in" to her. His stubbornness almost cost Joe, and his family, his life. The irony was that the things Joe needed to learn in order to turn his situation around were eminently teachable, small considerations practiced over and over again. The hard part was facilitating the initial shift in Joe's consciousness—getting him to see that it was in his interest to take up the study of relational caretaking to begin with. First, with Allie and Barbara, and then with Trish, Joe practiced D. H. Lawrence's "difficult repentance," "the freeing oneself of the endless repetition of the mistake." The Hannigan family proved to be winners.

My parents had not the resources, the help, nor the insight that was available, a generation later, to Joe and Barbara Hannigan. My parents lived unhappy lives, which were finally relieved by miserable deaths. In any given quest, not one but many knights venture forth. Some get further than others. Some do not make it at all.

When the wife or partner of a depressed man I am treating presents me with the same dilemma that faced my mother or Barbara Hannigan, I tell her that she has little real choice. She must confront the reality of her husband's condition. It is in her interests to insist that he behave responsibly inside their family. In overt depression, the man may express "feminine" vulnerabilities but, like Joe and his father, couple them with a "masculine" entitlement to behave irresponsibly. In covert depression, the man cannot afford to be relationally responsive either, for three reasons. First, his primary allegiance must be to the defenses he uses for self-regulation. Second, intimacy with another will inevitably trigger intimacy with himself—an intimacy many covertly depressed men prefer to avoid. Finally, because relational skills have frequently

317

lain dormant and unexercised, demands for intimacy initially exacerbate the feelings of inadequacy that may already plague him. Despite these dangers and difficulties, nothing positive will happen in a depressed man's relationships until the net of protectiveness is dropped. I tell the wives of depressed men: "If you directly confront this condition and do not back away from reasonable demands for intimacy, there may be a fifty-fifty chance your husband will leave you. But, if you do not honestly engage with these issues, there is a ninety percent chance your relationship will slowly corrode over time. Which risk would you prefer to take?"

In twenty years of practice, I have encountered many unfortunate women who, afraid to make reasonable demands on their depressed husbands, wound up, years later, being left anyway. Most wives do not fully contain the resentment that they rightfully feel. And even if they do, the relationship itself eventually loses vitality by virtue of the lack of honest engagement. Conversely, unless the patient has already decided to leave his family, I have rarely encountered a man who was willing to set foot in my office but unwilling, with coaching and help, to pick up the challenge of increased relational skill.

Work with depressed men and their partners has convinced me that men's much-vaunted fear of women and of intimacy is really not a fear of either. What men fear is subjugation. In the one up/one down, better than/less than, hierarchical world of traditional masculinity, one is either in control or controlled. Vulnerability, openness, yielding to another's wishes—many of the requisite skills for healthy relationships—can be experienced by men as invitations to be attacked. Men's fear of entrapment, of female engulfment, is not really about women at all. It is a transposition of a male model of interaction to the living room and the bedroom. When men fear that their women will "engulf" them, they fear that their women will act like men.

Most women have no more wish to "emasculate" their husbands than most mothers wish to "castrate" their sons. But neither men nor women have been taught basic skills for the tough negotiation of contrasting needs. Take the most ordinary of examples. Joe comes home late after a long day at the office. After dinner, he wants to go to bed. Barbara, who has been alone with the kids all day, is hungry for interaction. She launches into an account of her day, her feelings and problems. Joe is annoyed; he puts her off with a few terse grunts and heads for the bathroom. Both of them are angry. Neither has negotiated anything. Joe's caricatured image of his wife, at that moment, is that she is a bottomless pit of emotional need; that anything he does will be wrong anyway, and that she has no appreciation of either his needs or his contributions. Barbara's equally caricatured imagery holds Joe as an unresponsive cretin. They blame one another, rather than asking themselves what they might have done differently.

All that Joe and Barbara needed to do, in that simple example, was talk to each other. Rather than rushing in with a de facto demand for conversation, Barbara would have done better to tell her husband what she had in mind, and ask him if he were up to it. If Joe was too tired to listen to his wife, at that moment, he needed to say so in words, as opposed to grunts, to explain why, and offer her an alternative, such as "Honey, I'm just too drained to listen right now. But I'd be happy to hear more over breakfast tomorrow." These rudimentary skills of communication, direct assertion, and accountability, are easily learned, taught by therapists all over the country.

The good news is that once a man has a few of such elementary skills under his belt—particularly if he is working in conjunction with an equally committed partner—the relationship shows quick improvement. And improved relationships often help alleviate the man's depression. For many overtly depressed men, and virtually all covertly depressed men, therapeutic nurture alone is not enough. It is too passive. There must also be guidance. As healing as my work was with Frank Paolitto, it took years more of therapy before my depression began to yield. After my individual therapy, I went on to engage in couples therapy with Belinda for several years. And, over and above our couples work, I trained for countless hours in the theory and technique of family therapy. It was clear to me that, just as I learned about individual therapy in order to figure out what to do with my pain, I was now learning family therapy in order to figure out what a healthy relationship looked like. As is true of most of the men that I treat, my family certainly did not teach me what I needed to know in order to sustain satisfactory intimacy. And society at large had not taught me these skills either. While I do not believe that most depressed men need to devote their lives to learning various schools of psychotherapy as I did, I do believe that any man who has struggled in his life with a deep, core experience of depression will need help not only in learning how to cherish himself, but also in learning the art of cherishing others. Just as the beam of contempt, the internalized dynamic of violence, may sometimes turn inward in overt depression, sometimes outward in covert depression, the regenerative force of recovery must turn inward toward increased maturity, increased self-regulation, and outward toward increased relational skill. Recovery, at its deepest level, evokes the art of valuing, caring for, and sustaining. The relationship one sustains may be toward oneself, toward others, or even toward the world itself.

CHAPTER TWELVE

Conclusion:
Where We Stand

Why would a depressed man choose the hard work of reaccessing the very longings, skills, and responsibilities of mature relationship that were actively discouraged throughout his socialization? One reason may be that, like Joe Hannigan, he is being asked to in no uncertain terms. Another reason is that he will feel better for it.

When a depressed man steps up to the task of practicing full relational responsibility, he not only transforms the dynamics of his disorder, he also shifts to a more mature stage in his own development. I speak to men of this shift in life orientation as *the move into fathering*. Fathering, as I speak of it, can, but need not, involve the biological begetting of children. Fathering need not involve children at all. Fathering occurs when the essential question a man lives by changes. At the heart of the quest is a question. In *The Quest for the Holy Grail*, the young hero, Perceval, crosses the Wasteland, finds the hidden Castle of Wonders, meets the wounded Fisher King, and sees the awesome spectacle of the Grail. Everyone waits with baited breath for the young knight to ask the right question and free the king, the castle, and all of the people of the realm. But at the tale's beginning, the hero is too immature. Overwhelmed, he leaves the castle in disgrace, having failed. It takes the rest of his journey—the rest of his life, by some accounts—before Perceval is granted a second chance.

The essential shift in question that marks a depressed man's transformation is the shift from: *What will I get?* to: *What can I offer?*

Entering into a fathering relationship—to a child, a mate, an art, a cause, to the planet entire—means to become a true provider. Recovery demands a move into generativity.

The greatest cost of the less than/better than dynamic of traditional masculinity lies in its deprivation of the experience of communion. Those who fear subjugation have limited repertoires of service. But service is the appropriate central organizing force of mature manhood. When the critical questions concern what one is going to get, a man is living in a boy's world. Beyond a certain point in a man's life, if he is to remain truly vital, he needs to be actively engaged in devotion to something other than his own success and happiness. The word *discipline* derives from the same root as the word *disciple*. Discipline means "to place oneself in the service of." Discipline is a form of devotion. A grown man with nothing to devote himself to is a man who is sick at heart. What a great many men in this culture choose to serve is their own reflected value, which they often believe serves the needs of their family, even while their families may be crying out for something different from them.

What the ethic of man-the-breadwinner has ignored is the wisdom of relationship. That wisdom—shared by most human cultures throughout the globe—has as a central tenet that it is a source of one's own growth to care for the context one lives within. It is essentially an ecological wisdom, teaching that we are not objective observers standing above and acting upon a passive world. We do not stand apart from a system, like God, but within it—whether the system is our body, our psyche, our marriage, our state, or our planet. Tending to the well-being of contexts we live within is an exercise of mature self-care, self-interested sacrifice. This culture, with its reliance on performance-based esteem, gives men few models for healthy sacrifice. I often give the men I work with the following simple example: A small manufacturer finds himself in the position of being able to triple his profits by dumping toxic waste into a nearby stream. But he might also understand that his children and grandchildren would run an increased risk of getting cancer. Any sane man would forgo the immediate gain of increased profits for the long-term gain of safety and a clean conscience. This is not a dispute between selfishness and altruism. It is a dispute between shortsighted greed and farsighted wisdom. Similarly, when a man "gives in" to his wife's desire to stay at home and watch a video on a particular evening rather than to go out to the movies, he does so not because she has won and he has lost, but because he is caretaking a relationship that it is in his best interests to preserve.

Most men understand the wisdom of relationship, of sacrifice to larger goals, in relation to their careers. But it takes some effort to transpose this same wisdom to the care of their families, their marriages, their friendships, and even their own health. Yet it is the placing of oneself at the service of a larger context that drives a man deep into his own growth and fullest potential. Studies indicate that while fathering may or may not be necessary for the psychological adjustment of boys, it is highly advantageous for the psychological adjustment of the father. Men who were judged as having warm, nurturant relationships with their children were shown to be healthier, less depressed, and, surprisingly, more successful in their careers. In popular films, there is a spate of lost or damaged heroes who are redeemed by their relationships to real or surrogate sons. This may have less to do with boys' needs for fathers than with the men's need to be fathers, to live for something beyond performance, kudos, and acquisition.

As more and more women enter the work force, as decades of feminism and cultural change stimulate new demands from women for responsible, intimate partners, as business itself breaks out of traditional hierarchical management structures in favor of more cooperative models, polarized gender arrangements and gender characteristics are reshuffling once again. Man-the-breadwinner, woman-the-caretaker may be figures contained within the borders of the twentieth century. It is becoming increasingly apparent that the old paradigm of worth through dominance, of valor, is atavistic. It no longer fits our complex, interdependent world.

*　　*　　*

In *The End of Victory Culture*, political commentator Tom Englehardt posits that with the explosion of the first atom bomb on Hiroshima, European culture entered a new historical stage. Nuclear warfare made it abundantly apparent that conquest and frontier were not endless propositions. For the first time, Europeans were forced to understand the kind of ecological interconnectedness that was a principal wisdom of the indigenous peoples whom they had viewed as savages. A nation could no longer build larger and more effective arsenals without consequences to itself. The radiation unleashed over on the other side of the globe was quite capable of blowing back into its own people's faces. A culture of limitless resources and limitless conquest had reached an undeniable boundary.

Our interconnectedness to nature, and to one another, can no longer be denied. We live in a global economy. We share global resources. We face global threats. The paradigm of dominance must yield to an ethic of caretaking, or we simply will not survive.

The dynamic of dominance and submission, which has been at the heart of traditional masculinity, can play itself out inside the psyche of a man as depression, in his interpersonal relationships as irresponsibility and abuse, in one race's contempt for another people, or in humanity's relationship to the earth itself. We have abused the environment we live in as if it were an all-giving and all-forgiving mother, an endless resource, like the Grail.

In his book *Earth in the Balance*, subtitled *Ecology and the Human Spirit*, Al Gore likens the central ecological problem facing humankind to an addictive process in a dysfunctional family. Gore's formulation bears close resemblance to the dynamics of covert depression. Gore writes:

> I believe that our civilization is addicted to the consumption of the earth itself. This addictive relationship distracts us from the pain of what we have lost: a direct experience of our connection to the vividness, vibrancy, and aliveness of the rest of the natural

world. The froth and frenzy of industrial civilization masks our deep loneliness for communion . . . the price we pay is the loss of our spiritual lives.

The weakest and most helpless members of the dysfunctional family become the victims of abuse at the hands of those responsible for providing nurture. In a similar fashion, we systematically abuse the most vulnerable and least defended areas of the natural world.

Gore's prescription for the species is recovery:

If the global environmental crisis is rooted in the dysfunctional pattern of our civilization's relationship to the natural world, confronting and fully understanding that pattern . . . is the first step toward mourning what we have lost . . . and coming to terms with the new story of what it means to be a steward of the earth.

Gore's prescription is similar to my own. First, the addictive defenses must be confronted and stopped, then the pain beneath them must be allowed to surface. Finally, the skills and responsibilities of true intimacy—"stewardship" as Gore, among others, calls it—must be reestablished. The boy must become a steward, a husband-man. The earth is not our mother; she is our wife. We are married to her and, if we do not take care, we may soon be divorced. In his address to the environmental conference in Rio, Czechoslovakian president Václav Havel surveyed the environmental wreckage left by the reign of communism in his country, the ravages of unmitigated greed. He lamented "the arrogance of modern man, who believes he understands everything and knows everything, who names himself master of 'nature' and the world. Such was the thinking of man who refused to recognize anything above him, anything higher than himself."

What Havel describes is hubris, the delusion of control that lies at the heart of traditional masculinity. And it is this hubris that is transformed in the recovery process of depressed men.

In family therapy, we are trained to consider a symptomatic person as a signal that old mores and beliefs in the family no longer serve the present context. A symptomatic family member is the bearer of news that a change must come, a messenger of transformation. Other men, less pained in their lives, may have the luxury of experimenting with changing male roles in a voluntary, leisurely way. But for those of us who have wrestled with depression, healing from the wound of disconnection is a matter of urgent necessity. We must learn how to serve, to place ourselves inside relationships rather than above them, if we are to relieve our own suffering.

After close to a lifetime of wandering, Perceval is granted a second chance. Out of the clouds, the Castle of Wonders appears to him again. Once more, he sees the hurt Fisher King and he encounters the Grail. All ears bend toward him in expectation. And this time, the hero has learned enough to ask the right question.

"Who serves the Grail?" Perceval asks. Not whom does the Grail serve, but who serves it? Depressed men have been given the task of answering that question with their lives. "Who serves the Grail?"

We do.

Epilogue

My father died on September 15, 1989. My mother called us the day after he had been taken into intensive care. When the phone rang, Belinda and I were lying in bed after an exhausting, satisfying day. We were congratulating one another for, as we put it, "making the jump." Belinda was six months pregnant with Alexander. Justin was just over two years old. We two old reprobate hippies had somehow amassed the small fortune required to move from our beloved rent-controlled apartment in Coolidge Corner, Brookline, to a big old house in a prosperous suburb. We were in sudden possession of a great school system, neighborhood kids for our children to play with, a lawn that needed tending—even a flower garden. We had moved in. We had made a few months' mortgage. We had unpacked most of the boxes. We had arrived. On the Sunday afternoon preceding Mom's call, little Justin ran upstairs to get me.

"Mom's sad, Daddy," he told me, breathlessly. "Come quick!"

I followed Justin down into our flower garden where I found Belinda, a spade in her hands, in dirt up to her elbows, crying like a girl.

"What's the matter?" I put my arms around her, while Justin hovered.

Belinda waved the spade at the house, the terrace. Belinda, who had grown up in a family as psychotic as mine was incompetent, who still had marks on her body from where her father had struck her with a metal pipe.

"It's so *stupid*," she tells me. "I don't know if I'm happy or sad. It's just that we're so *normal!*"

I hold her, kiss her mud-streaked forehead, while she cries. Justin lays his head on her lap.

"It's okay, Mommy," he tells her. "It's okay to be normal." Except he says, "norbal," cracking us up.

There is a blackness that has lain inside the center of my being. When I have closed my eyes, it has been there. When I have been left alone for more than a few hours, I have returned to it. This jagged, empty, frightened feeling has been a part of my internal atmosphere for as long as I can remember. It has been my baseline, my steady state—the *me* I spent a good many years running from. I have come to understand that the dark, piercing unease at my center was my experience of emotional abandonment and fear growing up in a dangerous household. It is a little boy's loneliness, which I brought with me out into the world for the next thirty years.

I do not blame myself for running from those feelings. No one would deliberately subject himself to the discomfort I carried inside my skin unless he had a very good reason to. As a little boy fleeing into the streets and waiting neighborhood games, as an adolescent fleeing toward drugs that soothed me like a mother, I have taken flight throughout most of my life. Hurt, grandiose, blaming others for not filling me up, I was in search of the next big fix, in search of love without having the skills to love well in return. Like Perceval, I have spent a good portion of my life wandering, searching for the right question.

"They've taken him," Mom breathes into the phone, ever dramatic.

I dissociate immediately. I remember thinking, "What an odd phrase." "*They've taken him.*" Evocations of jackbooted authorities dragging Dad off, men in white coats. Or did Mom mean—*They've taken him off my hands?*

When I rouse myself from cerebral distractions, I realize that it feels exactly as though someone has punched me in the chest. I am winded and disorganized.

"What's his condition?" I snap at my mother.

"It's gotten into his lungs," she begins to cry. "It's got his lungs!"

I listen to Mom cry for a while, doing my best to soothe her. Beside me, Belinda watches, her hand on my arm. "Okay, Mom," I say. "There probably aren't any direct flights at this hour. I'll see what I can do about getting into Philly and I'll call you right back. Has Les been told?"

She tells me he has.

"Is there anything you need, Mom? Anybody I should call? You want someone to come be with you?"

"You come be with me, Terry. You and Les just get here as quickly as you can."

"I will, Mom," I tell her. "I'll call you right back."

There is something horrible, something overly vivid, about the snorting, chugging engine of the cab that waits for me in the stillness of our little street. I pass through the glare of its headlights in 3:00 A.M. summer blackness. The driver wants to talk. I am in a state of shock. We prattle about the weather, the Red Socks. I really don't feel like answering, but, having driven a cab myself for a year, I know how lonely 3:00 A.M. must feel to him.

"So, what brings you to such an early flight?" the driver chats.

"My father is dying," I answer and finally gain some silence.

On the ride to the airport, I try to think of my father, try to remember him walking, healthy. Nothing much comes to me. I overtip the driver out of guilt.

"I'm real sorry," he says, handing me my bag.

I just nod.

On the plane, I take refuge in details. There are patients to cancel, appointments to change. What will I say to people? How open should I be with my clients? What if they ask me about him? I start making lists.

Les meets me at the Philadelphia airport, a Styrofoam cup of lukewarm coffee in his hand.

"Here," he says. "Thought you could use this."

We hug. Les has been characteristically efficient. He has rented a car and booked rooms. We are ready to go.

In the car, speeding along the expressway to Atlantic City, I stare out at the window.

"Oh, did you take the Expressway down?" my uncle Matt asks in my mind.

"The expressway, eh?" a faceless male relative answers, a paper cup full of schnapps *in hand, "I always get stuck in traffic that way. I take the Pike."*

"Black Horse Pike or White Horse Pike?" my Dad asks, warming to one of his favorite conversations. *"I think the Black Horse Pike is a lot faster, even though it's a few miles longer."*

"I think the White Horse Pike is the definite choice," someone contends.

"I used to," says Dad. *"But not anymore."*

"You know, funny you should say that, Ed . . . "

And so, in my mind, the men of my family drone on and on, connecting to one another through endlessly stolid preoccupations.

"Black Horse Pike or White Horse Pike?" I quote aloud to my brother.

"Oh," he answers in mock solemnity, "I always take the expressway, these days. Those new automatic tellers they've added really speed things up."

We both look out at the road, good-willed, wanting to support one another. There doesn't seem much to say.

"Have you spoken to a doctor?" I ask him.

He shakes his head. "No time to," he tells me, and then adds, gratuitously, "There'll be plenty of time for all that."

"Do you have any idea how much—"

"No," he cuts me off, definitively.

I lean back into my seat, close my eyes. We pass the rest of the trip in silence.

Hooked up to monitors, IV's, and an oxygen tube, my dad doesn't quite look human. He does not seem to be made out of flesh anymore. Even at this juncture, he remains a big-looking man, with broad shoulders and a huge barrel chest. But his potbelly is gone, his face has sunken to the bone, his skin stretched tight over the aperture of his cheeks. His arms and legs have lost all of their muscle. Lying flat on the bed, they look like pieces of lumber, two-by-fours. I remember thinking that my father was turning into one of his own sculptures.

"Ah!" he says, seeing me arrive. By his inflection, the arch of an eyebrow, it feels as though Dad has risen to greet us. His "Ah!" is such a public-sounding hello, like reaching out a hand to a neighbor who has just rung the doorbell. For a moment, it feels as though we might have been at a cocktail party, but the illusion fades quickly. "Good you could come!" He lets me hug him. His voice is weak, a hoarse whisper, but somehow he manages not to seem enfeebled; the force of his personality remains strong. "I've been looking forward to this!" he adds.

Les comes to join me by the bed. We talk over small details—our lives, not Dad's.

"Hey," he asks. "So, how did you get here?"

"We took the expressway," Les answers.

Dad shakes his head. I can feel his finger digging into my chest, although it's as dead as a stick on top of his bedsheets. "Shoulda taken the Pike," he tells Les.

"Black Horse or White Horse?" Les deadpans.

"Cut the shit, wise ass," Dad answers.

"Dad"—I stroke his gray hair—"you should probably rest. Save your strength."

He angles his head so he can look at me. "What for?" he whispers. "My guys are here. Mom's here. My family. What should I be saving for? Am I going somewhere?"

From the foot of the bed, Mom quietly cries.

"Shit," Dad says.

"I'm all right, Edgar," Mom puts in, pugnaciously.

"Where's my kiss?" he croaks to her.

She walks to the head of the bed, bends down, and kisses him. "I've got you all wet," she says, wiping her tears from his face.

"I don't mind," he answers.

*   *   *

We while away the afternoon. I show Dad recent pictures of Justin. Les shows him pictures of his son, Daniel. In my briefcase, I have an ultrasound shot of Alexander, but it doesn't seem quite right to give it to him now. I am suddenly aware that Alexander will never meet his grandfather. I feel a pang, like a hand squeezing my heart, not too hard, just enough, a blush.

"So, Harvey says to Shirley, 'Darlink I'm leafink you for a younger woman!' " I am telling Dad a series of off-color jokes. My father has always been fond of a good dirty joke and he laughs appreciably. At last, he has become a receptive audience to me.

Over the course of his illness, Dad has become a nicer man to be around. The more ALS whittled his body, the more humble he became. Toward the end of his life, I heard him actually ask questions of other people—what they thought about things, what their experience was. The legions of orderlies and aides that trooped through his life all seemed to think him a likable fellow. He was considered a good assignment.

About a year earlier, I had worked up the courage to send Dad a copy of Sam Osherson's book *Finding Our Fathers*. "This is similar to the kinds of work I do with guys," I had explained.

Uncharacteristically, my father read it, cover to cover, with my mother sitting beside him, holding it for him, turning each page. Uncharacteristically, he called me to tell me how much he had liked it.

"Hold the phone, honey," Mom says. "Your dad wants to get on the line."

Encouraged by his thoughtful response, figuring there was limited time left between us, I decide to take a further risk. I ask Dad for his blessing. Ostensibly, I ask him to bless my work with other fathers and sons, but, for once in his life, Dad knows better.

Without demeaning my request, as he would have done throughout most of his life, he pauses. Then Mom accidentally dropped the phone on the floor.

"God *damn* it, Leah!" I hear him explode, followed by mad scramblings for the telephone.

"Don't you talk to me like that, Edgar!" she answers him back.

"All I *wanted*—"

"I don't care. I'm tired. I'm doing—"

"Guys," I try to interject, but they ignore me, going after one another for a few minutes more. *"Guys?"* I try again from time to time.

After more unintelligible wrangling, I finally hear, *"Damn it,* Leah. This is costing us *money!"* And, then the phone is brought back to Dad's ear.

"Sorry, son," he tells me.

"Its all right, Dad," I say.

"It's just that your mother—"

"Dad," I interrupt, "the blessing."

He takes a moment to gather his thoughts.

"Okay," he says, gruffly. "Here's the blessing." And, then he pauses. "May you and your brother reach your fullest potential in every regard. My blessing for you is this: May nothing in my past, or in the family's past, in any way hold you back or weigh you down. If there are any encumbrances on you, I release you from them. You hear me? I release you. I want you to be free. Happy, strong, and free. That is my blessing to you, son."

We sit for a moment in silence together.

"Thank you, Dad," I say.

"It's no small thing," he comments, almost belligerently.

"Dad?"

"What I said, just then. All that," he tells me. "It's no small thing."

"I know that, Dad," I reassure him.

"I know you do," he answers. "I know you do."

A friend takes Mother to the cafeteria downstairs and my brother and I are left alone with my father.

"Come here, boys." He beckons us.

We flank his bedside. My brother takes his right hand. I take his left.

I begin to speak, accessing the skills I have counseled others to use when approaching a dying parent, acknowledging, in Dad's final moments, the positive aspects of his legacy. Les falls right into step beside me. We take turns telling our father what we take from him, the gifts he has left to us. And then my brother and I, for perhaps the first time in our lives, celebrate one another in his presence.

"One of the things you have given me, Dad," Les says, "is your great love of science. The fact that I am a scientist now has a lot to do with you, Dad. I remember those stupid experiments you used to make us do. . . ."

Dad chuckles, then coughs.

"I take with me," I say, "a wonderful appreciation of nature. I think my happiest times, Dad, were camping together. Building a fire . . ."

And so we went on, with a certain ritual formality, like a warm, solemn processional.

"I don't know if you know this, yet, Dad," I tell him, "but Les has been asked to do a stint of teaching in England. Our little *schmuck* from New Jersey is going to be lecturing at Oxford University."

"Better work on my accent," Les demures.

"You'll do fine," Dad whispers. He is barely able to speak.

"And did you know, Dad," Les reciprocates, "that Terry's first article has been accepted?"

"Listen to me," Dad says, after a while. "Listen to me, children. I'm having more trouble talking." We both draw in closer. "I want to tell you something. It's important to me."

"Okay, Dad," we both tell him. "We're here."

It takes a while for my father to speak. I can't tell whether it's because he's losing ground, or because he has become emotional.

"I want you both to know that the one important thing, the most important thing, is love. That's what it is. The rest is bullshit. When you're where I am now. It's just like they say. All that matters is love."

He leans back, closes his eyes, concentrates on his breathing.

"Maybe you should rest a bit," I suggest.

"Listen," he says, ignoring me. "I didn't always know that. About love. I had a lot of barriers I built around me. I didn't let you love me like you might and even though I loved you—I always loved you—I didn't act like it, sometimes."

"Oh, Dad!" Les begins to cry.

"It's true, though," he tells us. "We all know it." He pauses, asks for water, swallows. "I'm sorry," he tells us. "I'm sorry for the things I did."

"You don't have to—" I begin.

"I do have to," he interrupts. "I do have to." He pauses, gathers strength. "Now, here's the thing," he says. "Here's the main thing. You can do better than me, you understand? You two. I want you two to do better than I did. You hear? Remember this. Don't get caught up in bullshit."

"Okay, Dad," we both tell him. "We'll try. We'll do our best."

"I know you will," he says. "I always knew you would. But I wanted you to know that . . . that I want it for you."

I wring out a face cloth and drape it over his forehead. He closes his eyes.

"Ah, that feels good," he says. "You're all being so nice to me. I don't deserve it."

I bend down and kiss him.

My father died the following morning. I stumbled into his room, a cheerful greeting on my lips, and bumped into the fact of his corpse. He must have died moments earlier. His head was thrown back, his mouth stretched wide open, his eyes shut. Whether it was my own physiological surge, or shock, or a spiritual sensibility, I felt an enormous rush of energy swirl through the room, a powerful vortex. It was as if a portal had blown open and I could palpably feel my father's life *whoosh* out of him, like a great wind.

"You'll have to leave now," the nurse in the room informs me, annoyed.

"In a minute," I answer. I stroke my father's silver hair one last time and kiss him, touch his cheek. "I will do better," I promise him. "It's all over, for you, now. You can rest."

"For as long as I can remember, my father identified with the figure of Prometheus," I address the motley knot of mourners who have gathered for my father's funeral. Aides and hospice workers, mostly. A handful of my mother's friends, no friends of his own. His brother, Phil.

"I remember," I continue my eulogy, "a statue of Prometheus and the Eagle by Dad's favorite sculpture, Jacques Lipchitz. In the sculpture, hero and nemesis merge and flow into one another, even as they lock together in combat."

"Like Prometheus, my father wrestled with the force of violence his whole life. Sometimes, he managed to gain the upper hand. Sometimes, he didn't. No one here blames you, Dad. No one here sits in judgment of your faults. You did the best you knew how. You are forgiven."

The humidity cloys, no wind to speak of. The sun beats down on my black suit and sweat pours off my body.

"Before he died," I continue, "my father gave me a benediction. I ask now that his own blessing become his eulogy. Dad said: May nothing of his past, or his family's past, impede the full realization of our gifts. I would ask you now to silently join me in that same prayer."

Without being asked, the people gathered stand to their feet.

"Father," I say, "may the violence you struggled with be buried with you here. May your children be released from it. May our children be released from it. And, may you be released from it.

"I pray that Prometheus has let go the eagle. I pray it returns to wherever it came from and does no one here harm. I pray that you have finally found peace. We who survive you, send love. Amen."

* * *

"You know," Uncle Phil says to me later that evening when I press him on it, "your dad told me that story about Abe in the car. But I don't remember it."

"You would have been pretty young, Phil."

"Well, I've actually asked and your grandfather denied it," he says.

"It's hardly the—"

"I just don't see it," Phil goes on. "Our parents were two of the nicest—"

"Your mother was dead," I interject.

"Well, I mean that, my memories of growing up were pretty normal, all things considered," he goes on. "You don't really know what it was like, back then, Terry."

I smile. "You sound just like Dad, Uncle Phil," I tell him.

Phil gives us all a warm hug, promises to stay in touch. We never hear from him again.

After the funeral, I am alone on a dock overlooking the bay a block and a half from our little house. I have come out to the ocean to cry, to feel my grief. Inside the house, it is all handshaking and sincere good wishes—formalities. I sense the presence of my father very strongly. I feel it surround me, up in the sky, in the birds flying overhead. I am filled with thoughts of him, conversations, memories.

As I sit on the dock, I ask him if he really meant it. If it was really all right with him for me to surpass him. A herring gull flies overhead, cawing, and lands on the stern of a boat moored dead ahead of me. I have to chuckle. On the stern of the weathered old fishing boat is painted the name: *Dad's Desire*.

There is a blackness that has lain in the center of my soul for as long as I can remember. Years of therapy with Paolito helped. Years more of family therapy helped. The week my courageous parents spent in Boston braving four consecutive days of therapy with me helped a great deal. The active reparenting techniques and the profound trauma recovery techniques of my colleague, Pia Mellody, have brought enormous relief.

The blackness inside me is mostly gone now. I feel a touch of it here and there. A bad day now and again, a tickle in the back of my mind, like a threat. But, as I go about my life, I am essentially free of it. That little boy who sat alone in such darkness and pain is with me now. I have learned how to attend to him, be responsible to him, as surely as I am responsible to the others in my life. Knowing his pain, I do not allow him to reach for a drug, or a woman, or one more gleaming award. We have learned to sit quietly together, he and I. We have learned to keep one another company.

My mother had a massive stroke six months after my father died. Disabled and virtually unable to speak, she was welcomed into the nursing home she had run for twenty-five years. They treated her with as much care and respect as they could. She had a second stroke a year later and died.

The evening of my mother's funeral, sitting in a favorite childhood diner, my brother and I confessed to one another, with some consternation and shame, that neither of us felt much of anything. Neither of us had cried.

I think of my parents often. I miss them sometimes. I am also deeply relieved.

I end this book as I began it: upstairs, in my third-floor study, listening below to my children at play. As I write, the sounds of their passions drift up to me, their ardent laughter, their voices. I look down at them, the way they hurl their strong little bodies through the bright air all uncaring, assured and innocent. Profoundly benevolent.

I know that my children will encounter pain. They must learn to handle life's sufferings, as hard as it may be to watch sometimes. I draw comfort from believing that the pain they encounter in life will be theirs alone. When they are old enough, if they are inter-

of Abnormal Psychology, 1977, vol. 86 (b) pp. 609–14. See also S. J. Oliver and B. B. Toner, "The Influence of Gender Role Typing on the Expression of Depressive Symptoms," *Sex Roles,* vol. 22 (11–12) pp. 175–262, 1990.

23 *handled in the same way by both sexes:* E. S. Chevron, D. M. Quinlan, and S. J. Blatt, "Sex Roles and Gender Differences in the Experience of Depression," *Journal of Abnormal Psychology,* 1978, vol. 87 pp. 680–83. See also A. F. Chino and D. Funabiki, "A Cross-Validation of Sex-Differences in the Expression of Depression," *Sex Roles,* 1984, vol. 11 pp. 175–87, and C. A. Padesky, "Sex Differences in Depressive Symptoms Expression and Help Seeking Among College Students," *Sex Roles,* vol. 7 1981, pp. 309–20.

23 *Traditional gender socialization:* The phrase "halve themselves" and many of my ideas on boys' socialization I owe to Olga Silverstein. See O. Silverstein and B. Roshbaum, *The Courage to Raise Good Men* (New York: Viking, 1994).

23 *Girls are allowed:* C. Gilligan, *In a Different Voice: Psychological Theory and Women's Development* (Cambridge: Harvard University Press, 1982).

24 *given the right mix of chromosomes:* D. L. Duner, "Recent Gender Studies of Bipolar and Unipolar Depression," in J. C. Coyne, ed., *Essential Papers on Depression* (New York: New York University Press, 1985). See also E. S. Gershon, W. E. Bunney, Jr., J. F. Lehman, "The Inheritance of Affective Disorders: A Review of Data and Hypothesis," *Behavioral Genetics,* 1976, vol. 6 pp. 227–61.

24 *inherited vulnerability with psychological injury:* P. Gilbert, *Depression: The Evolution of Powerlessness* (New York: Guilford, 1982).

27 *Bringing the scene palpably:* Enactment is a common technique used by several family therapy schools, and by practitioners as diverse as Virginia Satir, Peggy Papp, and Salvador Minuchin. At the Family Institute of Cambridge, a number of my colleagues, including Richard Chasin, Laura Chasin, Richard Lee, and Sally Ann Roth, have been in the forefront in applying complex theater techniques known as *psychodrama* to family therapy. For more on enactment, see A. Williams, *The Passionate Technique: Strategic Psychodrama with Individuals, Groups, and Families* (New York: Tavistock/Routledge, 1989); S. Minuchin, *Families and Family Therapy* (Cambridge: Harvard University Press, 1974); R. Chasin, S. Roth, M. Bograd, "Action Methods in Systemic Therapy: Dramatizing Ideal Futures and Reformed Pasts With Couples," *Family Process,* vol. 29(2) 1989, pp. 121–36; R. Chasin and S. Roth, "Past Perfect, Future Perfect: A Positive Approach to Opening Couple Therapy," in R. Chasin, H. Grunebaum, M. Herzig, eds., *One Couple, Four Realities: Multiple Perspectives on Couples Therapy* (New York: Guilford, 1990).

29 *"Fix this scene. Make it right":* The technique used here is called a "reform scene." First, the therapist has the family reenact a problematic encounter. The therapist then uses an "affect bridge" to surface the personal resonance of the scene for a family member (e.g., "What does this remind you of from your own past?"). The old scene is then reenacted and "fixed"—healed in some way—under the direction of the patient. The healing of "the scene beneath the scene" increases understanding and releases underlying emotions. Richard Chasin, Laura Chasin, and Sally Ann Roth have been my principal guides.

32 *And the fool replied.* [Lear] "Who is it that can tell me who I am?" [Fool] "Lear's shadow." *King Lear,* I, 4. *Shakespeare's Complete Works* (Baltimore: Penguin, 1969).

33 *"The mass of men lead lives of quiet desperation":* H. D. Thoreau, cited in *The Columbia Dictionary of Quotations* (New York: Columbia University Press, 1993).

ested, Belinda and I will tell them the facts, the details of our own childhoods. But, I realize, as I watch them dart and throw and laugh, that in a lived-through, visceral way, my children have little experience of, few reference points for, the violence their mother and father have come from.

We intend to keep it that way.

Notes

Chapter One: Men's Hidden Depression

21 *In the middle of the journey:* "Nel mezzo del cammin di nostra vita mi ritrovai per una selva oscura. . . ." Dante, *Inferno,* trans. J. D. Sinclair (London: Oxford University Press, 1972), pp. 22–23.

22 *depression was predominantly a woman's disease:* G. Klerman and M. Weissman, "Sex Differences and the Epidemiology of Depression," *Archives of General Psychology,* (vol. 34:98–111) Jan. 1977.

23 *a toll on a par with heart disease:* P. E. Greenberg, L. E. Stiglin, L. Finkelstein, S. Ernst, R. Berndt, "The Economic Burden of Depression in 1990," special report in *The Journal of Clinical Psychiatry,* vol. 54 (11) 408–418 1990: "The Economics of Depression," 1990. See also P. Greenberg, L. Stiglin, S. Finkelstein, "Depression: A Neglected Major Illness," *Journal of Clinical Psychiatry,* Nov. 1993, pp. 419–24. For reactions to and discussions of Greenberg's report, see D. Goleman, "Depression Costs Put At $43 Billion," *The New York Times,* Dec. 3, 1993.

23 *Somewhere between 60 and 80 percent:* D. A. Reiger, R. M. A. Hirschfeld, F. K. Goodwin, et al., "The NIMH Depression Awareness Recognition and Treatment Program: Structure, Aims, and Scientific Basis," *American Journal of Psychiatry,* 1988, vol. 145 pp. 1351–57.

23 *treatment has a high success rate:* L. Eisenburg, "Treating Depression and Anxiety in Primary Care: Closing the Gap Between Knowledge and Practice," *New England Journal of Medicine,* 1992–93, vol. 326 pp. 1080–84.

23 *between 80 and 90 percent of depressed patients:* Reiger, Hirschfeld, Goodwin, et al., "The NIMH Depression Awareness Recognition and Treatment Program." See also M. Weissman, "The Psychological Treatment of Depression: Evidence for the Efficacy of Psychotherapy alone, in Comparison with, and in Combination with Pharmacotherapy," *Archives of General Psychiatry,* vol. 36 Oct. 1979, pp. 1261–69.

23 *men tend to manifest depression differently:* I am neither the first nor the only person reviewing the research on depression and gender to posit this explanation. See, for example, epidemiologists Hammen and Padesky, who remark: "It is unclear whether women are in fact more depressed than men, or whether male and female experiences with depression differ in ways that lead women to express symptoms. . . . seek help, or receive labels of depression in ways [that are] different from men." C. L. Hammen and C. A. Padesky, "Sex Differences in the Expression of Depressive Responses on the Beck Depression Inventory," *Journal*

33 *The guidebook for diagnosis:* American Psychiatric Association, *Diagnostic and Statistical Manual of Mental Disorders,* 4th ed. (Washington, D.C.: American Psychiatric Association, 1994.)

33 *caused by an imbalance of black bile:* Stanley Jackson has written a remarkably comprehensive history of the idea of depression, from early Greek writers to the present. See S. Jackson, *Melancholia & Depression,* (New Haven: Yale University Press, 1986). See also P. Gilbert, *Depression.*

34 *Epidemiologists have found:* See D. Goleman, "A Rising Cost of Modernity: Depression," *The New York Times,* Dec. 8, 1992, science section.

34 *each successive generation has doubled its susceptibility:* Reiger, Hirschfeld, Goodwin, et al. "The NIMH Depression Awareness Recognition and Treatment Program," pp. 1351–57. See also N. M. Weissman, M. L. Bruce, P. J. Leaf, et al., "Affective Disorders," in L. N. Robbins, D. A. Reiger, eds., *Psychiatric Disorders in America: The Epidemiologic Catchment Area Study* (New York: The Free Press, 1991).

34 *depression in greater numbers and at earlier ages:* Goleman, "A Rising Cost of Modernity: Depression."

34 *between 6 and 10 percent of our population:* National Institute of Mental Health, *Number of U.S. Adults (in millions) with Mental Disorder, 1990,* March 25, 1992. See also E. S. Schneidman, "Overview: A Multidimensional Approach to Suicide," in D. Jacobs and H. N. Brown, eds., *Suicide: Understanding and Responding,* Harvard Medical Perspectives (Connecticut: International Universities Press, 1989).

34 *a sign of personal weakness:* See J. Brody, "Myriad Masks Hide an Epidemic of Depression," *The New York Times,* Sept. 30, 1992, for both surveys.

35 *"My head is bloody, but unbowed":* W. E. Henley, "Perseverance," cited in *The Columbia Dictionary of Quotations.*

35 *And I guess the ultimate wimp kills himself:* John Rush spearheaded the recent committee assigned with devising federal guidelines for the recognition of depression to be used by medical practitioners. He is interviewed in K. Cronkite, *On the Edge of Darkness: Conversations about Conquering Depression* (New York: Doubleday, 1994), p. 79.

36 *more likely than women to take their own lives:* National Center for Health Statistics, U.S. Department of Health and Human Services, 1993. USDH & HS (NCHS, Center for Disease Control, Division of Vital Statistics, Office of Mortality Statistics, Monthly Vital Statistics Report), vol. 40, no. (8), supp. 2, Jan. 7, 1992.

36 *men would rather place themselves at risk:* A. P. Douglas, D. Hull, J. Hull, "Sex Role Orientation and Type A Behavior Pattern," *Personality and Social Psychology,* 1981, vol. 9 (2) pp. 600–604; F. Conrad, "Sex Roles as a Factor in Longevity," *Sociology and Social Research,* 1962, vol. 46 pp. 195–202; D. McCelland, N. D. William, B. Kalen, K. Rudolph, *The Drinking Man* (Riverside, N.J.: Free Press, 1972).

36 *"They were too frightened to be cowards":* T. O'Brien, *The Things They Carried* (New York: Penguin, 1990), pp. 20–21.

37 *Men wait longer to acknowledge:* I. Waldron, "Why Do Women Live Longer than Men?" *Journal of Human Stress,* 1976, vol. 2 pp. 1–13; G. E. Good, D. M. Dell, and L. B. Mintz, "Male Role and Gender Role Conflict: Relations to Help Seeking in Men," *Journal of Counseling Psychology,* 1989, pp. 295–300; J. Harrison, "Warning: The Male Sex Role May Be Dangerous to Your Health," *Social Issues,* vol. 34 1978, pp. 65–86.

37 *obsessive concerns about the size and shape of their physiques:* On muscles, see B. Glasner,

"Men in Muscles," in M. Kimmel and M. Messner, eds., *Men's Lives* (New York: Macmillan, 1989). On bulimia, see R. Olivardia, G. Harrison, Jr., and B. Mangweth, "Eating Disorders in College Men," *American Journal of Psychiatry*, Sept. 1995, vol. 152 (9) p. 1279.

37 *"Above all else":* From the film version of P. Conroy's novel *The Great Santini* (New York: Bantam Books, 1987).

38 *Hammen and Peters tested hundreds of college roommates:* C. I. Hammen and S. D. Peters, "Interpersonal Consequences of Depression: Responses to Men and Women Enacting a Depressed Role," *Journal of Abnormal Psychology*, 1978, vol. 87 pp. 322–32.

38 *The "roommate study" was later repeated:* See Joiner for a review of both supporting and nonsupporting studies. Joiner and his colleagues conclude: "When men with low self-esteem are depressed, they may be expected to suffer in silence and take it like a man. Excessive reassurance seeking violates this expectancy, as well as stereotypical male behavior in general and consequently may result in rejection. In contrast, reassurance seeking by depressed women with low self-esteem may not violate stereotypic societal norms to the same degree and therfore may be less objectional." T. E. Joiner, Jr., M. S. Alfano, and G. I. Metalsky, "When Depression Breeds Contempt: Reassurance Seeking, Self-Esteem, and Rejection of Depressed College Students by Their Roommates," *Journal of Abnormal Psychology*, 1992, vol. 10 (1) p. 171.

38 *It is better just to "get on with it":* See R. Taffel, "The Politics of Mood," in M. Bogard, ed., *Feminist Approaches for Men in Family Therapy* (New York: Harrington Park Press, 1991), pp. 153–77.

39 *It's okay if you have a neurological disease:* John Rush quoted in K. Cronkite, *On the Edge of Darkness*, pp. 79–80.

40 *a tendency for mental health professionals to overdiagnose women's depression:* M. K. Potts, M. A. Burnam, and K. B. Wells, "Gender Differences in Depression Detection: A Comparison of Clinician Diagnosis and Standardized Assessment," *Psychological Assessment*, 1991, vol. 3(4) pp. 609–15. See also I. M. Werbrugge and R. P. Steiner, "Physician Treatment of Men and Women Patients. Sex Bias or Appropriate Care?" *Medical Care*, 1981, vol. 19 pp. 609–32.

40 *If it is unmanly to be depressed:* See J. Waisberg and S. Page, "Gender Role Noncomformity and Perception of Mental Illness," *Women and Health*, 1988, p. 3. See also J. Wallen and J. D. Waitzkin, "Physician Stereotypes about Female Health and Illness: A Study of Patient's Sex and the Informative Process During Medical Interviews," *Women and Health*, vol. 4 1979, pp. 135–46.

41 *"Masked depression is one of the most prevalent disorders":* M. K. Opler, "Cultural Variations in Depression: Past and Present," in S. Lesse, ed., *Masked Depression* (New York: J. Aronson, 1974).

Chapter Two: Sons of Narcissus

43 *He is the longed-for:* Ovid, *Metamorphoses*, trans. A. Mandelbaum (New York: Harcourt Brace, 1993), p. 94.

43 *"Narcissus was loved by many":* Ibid.

44 *"Let me at least gaze upon you":* This quote is from Thomas Bulfinch's rendition of the tale. T. Bulfinch, *Bulfinch's Mythology* (London: Springer, 1964), p. 75.

44 *"With this," the tale concludes, "and much more of the same":* Ibid.

44 *As the Renaissance philosopher:* M. Ficino, *Commentary on Plato's Symposium,* trans. J. Sears (Dallas: Spring, 1985).

44 *Healthy self-esteem presupposes:* This viewpoint on healthy self-esteem derives from the thinking of Pia Mellody. P. Mellody, with A. Miller and J. Miller, *Facing Codependence* (San Francisco: HarperCollins, 1987). See also H. Kohut, "Forms and Transformations of Narcissism," in A. P. Morrison, ed., *Essential Papers on Narcissism* (New York: New York University Press, 1986).

45 *the "gleam in the mother's eye":* The phrase belongs to the great child analyst D. W. Winnicot. For a discussion of the physiological aspects of self-esteem and their relationship to depression, see P. Kramer, *Listening to Prozac* (New York: Viking, 1993).

45 *This can never replenish:* See H. Kohut, E. Wolf, "The Disorders of the Self and Their Treatement: An Outline" in A. P. Morrison, ed., *Essential Papers on Narcissism.*

50 *in a state of deep relaxation:* See D. Kantor, "Critical Identity Image: A Concept Linking Individual, Couple and Family Development," in J. K. Pierce and L. J. Friedman, eds., *Family Therapy: Combining Psychodynamic and Family Systems Approaches* (New York: Grunet Stratton, 1980), ch. 9. See also M. Phillips and C. Frederick, *Healing the Divided Self: Clinical and Ericksonian Hypnotherapy for Post Traumatic and Dissociative Conditions* (New York: W. W. Norton, 1995).

50 *to reexperience rather than merely report:* P. Mellody, *Post Induction Training: A Manual for Psychotherapists* (Wickenburg, Arizona: Mellody Enterprises, 1994).

55 *"This picture of a delusion":* S. Freud, "Mourning and Melancholia," in J. C. Coyne, ed., *Essential Papers on Depression* (New York: New York University Press, 1985), p. 51.

55 *In psychiatry today, the self-attack Freud:* The current literature on shame and its relationship to depression is vast. Shame is one of a few concepts that has inspired acute interest in psychoanalytic theory, family systems theory, and addictions recovery theory. For reviews, see A. Morrison, *Shame: The Underside of Narcissism* (New York: Analytic Press, 1989). Also, F. Wright, J. O'Leary, and J. Balkin, "Shame, Guilt, Narcissism and Depression: Correlates and Sex Differences," *Psychoanalytic Psychology* 1989, vol. 6 (2) pp. 217–30.

55 *This experience of depression:* For more on alexithymia, see H. Krystal, "Alexithymia and Psychotherapy," *American Journal of Psychotherapy,* January 1979, vol. 33 (1) pp. 17–31. Also see R. Levant, *Masculinity Reconstructed* (New York: Penguin, 1995).

55 *They are like the souls:* Dante, *Inferno,* trans. M. Muse (Bloomington, Indiana: Indiana University Press, 1971).

56 *The central point:* For clarity's sake, I have taken the liberty of substituting the term *grandiosity* for the term *narcissism,* which was used by Wright and his colleagues to denote both unrealistic superiority and also any pathological state of self-esteem, either grandiose or shame ridden. I feared the double usage of the term, while familiar to therapists, would confuse the lay reader. F. Wright, J. O'Leary, and J. Balkin, "Shame, Guilt, and Depression," vol. 6 (2) pp. 223–24. For more on the dynamics of this defense, see A. Reich, "Pathological Forms of Self-Esteem Regulation," *Psychoanalytic Study of the Child,* 1960, pp. 215–32. See also A. Miller, "Depression and Grandiosity as Related Forms of Narcissistic Disturbance" in A. P. Morrison, *Essential Papers on Narcissism.*

56 *The flight from shame:* For both a review and important current research on the role of gender, see P. Gjerde, "Alternative Pathways to Chronic Depressive Symptoms in Young Adults: Gender Differences in Developmental Trajectories," *Child Development,* 1995, in press.

Chapter Three: The Hollow Men

59 *Remember us:* T. S. Eliot, "The Hollow Men," in *Selected Poems: The Centenary Edition* (New York: Harcourt Brace, 1988), p. 77.

59 *can be called an addictive process:* P. Mellody, *Facing Codependence* (San Francisco: HarperCollins, 1987).

60 *Like wheels within wheels:* The dynamics of a shame or dysphoria spiral have become a commonplace observation in the addictions field. See, for example, G. A. Marlat, "Alcohol the Magic Elixir: Stress, Expectancy, and the Transformation of Emotional States," in E. Gotthel, K. A. Druley, S. Pashko, and S. P. Weinstein, eds., *Stress and Addiction* (New York: Brunner/Mazel, 1987), p. 302.

60 "Alcohol was a central factor": William Styron interviewed in K. Conkrite, *On the Edge of Darkness: Conversations about Conquering Depression* (New York: Doubleday, 1994).

61 *The first to recognize these qualities:* In S. E. Jackson, *Melancholia and Depression from Hippocratic Times to Modern Times* (New Haven: Yale University Press, 1986).

62 *a topography of addictive choices.* For reviews, see E. Khantzian, "The Self-Medication Hypothesis of Addictive Disorders," *American Journal of Psychiatry,* Nov. 1985, v 142(11) pp. 1259–64. See also E. Khantzian, K. Halliday, and W. McAuliffe, *Addiction and the Vulnerable Self: Modified Dynamic Group Therapy for Substance Abusers* (New York: Guilford, 1990).

62 *Wachtler's compulsive behavior screened symptoms:* L. Wolfe, *Double Life: The Shattering Affair Between Chief Judge Sol Wachtler and Socialite Joy Silverman* (New York: Pocketbooks, 1994).

62 *In related work, researcher Lewis Staner:* L. Staner, "Sleep, Desamethasone Suppression Test, and Response to Somatic Therapies in an Atypical Affective State Presenting as Erotomania: A Case Report," *European Psychiatry,* pp. 269–71. See also D. J. Stein, E. Hollander, et al., "Serotonergic Medications for Sexual Obsessions, Sexual Addictions, and Paraphilias," *Journal of Clinical Psychiatry,* 1992, vol. 6 (5) pp. 267–71.

64 *In severe love addiction:* See P. Mellody, *Facing Love Addiction: Giving Yourself the Power to Change the Way You Love* (New York: HarperCollins, 1992).

65 *Perhaps the most unadorned form:* See D. Balcom, "Shame and Violence: Considerations in Couples' Treatment," *Journal of Independent Social Work,* vol. 5 (3–4) 165–181 1991.

65 *Ernst Becker called these two possibilities:* E. Becker, *The Denial of Death* (New York: Free Press, 1973). Also relevant is Heinz Kohut's formulations concerning the "mirroring" and "idealizing" transference phenonomon. See H. Kohut, *The Analysis of the Self* (New York: International University Press, 1971).

65 *Judith Herman shows in* Trauma and Recovery: J. Herman, *Trauma and Recovery* (New York: Basic Books, 1992).

67 *These are the common dynamics.* For a review, see D. Balcom, "Shame and Violence."

67 *When Jimmy lashed out:* P. Mellody, personal communication.

68 *As mythologist Joseph Campbell:* J. Campbell, *The Hero with a Thousand Faces* (Princeton, New Jersey: Princeton University Press, 1973).

69 *In fact, almost every recent Hollywood:* For an excellent analysis, see S. Jeffords, *Hard Bodies: Hollywood Masculinity in the Reagan Era* (New Brunswick, New Jersey: Rutgers University Press, 1994).

69 *not transmuted by spirit but inflated by violence:* Literary critic Richard Slotkin has written an engaging and thorough analysis of this recurring pattern and its link to frontier mythology in the United States: R. Slotkin, *Regeneration Through Violence: The Mythology of the American Frontier 1600–1860* (New York: Atheneum, 1973); *The Fatal Environment: The Myth of the Frontier in the Age of Industrialization 1800–1895* (New York: Atheneum, 1985); *Gunfighter Nation: The Myth of the Frontier in 20th Century America* (New York: Atheneum, 1992).

69 *one distinguishing characteristic of battering:* Donald Dutton, expert in work with male batters, writes: "In my research with Jim Browning, in which we showed men videotapes of women arguing with their husbands . . . I found that abusive men are more sensitive to and perceive more abandonment then do nonabusive men. And having done so, they react with elevated anger and anxiety to these scenes." D. Dutton, *The Batterer; a Psychological Profile* (New York: Basic Books, 1995), p. 45. For the original research, see D. Dutton and J. J. Browning, "Concern for Power, Fear and Intimacy and Aversive Stimuli for Wife Assault," in G. T. Hotaling, D. Finkelhor, J. T. Kirkpatrick, and M. A. Straus, eds., *Family Abuse and Its Consequences: New Directions in Research,* (Newbury Park, Calif.: Sage, 1988), pp. 163–75. Much of my thinking on batterers derives from the work of Fernando Maderos of Common Purpose, Inc., Somerville, Massachussets. Fernando is one of the lights in the field of domestic violence. See F. Maderos, *Differences and Similarities Between Violent and Nonviolent Men: An Exploratory Study.* Thesis presented to the faculty of the Graduate School of Education of Harvard University, 1995.

69 *When their partners "fail them":* See S. Krugman, "Male Development and the Transformation of Shame," in R. Levant and W. Pollack, eds., *A New Psychology of Men* (New York: Basic Books, 1995).

73 *"setting a sexual boundary":* On sexual boundaries, see P. Mellody, *Facing Codependence.* See also P. Carnes, *Out of the Shadows: Understanding Sexual Addiction* (Minneapolis: Compcare Publications, 1983). Carnes, the founder and director of the Dallamo Hospital, the only residential setting dealing exclusively with sex addiction issues, writes powerfuly about the disorder.

75 *Under my direction, on his knees:* Bringing the perpetrator literally to his knees in the family session helps break through denial and minimization and also offers some sense of spiritual expiation. I have borrowed and adapted the technique from its creator Cloe Madanes. Madanes has long been considered one of family therapy's most innovative clinicians and teachers. C. Madanes, *The Violence of Men . . . New Techniques for Working with Abusive Families: a Therapy of Social Action* (San Francisco: Josey Bass, 1995).

76 *Between the inordinate shame of depression:* P. Mellody, personal communication.

79 *Addiction experts have termed:* See, for example, M. Fossum & M. Mason, *Facing Shame: Families in Recovery* (New York: Norton, 1986).

79 *Research indicates that depressed people:* See E. Deykin, J. D. Levy, and V. Wells, "Adolescent Depression, Alcohol and Drug Abuse" in E. Khantzian, K. Halliday, and W. McAuliffe, eds., *Addiction and the Vulnerable Self: Modified Dynamic Group Therapy for Substance Abusers* (New York: Guilford, 1990). Also E. Khantzian, "The

Self-Medication Hypothesis of Addictive Disorders: Focus on Heroin and Cocaine Dependence," *American Journal of Psychiatry*, 1985, vol. 142 (11) pp. 1259–64; B. J. Rousanville, M. M. Weissman, K. Crits-Christoph, C. Wilber, and H. D. Kleber, "Diagnosis and Symptoms of Depression in Opiate Addicts: Course and Relationship to Treatment Outcome," *Archives of General Psychiatry*, vol. 139 pp. 151–56.

79 *alcohol* both *provides relief from depression and simultaneously creates more:* See, for example, F. Petty and H. Nasrallah, "Secondary Depression in Alcoholism: Implications for Future Research," *Comprehensive Psychiatry*, vol. 122 pp. 587–95; S. Nolen-Hoeksema, *Sex Differences in Depression* (Palo Alto, California: Stanford University Press, 1990). For a review of the debate itself, see E. J. Khantzian, "A Clinical Perspective of the Cause-Consequence Controversy in Alcohol and Addictive Suffering," *Journal of the American Academy of Psychonalysis*, 1987, vol. 15 (4) pp. 521–37.

80 *"And depression was the main cause of it all":* Jim Jensen interviewed in K. Cronkite, *On the Edge of Darkness.*

82 *Women rate high in internalizing, men in externalizing:* See P. Gjerde, J. Block, and J. H. Block, "Depressive Symptoms and Personality During Late Adolescence: Gender Differences in the Externalization-Internalization of Symptom Expression," *Journal of Abnormal Psychology*, 1988, vol. 99 (4) pp. 475–86; P. Gjerde and J. Block, "Preadolescent Antecedents of Depressive Symptomatology at Age 18: A Prospective Study," *Journal of Youth and Adolescence*, 1991, vol. 20 (2) 217–232 pp. 215–30; L. A. Sroufe and M. Rutter, "The Domain of Developmental Psychopathology," *Child Development*, 1984, vol. 55 pp. 17–29; A. Ebata, A. C. Peterson, *Patterns of Adjustment During Early Adolescence: Gender Differences in Depression and Achievement*, manuscript submitted for publication, 1988; See also P. Gjerde, "Alternative Pathways to Chronic Depressive Symptoms in Young Adults: Gender Differences in Developmental Trajectories," *Child Development*, 1995, in press.

82 *Internalizing has been found to have a high correlation:* See P. Gjerde, "Alternative Pathways." See also S. Nolen-Hoeksema, *Sex Differences in Depression.* Gjerde's work, with his colleague, Jack Block, carries great interest because his data has been drawn from a massive twenty-year prospective study of a large sample of children. Gjerde and Block administered a battery of personality inventories to this sample every few years and were able to correlate particular character traits early in life with various psychological conditions that emerged later on. Their work stands as one of the few large-scale studies that is prospective rather than retrospective, and, as such, its data is particularly convincing.

83 *leading one "Men's Movement" leader to quip:* Both the figure on prison population and the reported comment are cited in A. Kimbrell, *The Masculine Mystique: The Politics of Masculinity* (Ballantine Books, 1995). See also W. Farrell, *The Myth of Male Power* (New York: Simon & Schuster, 1993).

84 *balances the level of pathology in each sex:* R. C. Kessler, K. A. McGonagle, S. Zhao, et al., "Lifetime and 12-Month Prevalence of DSM III-R Psychiatric Disorders in the United States: Results from the National Comorbidity Survey," *Archives of General Psychiatry*, Jan. 1994, vol. 51 (1) pp. 8–19.

84 Chart, *"Lifetime Incidents of Mental Disorders":* Ibid.

Chapter Four: A Band Around the Heart

88 *He pushes past other people's boundaries:* For more on walls and boundaries, see P. Mellody, *Facing Codependence* (San Francisco: HarperCollins, 1987).

91 *"Doc, I was frustrated when the plane went down":* Men's use of such terms was first pointed out to me by my colleague Jack Sternbach, Ph.D.

93 *allowing me to guide him into light trance:* The technique of working with childhood trauma illustrated in the following vignette is called *debriefing.* It was conceived by P. Mellody, *Post Induction Training: A Manual for Psychotherapists* (Wickenburg, Arizona: Mellody Enterprises, 1994).

95 *"A dissociated memory is breaking into consciousness":* Ibid.

97 *depression as a kind of mourning:* The central role of early childhood trauma and deprivation in the etiology of depression has been a consistent formulation in virtually all of the psychoanalytic theories on depression from Freud through to the present day, including object relations theory and self psychology. For reviews, see S. W. Jackson, *Melancholia and Depression: From Hippocratic Times to Modern Times* (New Haven: Yale University Press, 1986), or P. Gilbert, *Depression: The Evolution of Powerlessness* (New York: Guilford, 1992). A few classic works on the subject are: S. Freud, "Mourning and Melancholia," in *Collected Works,* vol. 14 (London: Holgarth Press, 1917), pp. 243–58; E. Bibring, "The Mechanism of Depression," in P. Greenacre, ed., *Affective Disorders* (New York: International University Press, 1953); J. Bolby, *Loss: Sadness and Depression. Attachment and Loss,* vol. 3 (London: Hogarth Press, 1980); J. Deitz, "The Evolution of the Self-Psychological Approach to Depression," *American Journal of Psychotherapy,* 1989, vol. 43 (4) pp. 494–505; M. Klein, *Envy and Gratitude and Other Works* (1946–1963) (London: Hogarth Press, 1957); H. Kohut, *The Analysis of the Self* (New York: International University Press, 1971); H. Kohut, *The Restoration of the Self* (New York: International University Press, 1977).

97 *hospitalism:* R. Spitz, "Hospitalism: An Inquiry into the Genesis of Psychiatric Conditions in Early Childhood," *Psychoanalitic Study of the Child,* 1945, vol. 1 pp. 53–74. Spitz first coined the phrase *anaclytic depression,* which has since become the technical term in psychiatry for childhood depression. Spitz chose the word *anaclytic,* which means "clinging," to underscore his conviction that in early childhood, depression and attachment disturbances are essentially synonymous.

98 *Bolby's colleagues filmed a seventeen-month-old boy's reaction:* From the film *John at Seventeen Months,* C. Robertson and L. Robertson, producers. Distributed by Windsor Total Video, and available through the New York University Library Audio-Visual Department.

99 *"major depression" and "dysthymia":* While the *Diagnostic and Statistical Manual of Mental Disorders,* 3rd ed. (DSM III) warns against confusing dysthymia with "mild major depression," I find such distinctions tortured and misconceived. I agree with Goldberg and Bridges, who characterize dysthymia as "a new plastic box for some rather old wine." The major depression/dysthymia distinction seems little more than the old endogenous/exogenous distinction repackaged. In epidemiology, for two similar disorders to be classed as distinct entities, rather than one disorder manifesting itself with variations along a spectrum, there must be evidence of *a zone of rarity,* a territory devoid of overlapping characteristics. Distinct disease entities must be shown to be, in fact, distinct. No evidence has been brought forward that clearly demarcates depression in milder, chronic

forms from depression in more severe acute forms. See D. P. Goldberg and K. W. Bridges, "Epidemiological Observations on the Concept of Dysthymic Disorder," in S. W. Burton and H. S. Akiskal, eds., *Dysthymic Disorder* (London: Royal College of Psychiatrists, 1990), p. 104; *Diagnostic and Statistical Manual of Mental Disorders*, 3rd ed. (Washington, D.C.: American Psychiatric Association, 1989), p. 789.

99 *The distinction between major and minor depression:* For a sound and accessible review, see P. Kramer, *Listening to Prozac* (New York: Viking, 1993).

99 *the overall economic and quality-of-life costs.* For a review of the literature on this distinction as well as a review of studies detailing the long-term consequences of dysthymia, see P. Gilbert, *Depression: The Evolution of Powerlessness* (New York: Guilford, 1984). See also A. Lewis, " 'Endogenous' and 'Exogenous,' a Useful Dichotomy?" *Psychological Medicine*, 1971, vol. 1 pp. 191–96.

100 *a strong genetic component to major depression:* For reviews, see D. Dunner, "Recent Genetic Studies of Bipolar and Unipolar Depression," and R. Baldessarini, "A Summary of Biomedical Aspects of Mood Disorders," both appearing in J. C. Coyne, ed., *Essential Papers on Depression* (New York: New York University Press, 1985).

100 *Depression Spectrum Disease:* G. Winokur, "Controversies in Depression," or "Do Clinicians Know Something After All?" in J. C. Coyne, ed., *Essential Papers on Depression.*

101 *depression and alcoholism, with the former linked to women:* R. Cadoret and G. Winokur, "Depression in Alcoholism," *Annals of the New Academy of Sciences*, 1974, vol. 22 pp. 34–39; G. Winokur and P. Clayton, "Family History Studies: Sex Differences and Alcoholism in Primary Affective Illness," *British Journal of Psychiatry*, 1967, pp. 973–79; G. Winokur, J. Rimmer, and T. Reich, "Alcoholism: Is There More than One Type of Alcoholism?" *British Journal of Psychiatry*, 1971, vol. 113 pp. 525–31. For a review of the literature rebutting Winokur's research, see S. Nolen-Hoeksema, *Sex Differences in Depression* (Palo Alto: Stanford University Press, 1990), pp. 42–46.

101 *"The intense and sometimes comically strident factionalism":* W. Styron, *Darkness Visible: A Memoir of Madness* (New York: Vantage, 1992), p. 11.

102 *Fritz Henn and Emmeline Edwards looked at the effect:* Henn and Edwards's research is reported and discussed in D. Papolos and J. Papolos, *Overcoming Depression* (New York: HarperCollins, 1992).

103 *"lifelong psychobiological consequences":* Bessel van der Kolk, former president of the International Association of Trauma Studies Research, has been a pioneer investigator on the biological consequences of trauma. Much of my thinking on the nature of trauma owes a debt to his formulations. In Chapter 2 of *Psychological Trauma*, "The Separation Cry and the Trauma Response: Developmental Issues in the Psychobiology of Attachment and Separation," one of the best reviews of recent research, van der Kolk discusses virtually all of the studies mentioned in this chapter. B. van der Kolk, *Psychological Trauma* (Washington, D.C.: American Psychiatric Press, 1987), p. 33.

103 *Primate infants who are separated from their mothers:* C. L. Coe, S. Weiner, L. T. Rosenberg, et al., "Endocrine and Immune Responses to Separation and Maternal Loss in Non-Human Primates," in M. Reite and T. Fields, eds., *The Psychobiology of Attachment and Separation* (Orlando, Florida: Academic Press, 1985), and P. S. Timeras, "The Timing of Hormone Signals in the Orchestration of Brain

Development," in R. N. Emide and R. J. Harmon, eds., *The Development of Attachment and Affiliative Systems* (New York: Plenum, 1982).

103 *Adrenal enzymes also change with maternal separation:* See C. Coe, S. Medoza, and S. Levine, "Mother-Infant Attachment in the Squirrel Monkey: Adrenal Responses to Separation," *Behavioral Biology,* vol. 22 pp. 256–63; M. Konner (1982), "Biological Aspects of Mother-Infant Bond," in *The Development of Attachment and Affiliative Systems;* W. McKinney, "Separation and Depression: Biological Markers," in M. Reite and T. Fields, eds., *The Psychobiology of Attachment and Separation;* M. Reite, R. Short, et al., "Attachment, Loss and Depression," *Journal of Child Psychological Psychiatry,* 1981, vol. 22 pp. 141–69.

103 *"These changes are not transient or mild":* van der Kolk, *Psychological Trauma.*

104 *might prove a good working model for depression in humans:* S. Suomi, S. Seaman, J. K. Lewis, "Effects of Imipramine Treatment of Separation Induced Social Disorders in Rhesus Monkeys," *Archives of General Psychiatry,* 1978, vol. 35 pp. 321–25. H. Harlow and C. Mears, *The Human Model: Primate Perspectives* (New York: Wiley and Sons, 1979).

104 *increased sensitivity to amphetamines and opoids:* C. Anderson and W. Mason, "Competitive Social Strategies in Groups of Deprived and Experienced Rhesus Monkeys," *Developmental Psychobiology,* 1978, vol. 11. pp. 289–99. See also M. Mason, "Early Social Deprivation in the Non-Human Primates; Implications for Human Behavior," in D. Glass, ed., *Environmental Influences* (New York: Rockefeller University Press, 1968).

104 *he disbelieved and blamed them:* For the history of our culture's attitudes toward trauma, see J. Herman, *Trauma and Recovery* (New York: Basic Books, 1992).

105 *virtually all of the men interred:* K. Cullen, "Camp Horror Still Haunts WWII POWs," *Boston Globe,* May 28, 1995.

106 *some trauma experts called "Type I" trauma:* L. C. Terr, "Childhood Traumas: An Outline and Overview," *American Journal of Psychiatry,* 1991, vol. 148 pp. 10–21.

106 *males who appear, if anything, even more sensitive:* A. Green, *Child Maltreatment* (New York: Aronson, 1980).

107 *estimates that one in eleven children:* R. Gelles and C. Cornell, *Intimate Violence in Families* (Newbury Park, California: Sage, 1990). See also C. P. Widom, *Child Abuse Neglect and Adult Behavior,* American Orthopsychiatric Association, 1989, pp. 355–67.

107 *nurturing, limit setting, and guidance:* P. Mellody, *Facing Codependency* (San Francisco: HarperCollins, 1987).

110 *boys are spoken to less than girls, comforted less, nurtured less:* For a review, see P. Gerdje, "Alternative Pathways to Chronic Depressive Symptoms in Young Adults: Gender Differences in Developmental Trajectories," *Child Development,* 1995, in press.

Chapter Five: Perpetrating Masculinity

113 *Before they had attended school a week:* J. M. Barrie, *Peter Pan* (New York: Penguin, 1911), pp. 195–96.

113 *135,000 children take handguns to school:* S. Coontz, *The Way We Never Were: American Families and the Nostalgia Trap* (New York: Basic Books, 1992).

113 *the leading cause of death in black men:* J. Gibbs, "Young Black Males in America:

Endangered, Embittered and Embattled," in M. Kimmel and M. Messner, eds., *Men's Lives*, 2nd ed. (New York: Macmillan, 1992), pp. 50–66; J. Archer, "Violence Between Men," in J. Archer, ed., *Male Violence* (London: Routledge, 1994), pp. 1–22.

113 *most violent acts, both inside and outside the home:* J. Archer, "Male Violence in Perspective," Introduction in Archer, *Male Violence*.

116 *most ferocious attacks are reserved for other males:* Y. Ahmad and P. Smith, "Bullying in Schools and the Issue of Sex Differences," in J. Archer, *Male Violence*; K. Bjorkqvist, K. Lagersptz, and A. Kaukiainen, "Do Girls Manipulate and Boys Fight? Developmental Trends in Regard to Direct and Indirect Aggression," *Aggressive Behavior*, 1992, vol. 19 (2), pp. 117–27.

117 *The evolutionary value of dominance aggression:* K. Moyer, *The Psychobiology of Aggression* (New York: Harper & Row, 1976); G. Weisfeld (1994), "Aggression and Dominance in the Social World of Boys," in J. Archer, *Male Violence*, pp. 42–69.

117 *"The first man to hurl an epithet instead of a stick":* S. Freud, *Civilization and Its Discontents* (London: Hogarth Press, 1930).

117 *"rough and tumble play":* "Rough and tumble play" is a widely used term denoting boys' more physically vigorous play, a phenomenon so thoroughly documented that it stands as one of the few relatively noncontroversial observations about boys' and girls' differences.

118 *schooled in the training ground of their own abuse:* J. Beynon, "A School for Men: An Ethnographic Case Study of Routine Violence in Schooling," in J. Archer and K. Brown, eds., *Human Aggression: Naturalistic Approaches* (London: Routledge, 1989); R. Gelles and C. Cornell, *Intimate Violence in Families*, 2nd ed. (Newbury Park, California: Sage, 1990); B. Egeland, "A History of Abuse Is a Major Risk Factor for Abusing the Next Generation," in R. Gelles and R. Loseke, eds., *Current Controversies on Family Violence* (Newbury Park, California: Sage, 1993).

120 *"appropriate shame":* P. Mellody, *Facing Codependency* (San Francisco: HarperCollins, 1987).

121 *to see the boys as relational:* "The separate-and-different-worlds story is seductive. It gives full weight to the fact that girls and boys often *do* separate in daily interactions. . . . But as I've tried to line up that model with my own empirical observations and with the research literature, I have found so many exceptions and qualifications, so many incidents that spill beyond and fuzzy up the edges, and so many conceptual ambiguities, that I have come to question the model's basic assumptions. [The 'different cultures' model] embeds the experiences of dominants and marginalizes many other groups and individuals; and it collapses 'a play of differences that is always on the move' into static and exaggerated dualisms. The different cultures framework gains much of its appeal from stereotypes and ideologies that should be queried rather than built on and perpetuated as social fact. It is, I have concluded, simply inadequate as an account of actual experience and is, in many ways, a conceptual dead end." B. Thorne, *Gender Play: Girls and Boys in School* (New Brunswick, New Jersey: Rutgers University Press, 1993), pp. 90–91.

121 *This "pseudo-gifted" group:* R. Rosenthal, L. Jacobson, "Teacher Expectancies: Determinants of Pupil's IQ Gains," *Psychological Reports*, 1966, pp. 115–18.

121 *By not attending to boys' relational needs:* I am enormously indebted to the thinking of my friend and colleague Olga Silverstein for my understanding of the cultural forces pushing boys out of the relational. In many ways, I see this work as a com-

panion to her book *The Courage to Raise Good Men,* which explores many of the same conditions from the mother's perspective that I explore from the son's.

121 *"smaller, more fragile and prettier":* J. Rubin, F. Provenzano, and Z. Luria, "The Eye of the Beholder: Parent's Views on Sex of Newborns," *American Journal of Orthopsychiatry,* 1974, pp. 512–19.

122 *"If you think your child is* angry*":* J. Cundry and S. Cundry, "Sex Differences: A Study in the Eye of the Beholder," *Child Development,* 1976, pp. 812–19.

122 *relationship to their daughters as warmer:* J. Block, "Another Look at Sex Differentiation in the Socialization Behaviors of Mothers and Fathers," in F. Denmark and J. Sherman, eds., *Psychology of Women: Future Directions of Research* (New York: Psychological Dimensions, 1978).

123 *"parents are not fully aware of the methods":* B. Fagot, "The Influence of Sex of Child on Parental Reactions to Toddler Children," *Child Development,* 1978, vol. 49 pp. 459–65; quote on p. 464. A similar finding was the result of research reported in C. Tavris and C. Offir, *The Longest War: Sex Differences in Perspective* (New York: Harcourt Brace, 1977). Researchers Jerrie Will, Patricia Self, and Nancy Datan gave a small sample of mothers the choice of a fish, a truck, or a doll to give to a baby. The researchers described the baby as male to half of the mothers and female to the other half. Overwhelmingly, mothers tended to give the baby toys conforming to gender stereotypes. The "boy" babies got trucks; the "girl" babies got dolls. The subjects of the study were "virtually unanimous" in describing themselves as nondiscriminating in their treatment of male versus female children. The mothers' socially conforming behaviors appeared to be wholly outside of their conscious awareness. While parents may be unaware of the force of their socialization pressures, innumerable studies have confirmed differential parental response based on sex, as well as the children's intuitive grasp of their parents' preferences. Even young children appear quite aware of them. See, for example, B. Florisha, *Sex Roles and Personal Awareness* (Morristown, N.J.: General Learning Press, 1978).

123 *They cry more easily:* For a review of these studies, see R. Levant and G. Kopecky, *Masculinity Reconstructed* (New York: Penguin, 1995).

123 *"the expressive-affiliative mode":* J. Bardwick, *The Psychology of Women* (New York: Harper & Row, 1971).

123 *boys are subtly—or forcibly—pushed out:* For a review, see J. O'Neil, "Gender Role Strain in Men's Lives: Implications for Psychiatrists, Psychologists and Other Human-Service Providers," in K. Solomon and N. Levy, eds., *Men in Transition: Theory and Therapy* (New York: Plenum, 1982).

124 *" 'Agencies of socialization' cannot produce":* R. Connell, *Gender and Power: Society, the Person and Sexual Politics* (Palo Alto, California: Stanford University Press, 1987), p. 195. See also Silverstein and B. Roshbaum, *The Courage to Raise Good Men* (New York: Viking, 1994).

125 *"Boys never cry. Never":* Conroy, *The Prince of Tides* (New York: Bantam, 1991), p. 145.

127 *"nothing worse on earth than a boy who ain't":* Ibid., p. 116.

128 *"soul murder":* L. Shengold, *Soul Murder: Effect of Childhood Abuse and Deprivation* (New Haven: Yale University Press, 1989).

130 *being a man generally means not being a woman:* R. Levant, "Toward the Reconstruction of Masculinity," in R. Levant and W. Pollock, eds., *A New Psychology of Men* (New York: Basic Books, 1995), pp. 229–51. See also D. Levinson, C. Dar-

row, E. Klein, et al., *Seasons of a Man's Life* (New York: Knopf, 1978); H. Goldberg, *The New Male: from Self Destruction to Self Care* (New York: Morrow, 1979).

130 *Masculine identity development turns out to be:* Although I disagree with some of her analysis, Nancy Chodorow accurately summarizes the boy's masculinization process: "Dependency on his mother, attachment to her, and identification with her represent that which is not masculine; a boy must reject dependency and deny attachment and identification. Masculine gender role training becomes much more rigid than feminine. A boy represses those qualities he takes to be feminine inside himself and rejects and devalues women and whatever he considers to be feminine in the social world." N. Chodorow, *The Reproduction of Mothering* (Berkeley, California: University of California Press, 1978), p. 181.

131 *"the tyranny of the kind and nice":* L. M. Brown and C. Gilligan, *Meeting at the Crossroads* (New York: Ballantine Books, 1992).

131 *psychologists have blamed unstable masculine:* J. Pleck, *The Myth of Masculinity* (Cambridge, Massachusetts: MIT Press, 1984).

131 *this myth is easily disputed:* Ibid. To my knowledge, Joseph Pleck, who stands, in many ways, as the father of sociological research on masculinity, was the first to question this pervasive myth. I consider Pleck's *The Myth of Masculinity* as the single most important book written about men and their development. For a review of more recent applications of Pleck's ideas, see J. O'Neil, "Gender Role Strain." Also R. Levant and W. Pollack, *A New Psychology of Men.*

131 *a woman's basic femininity is never questioned:* B. Thorne, *Gender Play: Girls and Boys in School* (New Brunswick, N.J.: Rutgers University Press, 1993).

131 *Some sociologists now distinguish:* For a review, see J. O'Neil, "Gender Role Strain."

132 *Rigid notions about masculinity:* For both a good review and original research, see C. A. O'Heron and J. L. Orlofsky, "Stereotypic and Nonstereotypic Sex Role Trait and Behavior Orientation, Gender Identity and Psychological Adjustment," *Journal of Personality and Social Psychology,* vol. 58 (1) pp. 134–143. Also O. Silverstein and B. Roshbaum, *The Courage to Raise Good Men.*

133 *Suddenly, I heard the first boy cry out, 'Ndiyindoda!':* N. Mandela, *Long Walk to Freedom: The Autobiography of Nelson Mandela* (London: Little Brown, 1994), p. 28.

Chapter Six: The Loss of the Relational

137 *Sister, mother:* T. S. Eliot, *Selected Poems: The Centenary Edition* (New York: Harcourt Brace, 1988).

137 *"Therefore, it must be destroyed":* S. Freud, "Female Sexuality," cited by J. Swigart, *The Myth of the Bad Mother: The Emotional Realities of Mothering* (New York: Doubleday, 1991).

139 *"Don't let her put you in dresses and take you to teas":* P. Conroy, *The Prince of Tides* (New York: Bantam, 1991), p. 143.

140 *"When he finally manages to flee his mother":* M. Segell, "The Pater Principle," *Esquire,* March 1995, p. 121(7).

141 Bly himself regrets the unbalanced focus on his comments about "soft males" that have been made so much of by both his proponents and his detractors (personal communication). Along with his stress on the needed separation from mother—about which I obviously disagree—there is much in Bly's work that

invites and celebrates increased "feminine" traits in men, particularly the need for community, compassion, and the expression of grief.

141 *boys raised by women, including single women:* The best elucidation of this point is in Silverstein. For more on lesbian parents, see D. Goleman, "Studies Find No Disadvantage in Growing Up in a Gay Home," *The New York Times,* Dec. 2, 1992. See also C. J. Patterson, "Children of Lesbian and Gay Parents," *Child Development,* Oct. 1992, vol. 63 (5) pp. 1025–39, for a review of over three dozen studies, leading to the conclusion of no disadvantage in the child's development. On divorced and single mothers, see M. Heatherington, M. Cox, R. Cox, "Effects of Divorce on Parents and Children," in M. Lamb, et al., eds., *Nontraditional Families: Parenting and Child Development* (NY: L. Erlbaum, 1982). See also M. Heatherington, M. Cox, R. Cox, "Long Term Effects of Divorce and Remarriage on the Adjustment of Children," *Journal of the American Academy of Child Psychiatry,* 1985, vol. 24 (5) pp. 518–30.

141 *The boys who fare poorly:* For a rich twenty-year longitudinal study on the qualities determining good and bad fathering, along with their consequences for both father and son, see J. Snarey, *How Fathers Care for the Next Generation* (Cambridge: Harvard University Press, 1993).

142 *"Mother died today. Or, maybe, yesterday":* A. Camus, *The Stranger,* trans. S. Gilbert (New York: Vintage, 1976), p 1.

142 *Psychologist William Pollock suspects:* W. Betcher and W. Pollack, *In a Time of Fallen Heroes: The Re-Creation of Masculinity* (New York: Atheneum, 1993). See also O. Silverstein, and B. Roshbaum, *The Courage to Raise Good Men* (New York: Viking, 1994).

142 *mothers have allowed themselves to be silenced:* For a moving treatment of the issue of maternal silence, see K. Weingarten, *The Mother's Voice: Strengthening Intimacy in Families* (New York: Harcourt Brace, 1994).

142 *At least as damaging to the boy:* See O. Silverstein and B. Roshbaum, *The Courage to Raise Good Men.* See also G. Brooks and L. Silverstein, "Understanding the Dark Side of Masculinity: An Interactive Systems Model," in R. Levant and W. Pollack, eds., *A New Psychology of Men* (New York: Basic Books, 1995).

143 *The typical American father spends:* R. C. Barnett and G. K. Baruch, "Correlates of Father's Participation in Family Work," in P. Bonstein and C. Cowan, eds., *Fatherhood Today: Men's Changing Role in the Family* (New York: Wiley, 1989). See also J. Pleck, *Working Wives, Working Husbands* (Beverly Hills: Sage, 1985). Michael Lamb suggests differentiating between *engagement, accessibility,* and *responsibility.* While some men may be spending more time engaged with their children, few are aware of responsibility issues (stocking supplies, making appointments, keeping track of medical issues, and so on). See M. Lamb, *The Father's Role: Crosscultural Perspectives* (Hillsdale New Jersey: Lawrence Erlbaum, 1987). For an excellent history, see R. L. Griswold, *Fatherhood in America* (New York: Basic Books, 1993).

144 *As family therapist Olga Silverstein.* I am indebted to Olga Silverstein for this perspective. See Silverstein and B. Roshbaum, *The Courage to Raise Good Men.*

144 *poor Mom, seeing his dust, drops dead on the spot:* W. von Eschenbach, *Parzival* (Goppingen: Kummerle, 1989). For an analysis from a Jungian perspective of *Parzival* as a parable about male development see R. Johnson, *He* (New York: Harper and Row, 1974).

146 *The psychiatric term for this impairment is* alexithymia: See R. Levant and G. Kopecky, *Masculinity Reconstructed* (New York: Penguin, 1995). See also J. Bal-

swick, "Male Inexpressiveness: Psychological and Social Aspects," in K. Solomon and N. B. Levy, *Men in Transition; Theory and Therapy* (New York: Plenum, 1982). For more on alexithymia, see: H. Krystal, "Alexithymia and Psychotherapy," *American Journal of Psychotherapy*, Jan. 1979, vol. 33 (1) pp. 17–31.

146 *not by sedating him but rather by "revving him up"*: E. Khantzian, K. Halliday, and W. McAuliffe, *Addiction and the Vulnerable Self: Modified Dynamic Group Therapy for Substance Abusers* (New York: Guilford, 1990).

147 *"addiction to trauma."*: B. van der Kolk, *Psychological Trauma* (Washington, D.C.: American Psychiatric Press, 1987).

147 *their behavior is not equally dangerous:* B. Allgood Merten, P. M. Lewinsohn, and H. Hops, "Sex Differences and Adolescent Depression," *Journal of Abnormal Psychology*, 1990, pp. 55–63. See also P. T. Dimock, "Adult Males Sexually Abused as Children; Characteristic and Implication for Treatment," *Journal of Interpersonal Violence*, 1988, pp. 203–21; A. Green, "Dimensions of Psychological Trauma in Abused Children," *Journal of American Medical Association Child Psychiatry*, 1983, vol. 22 pp. 231–37. E. H. Carmen, P. P. Reiker, T. Mills, "Victims of Violence and Psychiatric Illness," *American Journal of Psychiatry*, 1984, vol. 141 (3) pp. 378–79.

147 *self-mutilation as bringing a sense of relief:* I am grateful to Dr. Carl Fulwiler for his insights on self-mutilation in incarcerated men. For more on this topic, see M. P. Hillbrand, (1993) "Self-Injurious Behavior in Correctional and Noncorrectional Psychiatric Patients," *Journal of Offender Rehabilitation*, 1993, vol. 19 pp. 95–102. See also R. T. Rada and J. Williams, "Urethral Insertion of Foreign Bodies," *Archives of General Psychiatry*, 1982, vol. 39 pp. 423–29; G. Rita-Y-Bach, "Habitual Violence and Self-Mutilation," *American Journal of Psychiatry*, 1974, vol. 50 pp. 1018–20.

148 *an extreme form of the way in which society truncates:* For a discussion of the effects of deadening socialization on men, see D. Lisak, "Integrating a Critique of Gender in the Treatment of Male Survivors of Childhood Abuse," *Psychotherapy*, (in press).

148 *vulnerability of depression unacceptable even to himself:* See L. W. Warren, "Male Intolerance of Depression: A Review with Implications for Psychotherapy," *Clinical Psychology Review*, 1983, vol. 3 (2) pp. 147–56.

148 *Research teaches us that the capacity to reach out:* I. McCann and L. Pearlman, *Psychological Trauma and the Adult Survivor: Theory, Therapy, and Transformation* (New York: Bruner Mazel, 1990).

157 *while the fox gnawed away his side:* The story is attributed to Cato and retold by Michel de Montaigne. M. Montaigne, *The Complete Works of Montaigne*, trans. by Donald Frame (Palo Alto, California: Stanford University Press, 1958).

158 *Linguist Deborah Tannen, analyzing women's:* D. Tannen, *You Just Dont Understand: Women and Men in Conversation* (New York: Ballantine, 1990).

Chapter Seven: Collateral Damage

161 *lose his immortal soul:* New Testament, Mark 8:36, King James Version.

161 *"pretty, polite, not too smart":* The phrase was used by David Halberstam in his review of Peggy Ornstein's *Schoolgirls*, an account of girls' inhibitions in secondary education. For Halberstam's review see: *The New York Times Book Review*, September 11, 1994, pp. 15–18. The review is of *Schoolgirls: Young Women, Self-*

Esteem, and the Confidence Gap by Peggy Ornstein in association with the American Association of University Women (New York: Doubleday, 1994).

161 *Studies like those of Peggy Ornstein or Lyn Brown and Carol Gilligan:* Ornstein, *Schoolgirls.*

162 *some of the advantages boys come to expect:* L. M. Brown, C. Gilligan, *Meeting at the Crossroads* (New York: Ballantine, 1992).

162 *Rape can been seen . . . as an act of aggression:* S. Brownmiller, *Against Our Will; Men, Women and Rape* (New York: Bantam, 1976).

162 *The ritual wounds are often physical, sometimes sexual:* All of the examples cited are from Gilmore's sobering anthropological study. D. Gilmore, *Manhood in the Making: Cultural Concepts of Masculinity* (New Haven: Yale University Press, 1990). See also B. McCarthy, "Warrior Values: A Socio-Historical Survey," in J. Archer, ed., *Male Violence* (London: Routledge, 1994), pp. 105–20.

164 *American child watches twenty-eight hours of television:* Nielsen ratings are the source of this figure. For discussion of impact, see D. Levin and N. Carlsson-Paige, "Developmentally Appropriate Television: Putting Children First," *Young Children,* July 1994.

164 *on average twenty-six thousand television murders:* The source here is The National Coalition on Television Violence, cited in M. Miedzian, *Boys Will Be Boys* (New York: Anchor Books, 1991). The coalition estimates that children with cable TV and/or home VCRs will witness around 32,000 murders and 40,000 attempted murders by the age of eighteen. See also N. Minow and C. LaMay, *Abandoned in the Wasteland: Children, Television, and the First Amendment* (New York: Hill and Wang, 1995).

164 *There is a wide-ranging consensus:* See Miedzian, *Boys Will Be Boys.* See also T. Gore, *Raising PG Kids in an X-Rated Society* (New York: Bantam Books, 1988).

164 *An NIMH report found:* National Institute of Mental Health, *Television and Behavior: Ten Years of Scientific Progress and Implications for the Eighties* (Rockville, Maryland: National Institute of Mental Health, 1982).

165 *"the single best predictor of how aggressive":* L. Eron, R. Huesmann, "Adolescent Aggression of Children," *Annals of the New York Academy of Sciences,* June 20, 1980, vol. 347 pp. 310–31. L. Eron, "Parent-Child Interaction: Television Violence and Aggression and Television," *American Psychologist,* Feb. 1982, vol. 37 pp. 197–211. L. Eron, "Television Violence and Aggressive Behavior," in B. B. Lahey and A. E. Kazdin, eds., *Advances in Clinical Child Psychology* vol. 7 (New York: Plenum, 1984).

165 *extreme forms of traditional sex stereotyping:* See National Association for the Education of Young Children (NAEYC) in 1991 NAEYC position statement on media violence in children's lives. Adopted April 1990. *Young Children,* July 1994, pp. 18–21.

166 *both styles of inappropriate parenting:* P. Mellody, *Facing Codependence* (San Francisco: HarperCollins, 1987).

167 *As baseball legend Vince Lombardi.* Cited in M. Messner, "The Meaning of Success: The Athletic Experience and the Development of Male Identity," in H. Brod, ed., *The Making of Masculinities* (New York: Routledge, 1987).

167 *In the medieval Song of Roland: The Song of Roland,* trans. J. O'Hagan (Boston: Lothrop, Lee and Shepard, 1904).

167 *when Lancelot vanquished all foes:* For more on valor and courtesy, see E. R. Curtis, *European literature and the Latin Middle Ages,* trans. W. Trask (New York: Pantheon Books, 1953) (PB, Harper Torchbooks); W. T. H. Jackson, *The Anatomy of Love: A*

Study of the Tristan *of Gottfried Von Strassburg* (New York: Columbia University Press, 1966).

168 *As Joseph Campbell reminds us:* Campbell, *The Hero with a Thousand Faces* (Princeton, New Jersey: Princeton University Press, 1973).

169 *The statistical chance, for example, of a boy's:* D. W. Ball, "Failure in Sport," *American Sociological Review,* vol. 41 1976.

169 *Sociologist Michael Messner sums up the research:* Messner, "The Meaning of Success." See also J. J. Coakley, *Sports in Society* (St. Louis: Mosby, 1978); W. E. Schafer, "Sport and Male Sex Role Socialization," *Sport Sociology,* Fall 1975; R. C. Townsend, "The Competitive Male as Loser," in Sabo and Runfola, eds., *Jock: Sports and Male Identity* (Englewood Cliffs, NJ: Prentice Hall, 1980); T. Tutko, W. Bruns, *Winning Is Everything and Other American Myths* (New York: Macmillan, 1976).

169 *Young athletes who "fail":* H. Edwards, "The Collegiate Athletic Arms Race; Origins and Implications of the Rule 48 Controversy," *Journal of Sport and Social Issues,* Winter–Spring vol. 8 (1) 1984. The documentary film *Hoop Dreams* conveys the anguish often wrought by sports in the lives of urban black males.

169 *"On play after play":* M. Oriard, *The End of Autumn* (Garden City, N. Y.: Doubleday, 1982), pp. 97–98. Cited in Miedzian, *Boys Will Be Boys.* I am enormously indebted to Myriam Miedzian for her excellent book and trenchant analysis. *Boys Will Be Boys* was one of the first studies, and is still the most comprehensive, of the relationship between boys' socialization and violence. The discussion that follows owes a great deal to her work, both her thoughts and the resource material she gathered to support them.

170 *"And I was one of the lucky ones.":* D. Meggyesy, *Out of Their League* (Berkeley: Ramparts Press, 1970), pp. 81–82. Cited in Miedzian, *Boys Will Be Boys.*

170 *78 percent of professional football players:* M. Messner, "When Bodies Are Weapons: Masculinity and Violence in Sports," *International Reivew of Sociology of Sport,* Aug. 1990.

170 *An estimated 60 to 87 percent:* G. Lundberg, "Boxing Should Be Banned in Civilized Countries—Round 3," *Journal of American Medical Association,* May 9, 1986, pp. 2483–85.

170 *Sports, like scouting, were conceived of as:* P. G. Filene, *Him/Her/Self: Sex Roles in Modern America* (New York: Harcourt Brace Jovanovich, 1975). J. Hantover, "The Boy Scouts and the Validation of Masculinity," *Journal of Social Issues,* 1978, vol. 34 (1) 1978, p. 1.

171 *"I've seen it, Ben, I've seen it a thousand times":* A. Miller, *Death of a Salesman* (New York: Viking, 1994), p. 86.

171 *"I mean I can outbox, outrun, and outlift anybody":* Ibid., p. 24.

171 *"anytime I want, Biff. Whenever I feel disgusted":* Ibid., p. 25.

171 *Fine reports that in Little League:* G. Fine, *With the Boys: Little League Baseball and Preadolescent Behavior* (Chicago: University of Chicago Press, 1987), p. 114.

172 *Athlete Dave Meggyesy writes:* Meggyesy, *Out of Their League,* cited in Miedzian, *Boys Will Be Boys.* I am indebted to Miedzian for the quotes from Fine, Meggyesy, and many of the other athletes cited in this chapter.

172 *When displeased with a particular student's performance:* Reported by I. Berkow in *The New York Times,* May 16, 1988. Cited in Miedzian, Ibid.

174 *"That," writes Wiesel, "is what concentration camp":* E. Wiesel, *Night,* trans. S. Rodway (New York: Hill and Wang, 1960), p. 61. Cited in J. Herman, *Trauma and Recovery* (New York: Basic Books, 1992).

175 *Finally, terrorized beyond all reason:* The exact excerpt is: "But he had suddenly understood that in the whole world there was just one person to whom he could transfer his punishment—one body that he could thrust between himself and the rats. And he was shouting frantically, over and over: 'Do it to Julia! Do it to Julia! Not Me!' G. Orwell, *1984* (New York: Harcourt, Brace, 1949), p. 289.

176 *John McMurty, former Canadian football player, writes:* McNurty is quoted in M. Smith, *Violence and Sports* (Toronto: Butterworth, 1983), p. 28.

176 *Michael Oriard states:* M. Oriard, *The End of Autumn* (Garden City, New York: Doubleday, 1982). Cited in Miedzian, *Boys Will Be Boy.*

176 *Robert J. Lifton has called this process of self-alienation:* R. J. Lifton, *The Nazi Doctors; Medical Killing and the Psychology of Genocide* (New York: Basic Books, 1986). For more on male socialization as mitigating against empathy, see D. Lisak, "Integrating a Critique of Gender in the Treatment of Male Survivors of Childhood Abuse," *Psychotherapy,* in press; N. Eisenberg and R. Lennon, "Sex Differences in Empathy and Related Capacities," *Psychological Bulletin,* 1983, vol. 34 pp. 100–31; L. R. Brody (1985), "Gender Differences in Emotional Development: A Review of Theories and Research," *Journal of Personality,* 1985, pp. 102–49.

177 *"Just a crunchie munchie":* T. O'Brien, *The Things They Carried* (New York: Penguin, 1990).

177 *"They had never picked up":* R. Kovic, *Born on the Fourth of July* (New York: Pocket Books, 1977), pp. 166–67. Cited in Miedzian, *Boys Will Be Boys.*

177 *leaders who order them to kill:* Miedzian, *Boys Will Be Boys.*

179 *the connection to Dad had not been renounced:* S. Bergman, "Men's Psychological Development: A Relational Perspective," in R. Levant and W. Pollock, eds., *A New Psychology of Men* (New York: Basic Books, 1995).

179 *This tripartite cycle—the boy's renunciation:* J. Campbell, *The Hero with a Thousand Faces.*

180 *Their deepest vulnerabilities:* See A. Miller, *The Drama of the Gifted Child* (New York: Basic Books, 1981). Pia Mellody has called this role the "slave/god."

182 *Most men are not far behind Colonel Catcart:* The exact quote reads: "Colonel Catcart lived by his wits in an unstable, arithmetical world of black eyes and feathers in his cap, of overwhelming imaginary triumphs and catastrophic imaginary defeats. He oscillated hourly between anguish and exhilaration, multiplying fantastically the grandeur of his victories and exaggerating tragically the seriousness of his defeats." J. Heller, *Catch-22* (New York: Simon & Schuster, 1961), p. 186.

184 *when men are placed in empathy-demanding situations:* For a review of these studies, see C. Tavris, *The Mismeasure of Women* (New York: Simon & Schuster, 1992).

184 *"riding on a smile and a shoeshine":* A. Miller, *Death of a Salesman,* p. 138.

185 *"Will you take that phony dream and burn it":* Ibid., pp. 132–33.

185 *"He fought it out here":* Ibid., p. 139.

Chapter Eight: Two Inner Children

197 *"and it came at me screaming":* P. Knauth, *A Season in Hell* (New York: Harper & Row, 1975), pp. 33–35.

198 *What kind of relationship does he have with himself?* The relational perspective to which I refer is most closely associated with the relational theory currently espoused by some feminist researchers and theorists. As such, it has been most com-

monly applied to women's issues with only a glancing nod toward men. See A. Kaplan, "The Self-in-Relation: Implications for Depression in Women," in J. Jordan, A. Kaplan, J. Baker Miller, I. Stiver, and J. Surrey, *Women's Growth in Connection* (New York: Guilford, 1991); C. Gilligan, *In a Different Voice: Women's Conception of Self and of Morality* (Cambridge: Harvard University Press, 1982); D. C. Jack, *Silencing the Self: Depression and Women* (Cambridge: Harvard University Press, 1991). A growing body of analysis and research based on Joseph Pleck's debunking of the masculine identity theory is emerging as the predominant new theory on men's psychology. This new orientation toward male psychology freely acknowledges its debt to the feminist relational perspective. I view my own work as a part of this movement. An excellent compilation of this perspective can be found in R. Levant and W. Pollack, eds., *A New Psychology of Men* (New York: Basic Books, 1995).

198 *"pure psychical anguish"*: W. James cited in W. Styron, *Darkness Visible: A Memoir of Madness* (New York: Vantage, 1992).

204 *Both are instances of boundary dysfunction:* Appropriate boundaries require that the psychological membrane between people be neither too closed and rigid nor too open and porous. In family therapy we think of a too rigid boundary as creating *disengagement,* a too open boundary as creating toxic fusion or *enmeshment.* This concept, first adapted from general systems theory by structural family therapy, has been reiterated by the recovery movement. See S. Minuchin, *Families and Family Therapy* (Cambridge: Harvard University Press, 1974); M. Fossum and M. Mason, *Facing Shame: Families in Recovery* (New York: Norton, 1986); P. Mellody, *Facing Codependence* (San Francisco: HarperCollins, 1987); J. Bradshaw, *Healing the Shame that Binds You* (Deerfield, Florida: Health, Communication, 1988).

205 *"even at the sacrifice of their own welfare"*: J. Herman, *Trauma and Recovery* (New York: Basic Books, 1992), p. 98. See also A. Miller, *The Drama of the Gifted Child* (New York: Basic Books, 1981); C. Malone, "Safety First: Comments on the Influence of External Danger in the Lives of Children of Disorganized Families," *Orthopsychiatry,* 1966 vol. 36 (6). J. Bowlby, "Violence in the Family as a Disorder of the Attachment and Caregiving Systems," *American Journal of Psychoanalysis,* 1984 vol. 44 (1):9–27.

205 *Increased imprinting to abusing objects:* A. M. Ratner, "Modifications of Duckling Filiar Behavior by Aversive Stimulation," *Journal of Experimental Psychology* (Animal Behavior), 1976, vol. 2 pp. 266–84; H. F. Harlow and M. K. Harlow, *Psychopathology in Monkey Experimental Psychopathology,* H. D. Kimmel, ed. (New York: Academic Press, 1971); W. C. Stanley and O. Elliot, "Differential Human Handling as Reinforcing Events and as Treatments Influencing Later Social Behavior in Basenji Puppies," Psychology Reports, 1962, vol. 10 pp. 775–88.

206 *take upon themselves the shame and guilt:* J. Herman, *Trauma and Recovery,* pp. 102 and 105.

206 *and carried shame are the psychological seeds of depression:* P. Mellody, *Facing Codependence* (San Francisco: HarperCollins, 1987). See also Bradshaw, *Healing the Shame;* A. Morrison, *Shame: the Underside of Narcissism* (New York: Analytic Press, 1989); Follsom, *Shame:* A vivid example of transmitted shame is rape victims oft-reported urgent wish to shower. Rape victims characteristically describe a sense of having been sullied, dirtied, of wanting to rid themselves of a coating, a slime. This is a physical correlate to carried sexual shame.

207 *"felt it scream out its birth in a black, forbidden ecstasy"*: Conroy, *The Prince of Tides* (New York: Bantam, 1991), p. 116.

208 *Billy, feeling sorry for his parents:* On the abused child's need to blame himself rather than face the terrifying prospect of a hostile environment see M. Symonds, "Victim Responses to Terror: Understanding and Treatment," in F. M. Ochberg & D. A. Soskis, eds., Victims of Terrorism, (Boulder, Col.: Westview, 1982), pp. 5–103; T. Strenz, "The Stockholm Syndrome: Law Enforcement Policy and Hostage Behavior," Ibid., pp. 149–63; D. L. Graham, E. Rawling, and N. Rimini, "Survivors of Terror; Battered Women, Hostages and the Stockholm Syndrome: in Yllo and Bograd," Feminist Perspectives, 2178–33; D. Dutton and S. L. Painter, "Traumatic Bonding: The Development of Emotional Attachment in Battered Women and Other Relationships of Intermittent Abuse," *Victimology,* 1981, pp. 139–55.

212 If empathic reversal . . . *is the process:* I am profoundly indebted to Pia Mellody for this formulation.

213 *a functioning internal adult:* The division of the adult psyche into functioning adult, vulnerable boy, and harsh boy is an adaptation of Mellody's concepts of the functional adult, wounded child, and adaptive adult child. Mellody, *Facing Codependence.*

214 *envisioned mothers, fathers, bullies, and molesters:* Jack and I used a variety of formats and techniques in the gathering of which this is but one. For more of Jack's thoughts on group work with men, see J. Sternback, "The Father Theme in Group therapy with Men" in *Men In Groups,* ed. M. Adronico *American Psychological Association,* Wash. DC. 1996, pp. 219–229.

215 *"go down into that agitated feeling in your gut":* This is "inner child work" as taught to me by Pia.

225 *pharmacological help in some cases of traumatic disorders, addictions:* A. T. Butterworth, "Depression Associated with Alcohol: Imipramine Therapy Compared with Placebo," *Quarterly Journal Stud Alcohol,* 1971, vol. 32 pp. 343–48. J. E. Overall, D. Brown, J. D. William, et al., "Drug Treatment of Anxiety and Depression in Detoxified Alcholic Patients," *Archives of General Psychiatry,* 1973, pp. 218–21; F. H. Gawin, H. D. Kleber, "Cocaine Abuse Treatment," *Archives of General Psychiatry,* 1984, vol. 41 (9) pp. 903–9; G. E. Woody, C. P. O'Brien, K. Rickels, "Depression and Anxiety in Heroin Addicts: A Placebo-Controlled Study of Doxepin in Combination with Methadone," *American Journal of Psychiatry,* 1975, vol. 142 pp. 447–50. B. Eichelmann, "Neurochemical and Psychopharmacologic Aspects of Aggressive Behavior," in H. Meltzer, ed., *Psychopharmacology: The Third Generation of Progress* (New York: Raven Press, to be published).

227 *"which mankind at large has chosen to sanctify":* D. H. Lawrence, "Healing," in R. Bly, J. Hillman, M. Meade, eds., *The Rag and Bone Shop of the Heart: Poems for Men* (New York: HarperCollins, 1992), p. 113.

Chapter Nine: Balance Prevails

234 *complication of the man's "crisis in masculinity.":* See P. T. Dimock, "Adult Males Sexually Abused as Children: Characteristic and Implication for Treatment," *Journal of Interpersonal Violence,* 1988, vol. 3 (2) pp. 203–21; M. Lew, *Victims No Longer* (New York: Nevramont, 1988); D. Lisak, "The Psychological Consequences of Childhood Abuse: Content Analysis of Interview with Male Survivors," *Journal of Traumatic Stress,* 1988, p. 7; B. Watkins and A. Bentovim, "The Sexual Abuse of

Male Children and Adolescents: A Review of Current Research," *Journal of Child Psychology and Psychiatry,* 1992, vol. 33 pp. 197–248.

235 *when Lisak applied this variable.* David Lisak's research is reported in: D. Lisak, J. Hopper, and P. Song, *Factors in the Cycle of Violence: Gender Rigidity and Emotional Constriction,* manuscript in publication. Lisak described the course of his research in "Characteristics of Abused and Non-Abusing Men," Presentation to the Massachusetts General Hospital Conference on Men and Trauma, Boston, Mass., 1994.

235 *"unmanned," these men rewrite the criteria for manhood:* Lisak writes, "One way to understand these findings is to conceptualize two developmental pathways diverging from a history of childhood abuse. In one path, the male victim may appear conflicted and preoccupied by gender identity issues, but this preoccupation may indicate a lack of conformity to gender norms necessitated by his coping with the legacy of abuse. In the other path, the male abuse victim strives to be stereotypically masculine, and must therefore suppress the high magnitude emotional states that are a legacy of his abuse. The suppression required to hold at bay the emotional legacy of abuse may also suppress his capacity to empathize with others. Having sealed himself off from his own pain, the perpetrator may well seal off his capacity to feel the pain of others, and thereby diminish a crucial inhibition against interpersonal violence." Lisak, Hopper, and Song, *Factors in the Cycle of Violence,* p. 17.

236 *traumatized boys are shown to "act out":* For example, in a study of hospitalized psychiatric patients who had been victims of abuse and incest: 33 percent of the males had histories of becoming physically aggressive, compared with 16 percent of the females. 66 percent of the females turned hostility inward and had histories of self-destructive behavior, compared with only 20 percent of the males. E. H. Carmen, P. P. Reiker, T. Mills, "Victims of Violence and Psychiatric Illness," *American Journal of Psychiatry,* 1984, vol. 141 (3) pp. 378–79. For other studies and reviews, see A. H. Green, "Dimensions of Psychological Trauma in Abused Children," *Journal of the American Association of Child Psychiatry,* vol. 22 1983, pp. 231–37; B. Allgood Merten, P. M. Lewinsohn, and H. Hops, "Sex Differences and Adolescent Depression," *Journal of Abnormal Psychology,* 1990, pp. 55–63; Bluhmberg and Igard, "Affective and Cognitive Characteristics of Depression in 10–11 Year Olds," *Journal of Personality and Social Psychology,* 1985, vol. 91 (1) pp. 194–202; Ingram, Cruet, Hohnson, and Wisnicki, "Self-Focused Attention, Gender, Gender Role and Vulnerability to Negative Affect," *Journal of Personality and Social Psychology,* 1988, pp. 967–78; Panter and J. S. Tanaka (1987), "Cognitive Activity and Dysphonic Affect: Gender Differences in Information Processing," Paper presented at the 95th Annual Convention of the American Psychological Association, New York, August 1987; Edelbrock and Achenbach, "A Typology of Child Behavior Profile Patterns: Distribution Patterns and Correlates for Disturbed Children Aged 6–16 Years," *Journal of Abnormal Child Psychology,* 1980, vol. 8 pp. 441–70; R. Kobak, N. Sudler, and W. Gamble, "Attachment and Depressive Symptoms During Adolescence: A Developmental Pathways Analysis," *Development and Psychopathology,* 1992, vol. 3 (4) pp. 461–74; Ostrov, Offer, and Howard "Gender Differences in Adolescent Symptomatology: A Normative Study," *Journal of the American Academy of Child and Adolescent Psychiatry,* 1989, pp. 394–98; Puig-Antich, "Major Depression and Conduct Disorder in Prepuberty," *Journal of the American Academy of Child Psychiatry,* 1982, vol. 21 pp. 118–28.

236 *not to become abusive fathers:* I would like to stress that I am not arguing nor does the current research support the idea, that all abused men become abusive to others. Some men seem to demonstrate a high degree of resilience for reasons that remain a matter of speculation. Others work through their trauma experience. Still others turn aggression inward, as in overt depression, and/or in social withdrawal. Current research would place the ratio of abusing adults (both men and women together) at about one-third of all those who have been abused as children. This estimate means that an adult with an abuse history is about five to six times more likely to become abusive than one without such a history. On the other hand, this estimate also means that fully two-thirds of those with an abuse history—the vast majority—do not repeat their treatment.

My only quarrel with current research, which justifiably critiques simplistic notions of victimized-victimizers, is that, by and large, the issues of abuse and neglect upon which these studies focus tend to be extreme and abject. A man who has been beaten may not beat his son—particularly given changes in cultural norms about corporal punishment. But, unless that man deals with his own psychological and physical trauma, I remain unconvinced that he will not inflict harm. Perhaps it will be psychological rather than physical. Perhaps it will be passive rather than active. Perhaps it will be milder. But once we broaden the range of psychological damage to include less flagrant forms of injury, it becomes easier to understand why, in my years of practice, I have found it rare to encounter a man who can be truly available to his children while he is burdened with an unaddressed trauma history himself. Such a situation is possible. Some men evidence levels of resilience that one can not easily explain. They seem to have walked through horrible situations unscathed. Personally, I have found such instances by far the exception, not the rule.

For more on this topic, see D. Otnow, "From Abuse to Violence: Psychophysiological Consequences of Maltreatment," *Journal of the American Academy of Child Adolescent Psychiatry,* May 1992, vol. 31 (3) p. 3; C. P. Widom, "Child Abuse, Neglect, and Adult Behavior," *Journal American Orthopsychiatric Association,* July 1989, vol. 59 (3) 355–67.

236 *Boys with abusive or neglectful fathers:* See J. Snarey, *How Fathers Care for the Next Generation* (Cambridge: Harvard University Press, 1994) for a discussion of the Glueck study, an analysis of father-son relations that followed 240 Boston fathers for close to four decades. Silverstein and B. Roshbaum, *The Courage to Raise Good Men* (New York: Viking, 1994); M. Heatherington, M. Cox, R. Cox, "Effects of Divorce on Parents and Children,"; in *Nontraditional Families* ed. M. Lamb (Hillside, N.J.: Erlbaum Pub, 1982).

240 *"Dad, this one's for you!":* For work with batterers that employs similar techniques, see M. Scheinburg, "Gender Dilemmas, Gender Question and the Gender Mantra," *Journal of Family Therapy,* Jan. 1991, vol. 17 (1) pp. 33–44.

241 *quotes T. S. Eliot:* Henry's quote is from "The Wasteland." The original is from *The Confessions of Saint Augustine. T. S. Eliot,* Selected Poems *(New York: Harcourt, Brace, 1962).*

243 *toward that same church, which he forgot:* R. M. Rilke, "Sometimes a Man Stands up During Supper," trans by R. Bly in R. Bly, J. Hillman, and M. Meade, eds., *The Rag and Bone Shop of the Heart, Poems for Men* (New York: HarperCollins, 1992).

249 *while the kingdom around him decays:* For more on Percevale and the Grail legend, see E. Jung and M. L. von Franz, *The Grail Legend* (New York: Putnam 1970); R.

Johnson, *He!: Understanding Masculine Psychology* (New York: Harper & Row, 1989); J. Weston, *From Ritual to Romance* (Garden City, N. Y.: Doubleday, 1957). (Weston's book was Eliot's principal source for *The Wasteland*).

Chapter Ten: Crossing the Wasteland

270 *the distinction between abusive and addictive dependency:* Currently, addictions experts make a huge distinction between those who self-medicate an underlying depression, those who are alcoholic, and those who may be both—depressed and alcoholic. The addictions field and traditional psychiatry both utilize a discrete disease model, in which discrete disease "x" (in this case, depression) needs to be distinguished from discrete disease "y" (in this case, alcoholism). I believe that the discrete disease model is, and should be, breaking down.

Before the revolution of AA, thousands of lives were ruined when the psychiatric establishment attempted to treat addictions as if they were like any other neurosis or character problem, that is, as if addictions would yield to conventional therapy. As a rule, the results of such therapy were stunningly ineffective. One of the critical contributions of AA was its refusal to engage in the search for an "underlying" disorder. Drinking itself was the disorder! The need to treat addiction *as a disease unto itself* was first recognized, and millions of people have been helped by this shift in perspective.

While I sympathize with the shudder passing through addictions counselors at the thought of revivifying the idea that addicts and alcoholics have an underlying depression and underlying personality problems, my own clinical practice draws me away from simple either/or polarities. The abusive use of substances, persons, or processes—by definition concerns the self-medication of depressive feelings. Addictive use—as opposed to abusive use—also concerns the self-medication of depressive feelings. The latter, however, exists within the context of a progressive process with a predictable course, one that demands treatment in its own right. For my purposes, the only real difference between abusive and addictive self-medication is that once I evaluate someone's use as truly addictive, I know that stronger measures will be required to deal with it.

271 *Jeffrey began working out:* I have been struck by the frequency of my clients' reports of the salutary effects of exercise on depression. I am not aware of scientific studies on the subject, but anecdotal evidence suggests regular, physical exercise may have a mood-brightening capacity.

275 *his emotional "prosthesis":* The term comes from H. Weider, E. H. Kaplan, "Drug Use in Adolescents: Psychodynamic Meaning and Pharmacogenic Effect," *Psychoanalytic Study of the Child* vol. 24 (1969): 399–431.

275 *strategy for dealing with self "dysregulation":* E. J. Khantzian, "The Self-Medication Hypothesis of Addictive Disorders: Focus on Heroin and Cocaine Dependence," *American Journal of Psychiatry,* 1985 vol. 142 (11) pp. 1259–64; E. J. Khantzian, "Self-Regulation and Self-Medication Factors in Alcoholism and the Addictions; Similarities and Differences, in *Recent Developments in Alcoholism, vol. 8, Combined Alcohol and Other Drug Dependence,* Marc Galanter, ed. (New York: Plenum, 1990).

276 *four cardinal areas of dysregulation:* E. Khantzian, K. Halliday, and W. McAuliffe *Addiction and the Vulnerable Self: Modified Dynamic Group Therapy for Substance Abusers* (New York: Guilford, 1990).

277 *a moment of* relational heroism: I am endebted to my wife, Belinda Berman, for both the concept and the term *relational heroism.*

There seems to be a growing awareness that psychotherapy with men demands a more active, instructional approach than traditional therapy models. See, for example, Ron Levant's excellent work on teaching men how to feel and express their emotions. R. Levant and G. Kopecky, *Masculinity Reconstructed* (New York: Penguin, 1995).

278 *a five-point grid that I find practical:* P. Mellody, *Facing Codependence* (San Francisco: HarperCollins, 1987).

279 *extruding them, unburdening himself of them: Shame reduction work* and *feeling reduction work* are the terms given by Pia Mellody to these techniques for extruding internalized introjects. By focusing on the precise moment when the traumatic interaction becomes internalized, Mellody's work unites both an individual and a family systems perspective and it offers a powerful set of therapeutic tools. I have little doubt that hosts of new, effective techniques for healing will emerge as trauma study continues to expand.

For other innovative techniques on trauma release work, see R. Janov-Bulman, *Shattered Assumptions: Towards a New Psychology of Trauma* (New York: The Free Press, 1992); J. Jensen, "An Investigation of Eye Movement Desensitization and Reprocessing (EMD/R) as a Treatment for Posttraumatic Stress Disorder (PTSD) Symptoms in Vietnam Combat Veterans," *Behavior Therapy,* 1994, vol. 25 (2) pp. 311–25.

285 *The bad weather blows away:* See P. Gilbert, *Depression: The Evolution of Powerlessness* (New York: Guilford, 1984).

286 *our numbing attempts to avoid [feelings] can last a lifetime:* See B. Miller, *From Depression to Sadness in Women's Psychotherapy* (Cambridge: Stone Center for Developmental Series and Studies, Wellesley, 1988). On grief and mourning in the therapeutic process, see A. Miller, *Drama of the Gifted Child* (New York: Basic Books, 1981).

286 state dependent recall: American Psychiatric Association, *Diagnostic and Statistical Maunual of Mental Disorders,* 4th ed. rev. (Washington, D.C., American Psychiatric Association, 1994).

287 *in response to minor stress:* B. van der Kolk, "The Body Keeps the Score: Memory and the Evolving Psychobiology of Posttraumatic Stress," *Harvard Review of Psychiatry,* Jan./Feb., 1994, p. 259.

287 *Limbic system activity quieted again:* van der Kolk, Personal communication.

287 *the explicit and implicit memory systems:* van der Kolk summarizes: "In 1987 Kolb postulated that patients with PTSD suffer from impaired cortical control over subcortical areas responsible for learning, habituation, and stimulus discrimination . . . delayed-onset PTSD may be the expression of subcortically mediated emotional responses that escape cortical, and possibly hippocampal, inhibitory control." Van der Kolk, "The Body Keeps the Score," p. 261. Also see L. C. Kolb, "Neurophysiological Hypothesis Explaining Posttraumatic Stress Disorder," *American Journal of Psychiatry,* 1987, pp. 989–95; J. E. LeDoux, L. Romanski, and A. Xagoraris, "Indelibility of Subcortical Emotional Memories," *Journal of Cognitive Neuroscience,* vol. 1 (3) pp. 238–43; L. R. Squire, S. Zola-Morgan, "The Medial Temporal Lobe Memory System," *Science,* 1991, pp. 2380–86.

288 *differentiated from current reality:* B. van der Kolk, "The Body Keeps the Score," p. 261.

288 *They are Prozac and its family:* Ibid.

288 *a cluster of possible disorders and symptoms:* Robert Golden and his colleagues sum up the research spearheaded by van Praag: "{There are] compelling arguments for avoiding the limitations that are imposed by our current nosology [i.e., set of diagnostic criteria]. Biological markers, including measures of serotonergic function, may be more closely related to basic psychopathological dimensions such as impulsivity, sadness, and aggression dysregulation, than to specific current diagnostic categories. In support of this perspective, [Van Praag's group] has recently demonstrated significant intercorrelations between several psychopathologic dimensions that are felt to be linked to serotonin, including suicide, violence potential, impulsivity, depressed mood, and anxiety." R. N. Golden, M.D., J. H. Gilmore, M. H. N. Corrigan, "Serotonin, Suicide and Aggression: Clinical Studies," *Journal of Clinical Psychiatry,* Dec. 1991, suppl. See also H. M. Van Praag, R. S. Kahn, G. M. Asnis, et al., "Denosologization of Biological Psychiatry or the Specificity of 5-HT Disturbances in Psychiatric Disorders," *Journal of Affective Disorders,* 1987, vol. 13 (1) pp. 1–8; A. Apter, H. M. van Praag, R. Plutchik, et al., "Interrelationships Among Anxiety, Aggression, Impulsivity and Mood. A Serotonergically Linked Cluster?" *Psychiatry Research,* 1990, pp. 191–99.

289 *"chronic affect dysregulation . . .":* The quote is from van der Kolk, the concept Complex PTSD is fully developed by van der Kolk's colleague and sometime collaborator, Judith Herman. B. van der Kolk, "The Body Keeps the Score," p. 258; J. Herman, *Trauma and Recovery* (New York: Basic Books, 1992).

290 *a complex web of nature and nurture:* For a review, see P. Gjerde, "Alternative Pathways to Chronic Depressive Symptoms in Young Adults: Gender Differences in Developmental Trajectories," *Child Development,* 1995, in press. For an accessible review that leans more heavily on the biology of gender differences, see R. Pool, *Eve's Rib: Seaching for the Biological Roots of Sex Differences* (New York: Crown, 1992).

Chapter Eleven: Learning Intimacy

291 *" 'Farewell!' was just what Echo mimed":* Ovid, *Metamorphoses,* trans. A. Mandelbaum (New York: Harcourt Brace, 1993), p. 97.

292 A central paradox for boys is that they must earn connection through performance-based esteem by going one-up, which intrinsically erodes connection. A complimentray paradox for girls is that they must repudiate their voices, the expression of many legitimate ambitions, conflicts, truths, in the service of affiliation. Such servitude may, on the surface, appear "related" but, as Carol Gilligan and others forcefully agree, such tyranny also erodes deep, authentic relationships.

292 *a culturally sanctioned pas de deux:* R. Taffel, "The Politics of Mood," in M. Bogard, ed., *Feminist Approaches for Men in Family Therapy* (New York: Harrington Park Press, 1991, pp. 153–77); P. Papp, "Gender Differences in Depression Presentation," *American Marriage and Family Therapy Association,* 1994.

300 *begin to map out depression's influence.* These are "relative influence questions," a technique pioneered by family therapist Michael White. See M. White, *Narrative Means to Therapeutic Ends* (New York: Basic Books, 1992).

300 *stand up and beat the enemy back.* Again, from Michael White. I have been deeply

affected by White's work, which enlists clients in a collaboration with the thera-pist against cultural stories and myths that plague them—stories about the sub-jugation of womens' bodies expressed as anorexia, myths of patriarchy played out as domestic violence. See White, *Narrative Means*. A narrative, *externalizing* approach to male violence is elaborated in A. Jenkins, *Invitations to Responsibility, The Therapeutic Engagement of Men Who Are Violent and Abusive* (Adelaide, South Australia: Dulwich Centre Publications, 1990).

302 *at this moment that many of the divisions:* For more detailed histories, see J. Demos, *Myths and Realities in the History of American Family-Life,* in H. Grunebaum and J. Christ, eds., *Contemporary Marriage: Structure, Dynamics, and Therapy* (Boston: Lit-tle, Brown, 1976). H. Braverman, *Labor and Monopoly Capital; the Degradation of Work in the Twentieth Century* (New York: Monthly Review Press, 1975).

303 man-the-breadwinner *and* woman-the-caretaker: O. Silverstein, the *Courage to Raise Good Men.*

303 *"the cheerleaders of industrial society":* Matt Dumont writing as H. Drummond, "Diagnosing Marriage," *Mother Jones,* July 1979, pp. 16–17.

306 *They were signed Love, Martha:* T. O'Brien, *The Things They Carried* (New York: Penguin, 1990).

306 *Men have enjoyed the "privilege":* While I vehemently disagree with Farrell's attempt to stand sexism on its head with his claim that men are women's victims, Farrell does manage to point out many of the costs to men of their traditional roles. W. Farrell, *The Myth of Male Power: Why Men Are the Disposable Sex* (New York: Simon & Schuster, 1993).

309 *Male babies have been shown:* For a review of the literature, see J. J. Haviland and C. Z. Malatesta, "The Development of Sex Differences in Nonverbal Signals: Fal-lacies, Facts, and Fantasies," in C. Mayo and N. M. Henly, eds., *Gender and Non-verbal Behavior* (New York: Springer, 1981), pp. 183–208. Also, Levant, "Toward the Reconstruction of Masculinity."

309 *physiologically overwhelming:* J. Gottman and R. Levenson, "The Social Psy-chophysiology of Marriage," in P. Noller and M. A. Fitzpatrick, eds., *Perspectives on Marital Interaction* (Clevendon, U.K.: Multilingual Matters, 1988), pp. 182–200; C. L. Notorius and J. Johnson, "Emotional Expression in Husbands and Wives," *Journal of Marriage and Family Therapy,* 1982, vol. 44 pp. 482–89.

310 *rates of attack toward the proximate offspring:* M. Daly and M. Wilson, "Evolutionary Social Psychology and Family Homicide," *Science,* Oct. 1988 vol. 242 (4878) 519–524.

312 adult-to-adult carried feelings: The term matching Pia's "carried feelings" in analytic psychology would be "projective identification," Mellody, *Post Induction Therapy;* T. Ogden, *Projective Identification and Psychotherapeutic Technique* (New York: J. Aranson, 1982).

312 *Hafner's research supplies empirical evidence:* J. Hafner, "Sex Role Stereotyping in Women with Agoraphobia and Their Husbands," *Sex Roles,* June 1989 vol. 20 (11–12) 705–711, p. 705; Hafner, *End of Marriage: Why Monogamy Isn't Working* (London: Century, 1993).

312 *contemporary marriage appears to be beneficial:* J. Bernard, *The Future of Marriage* (New York: Bantam, 1972).

313 *"So, you've found a way to keep him company":* In family therapy this technique is called, "positively reframing" the symptom, that is, looking at the negative con-sequence of change for the entire system. No one uses this technique more adeptly than one of its architects, Olga Silverstein. See P. Papp, *The Process of*

Change (New York: Guilford, 1993) O. Silverstein and B. Keeney, *The Therapeutic Voice of Olga Silverstein* (New York: Guilford, 1986).

313 *the "dysfunction" of vulnerability itself:* J. B. Miller, *Toward a New Psychology of Women* (Boston: Beacon, 1986).

316 *step up to increased relational responsibility:* An adaption of A. Jenkins, *Invitations to Responsibility.*

Chapter Twelve: Where We Stand

322 *A grown man with nothing to devote himself to:* Psychiatrist Victor Frankl constructed an entire school of psychology around this shift. In the moving account of his own internment in a Nazi concentration camp, Frankl recalls how he saved many lives by directing other inmates toward the question What is life asking of you? In that hopeless environment, the question What does life hold for you? would yield no useful answer. For one man, life required that he survive to search for a relative; for another, that he honor a God-given talent; for another, that he exact revenge, or bear witness. Frankl recounts that those who could find nothing that life required of them died. V. Frankl, *Man's Search for Meaning* (New York: Pocket Books, 1985).

323 *surprisingly, more successful in their careers:* J. Snarey, *How Fathers Care for the Next Generation* (Cambridge: Harvard University Press, 1993).

324 *A culture of limitless resources:* T. Engender, *The End of Victory Culture* (New York: Basic Books, 1995).

325 *"least defended areas of the natural world":* A. Gore, *Earth in the Balance: Ecology and the Human Spirit* (New York: Penguin, 1993).

325 *"a steward of the earth":* Ibid, 236.

325 *"stewardship" as Gore, among others, calls it:* Ibid. See also A. Kimbrell, *The Masculine Mystique* (New York: Ballantine Books, 1995).

325 *"refused to recognize anything above him":* V. Havel, "Rio and the New Millennium (Earth Summit, 1992)," *The New York Times,* June 3, 1992.

Index

physique and, 37, 56-58
techniques for management of, 278-79
self-medication hypothesis, 61, 274, 275-76
self-mutilation, 24, 147-48
self-reliance, vulnerability vs., 148
sensation seekers, 147, 275
separation, 143-44, 165
septohippocampal system, 288
serotonin, 103
serotonin reuptake inhibitors, 288
service ethic, 322, 326
Sesame Street, 163
sex, television references to, 165
sex addiction (erotomania; love addiction), 62
  domestic violence linked to, 67, 69
  intoxication experienced in, 64, 65
  within marriage, 70-73, 75-76, 151
  withdrawal experiences from, 89, 101
sex role identity:
  gender identity vs., 132
  marital difficulties of, 300-305, 307-19
sexual abuse:
  of children by adults, 104
  Freudian rejection of reports on, 104, 289
  among siblings, 74-76
sexual mother archetype, 306-7
sexual obsession, 64
Shakespeare, William, 32, 128
shame:
  appropriate feelings of, 76, 120
  carried, 206, 207
  in cyclic pattern of addiction, 79-80
  of depression for men, 22, 35
  grandiosity as compensation for, 55-56
  in manic-depressive illness, 65
  military participation as avoidance of, 36
  of oppression, 181
  as self-attack, 55
  traumatic transmission of, 206
  of vulnerability, 148
shell shock, 104-5

siblings:
  physical abuse from, 56
  sexual abuse among, 74-76
Silverstein, Olga, 11, 144
Simon, Paul, 166-67
single mothers, 141
Sleeping Beauty, 164
social situations, dominance behaviors in, 178
soldiers:
  empathy loss experienced by, 176-77
  fear of shame as motivation for, 36
  trauma reactions of, 104-5, 106, 234, 286, 287, 289
solitary confinement, 147
Song of Roland, 167
soul murder, 128, 189
specialness, relational needs and, 184-91
spending, addiction to, 62
Spitz, Rene, 97
Spitzer, Robert, 62
sports:
  coaches as role models in, 172-74
  dominance values perpetuated through, 167, 169, 171, 173-76, 178, 183
  feminine traits ridiculed in, 171-72, 173
  heroic moral tradition vs., 167-69
  permanent physical disability from, 169-70
  success ideology and, 167, 168, 170-71, 185-91
  teamwork vs. individual achievement in, 168-69
Springle, Ira, 194, 195
stalking behavior, 62
Stallone, Sylvester, 69
Staner, Lewis, 62
Star Trek, 163
Star Wars trilogy, 144, 163, 168
state dependent recall, 286
stepfathers, 310
Sternbach, Jack, 11, 213-14
steroid abuse, 57
stoicism, 35
Stranger, The (Camus), 142
stress, 32
Styron, William, 60-61, 84-85, 101-2, 198